The Advanced Practitioner

The Advanced Practitioner

A Framework for Practice

Edited by

Ian Peate,

OBE, FRCN

Visiting Professor, St George's University of London and Kingston University London
Visiting Professor, Northumbria University
Senior Clinical Fellow, University of Hertfordshire
Professorial Fellow, University of Roehampton
Editor-in-Chief, British Journal of Nursing
Consultant Editor for the Journal of Paramedic Practice and the International Journal for Advancing Practice

Sadie Diamond-Fox,

MCP, ACCP, BSc (Hons), RN, PGC AHP, NMP (V300), FHEA

Advanced Critical Care Practitioner (FICM member) and ACCP Programme Co-Lead
at Newcastle upon Tyne NHS Hospitals
Subject Lead for Advanced Practice Programmes and Assistant Professor
in Advanced Critical Care Practice (Fellow – HEA)
at Northumbria University
Speciality Advisor for Critical Care at Regional Faculty for Advancing Practice
NHS England North East & Yorkshire Honorary Assistant Professor in Advanced
Clinical Practice at Nottingham University Member (& Past Chair) of the Advanced Practitioners
in Critical Care (APCC) Professional Advisory Group (PAG) at the Intensive Care Society (ICS).
External Examiner for MSc ACCP Programmes at Southampton University.
Editorial Board Member of the International Journal of Advancing Practice

Barry Hill,

MSc, AP, PGCAP, BSc (Hons), DipHE/OA, Dip SFHEA, TEFL, NMC, RN, RNT/TCH, V300

Associate Professor of Nursing Science and Critical Care; Director of Nursing
Midwifery and Health Employability, Northumbria University
Consultant Editor for the International Journal for Advancing Practice
Clinical Series Editor for the British Journal of Nursing

WILEY Blackwell

Registered Offices
John Wiley & Sons, Inc., 111 River Street, Hoboken, NJ 07030, USA
John Wiley & Sons Ltd, The Atrium, Southern Gate, Chichester, West Sussex, PO19 8SQ, UK

For details of our global editorial offices, customer services, and more information about Wiley products visit us at www.wiley.com.

Wiley also publishes its books in a variety of electronic formats and by print-on-demand. Some content that appears in standard print versions of this book may not be available in other formats.

Library of Congress Cataloging-in-Publication Data
Names: Peate, Ian, editor. | Diamond-Fox, Sadie, editor. | Hill, Barry
   (Lecturer in nursing) editor.
Title: The advanced practitioner : a framework for clinical practice /
   [edited by] Ian Peate, Sadie Diamond-Fox, Barry Hill.
Description: Hoboken, NJ : Wiley-Blackwell, 2024. | Includes
   bibliographical references and index.
Identifiers: LCCN 2022059953 (print) | LCCN 2022059954 (ebook) | ISBN
   9781119882039 (paperback) | ISBN 9781119882046 (adobe pdf) | ISBN
   9781119882053 (epub)
Subjects: MESH: Advanced Practice Nursing
Classification: LCC RT41 (print) | LCC RT41 (ebook) | NLM WY 128 | DDC
   610.73–dc23/eng/20230302
LC record available at https://lccn.loc.gov/2022059953
LC ebook record available at https://lccn.loc.gov/2022059954

Cover Design: Wiley
Cover Images: © Martin Barraud/Getty Images, traffic_analyzer/Getty Images

Set in 10.5/13pt STIXTwoText by Straive, Pondicherry, India
Printed and bound by CPI Group (UK) Ltd, Croydon, CR0 4YY

C9781119882039_230524

Contents

Contributors

Ihab Ali, MRPharmS, ASTEM, SFHEA, PGDip, IP

Lead Pharmacist for urgent care, Stockport NHS Foundation Trust. Ihab's career began in 2013 as a Community Pharmacist before transferring to a clinical role in an NHS hospital in 2014. He has experience in many different clinical areas but decided to specialise in acute medicine when completing his independent prescribing qualification. He side-stepped into becoming a teacher practitioner in 2019 before returning to work as Lead Pharmacist for urgent care in 2020. He has worked as unit lead for both undergraduate and postgraduate pharmacy courses, at the University of Manchester and Aston University. He is now working purely in the emergency department as a Clinical Pharmacist with the intention of becoming an advanced clinical practitioner and then eventually a Consultant Pharmacist.

Clare Allabyrne

Associate Professor and professional lead for advanced clinical practice mental health at London Southbank University and a fellow of the Higher Education Academy. A dual qualified nurse (Adult and Mental Health) by profession, her areas of expertise include advanced clinical practice in mental health, child and adolescent mental health services (CAMHS), forensic psychiatry, liaison psychiatry; mental health in adult and child physical health services, substance use, physical health care in mental health, service user involvement/people participation, multi-agency/partnership working, leadership and service creation and innovation. Clare worked for 35 years in the NHS across physical and mental healthcare services in clinical, therapeutic, senior operational, clinical academic and corporate/strategic leadership roles.

Sarah Ashelford, BSc (Hons), PhD

Sarah started her career as a researcher at Edinburgh University, Centre for HIV Research. This was followed by a move into teaching secondary level science in schools in Wakefield and Leeds. Sarah moved back into teaching biosciences on various healthcare professional courses at Bradford University and the University of Lincoln, and now works at the University of York. Sarah specialises in teaching physiology and pathophysiology relating to healthcare, and research in biosciences education.

Jill Bentley, mFICM, ACCP MSc

Lecturer in advanced clinical practice, non-medical prescribing and nursing, University of Salford, Salford, UK. Jill is an experienced practitioner with a demonstrated history of working in the hospital and healthcare industry. She is skilled in critical care, clinical research, medical education, medical-surgical, paediatrics and critical thinking. Jill is a strong healthcare services professional with a MSc focused in advanced practice from the University of Salford, and an MSc in pain management.

Roberta Borg, BSc (Hons), MSc

Roberta obtained a BSc (Hons) in nursing studies from the University of Malta (2008). Shortly afterwards, she moved to the UK and started her career in critical care at Cambridge University Hospitals.

Roberta has always enjoyed a side hustle in academia alongside her clinical work, engaging in research, teaching and advancing her own academic studies. She completed a PGCert in critical care and later an MSc in advanced clinical practice. The latter was in parallel with a two-year clinical training programme, which saw her qualify as an Advanced Critical Care Practitioner (mFICM) in 2015 and she continued to work in this role. She has recently taken a break from clinical work to spend time with her young family and move to the United States. During this time, she continues to contribute to the academic nursing world through various book chapters and has expanded her readership to a younger audience through a book that she wrote for children to understand the value of healthcare workers.

Phil Broadhurst, RN, BSc (Hons) (Nursing Practice), MSc (Advanced Clinical Practice), PGCE (Medical and Health Education)

Phil is a FICM-registered Advanced Critical Care Practitioner at Stockport NHS Foundation Trust. He started his career as a ward volunteer before working as an auxiliary nurse while completing his nurse training. He has significant experience in intensive care, where he has worked as a staff nurse and team leader, before qualifying in advanced practice. Phil has a special interest in professional education and around his clinical work he is actively involved in training and education of both medical and nursing colleagues, taking a lead on Trust-wide acute illness management training. Phil spent several years working in the international humanitarian sector co-ordinating relief and development projects, and he maintains a special interest in this field.

Mark Cannan, MSc, BSc (Hons), Dip HE

Mark is an Advanced Critical Care Practitioner in intensive care, at the North Cumbria University Hospitals Foundation Trust. Mark entered the healthcare profession as an Operating Department Practitioner (ODP) in 2013 with the University of Central Lancashire, having witnessed the work of an ODP first-hand in the theatres of Camp Bastion, Afghanistan. On qualification, he rotated through anaesthetic and scrub practice, in both elective and emergency surgical procedures in two busy district general hospitals. While qualifying with a diploma, he continued in education by completing an Honours degree in acute and critical care at the University of Cumbria, which is where he discovered the Advanced Critical Care Practitioner (ACCP) role. Having excluded career progression in managerial or educational roles, the ACCP role seemed to best fit his aspirations by being retained at the bedside, performing clinical duties. Mark started his ACCP training with Northumbria University in 2017 and qualified in 2019 with a post-graduate diploma and works across two general intensive care units which increased to four during the COVID-19 pandemic. Mark has since completed his Master's degree and has specialist interests in advanced airway management, regional anaesthesia and transfer of the critically ill patient. He is also on the national working group for legislation change in allowing ODPs who have progressed into advanced practice the ability to undertake non-medical prescribing.

Colin Chandler, BSc (Hons) Physiology, PhD, FHEA

Colin is a Lecturer in life science at the School of Health in Social Science (Nursing Studies), Programme Director MSc Advanced Nursing (online) and Programme Director PGCert Neurological Rehabilitation and Care (online) at the University of Edinburgh. Colin has extensive experience in life science education for nurses and allied health professional at both undergraduate and postgraduate levels. He has recently been involved in projects that have defined undergraduate anatomy and physiology curricula for nurses. He has wide experience of designing and delivering Master's and doctoral education and support for health, education and social care professionals to support their advanced practice.

Esther Clift, PhD, BSc (Hons), MSc

Consultant Practitioner – frailty, Chair of the Geriatric Society, National Speciality Advisor for NHSE, visiting lecturer at the University of Winchester, Winchester, UK.

Esther is currently working as a Consultant Practitioner in frailty for the Southern Health NHS Foundation Trust. She undertakes research in physiotherapy, geriatrics and allied health science. Her most recent publication is 'Use of the electronic Frailty Index to identify vulnerable patients: A pilot study in primary care'.

Rebecca Connolly, BA (Hons), BSc, MSc

Consultant ACP in emergency and critical care medicine, United Lincolnshire Hospitals NHS Trust, Associate Lecturer, University of Lincoln, Lincoln, UK, co-creator of the College of Paramedics national peer support programme, founding member of the College of Paramedics Diversity Steering Group. Rebecca specialises in Emergency and Critical Care Medicine. Before entering healthcare, she gained her undergraduate degrees in Japanese and Marketing, lived in Japan and studied at Kwansei Gakuin University. Returning to the UK, she worked as a police officer where her areas of specialism and interest were in deception and body language. Her passion for social psychology, body language, executive function and the neuropsychological processes that mediate decision making led her to complete her MSc in psychology where she researched psychopathy and success, together with facial microexpressions in psychopaths.

Stuart Cox, RN, BSc (Hons), MSc

Stuart works as an Advanced Critical Care Practitioner (ACCP) at University Hospitals Southampton NHS and Dorset and Somerset Air Ambulance. Prior to this, he was employed as a senior charge nurse ICU at Southampton and senior nurse CEGA Air Ambulance. He graduated with a BSc (Hons) in nursing science and completed his MSc in ACCP in 2018. Stuart is a registered nurse with the Nursing and Midwifery Council and an ACCP with membership with the Faculty of Intensive Care Medicine. Stuart is actively involved in national groups on advanced practice for the Intensive Care Society.

Rachael Daw

Senior Educationalist, Royal College of Physicians, London, UK.

Jo Delrée

Jo is a learning disability nurse with many years' experience as an Associate Professor in mental health and learning disability nurse education. She works as an educator and consultant for the NHS and higher education, including London South Bank University, specialising in issues affecting autistic people and people with learning disabilities.

Joanna De Souza, MSc, PATHE, RNT, AKC

Joanna is a Senior Lecturer at the Florence Nightingale Faculty of Nursing, Midwifery and Palliative Care, King's College London, UK. She has a nursing background in haemato-oncology and palliative care in the UK and New Zealand and is currently completing her doctorate in end-of-life family conversations with Lancaster University. She has taught the merits and skills of using evidence to inform practice since 2000 in the UK, China, Singapore and Somaliland.

Sadie Diamond-Fox, MCP, ACCP (mFICM), BSc (Hons), RN, PGCAHP, NMP (V300), FHEA

Sadie qualified as an adult nurse in 2008 and has since worked in various critical care departments. She progressed to her current advanced practice roles which include Advanced Critical Care Practitioner (ACCP),

Assistant Professor in Advanced Critical Care Practice (FHEA) and Speciality Advisor for Critical Care for the North East and Yorkshire's Regional Faculty of Advancing Practice, NHS England. Sadie is also currently a second-year Doctor of Philosophy (PhD) candidate and sits on various national and local advancing practice and critical care committees. She has an extensive teaching portfolio spanning multiple disciplines within postgraduate healthcare education, making a wide range of contributions at local and international levels. Her key areas of interest are postgraduate healthcare education, acute, emergency and critical care, physiology and pharmacology, advanced-level practice and simulation and virtual reality education modalities.

Leanne Dolman, RN, MSc, PGDip, BSc
Leanne is Lecturer (Adult Nursing), King's College, London, UK.

Christine Eade, MSc, PGCE, PgC, BSc (Hons)
Christine is a Consultant Plain Film Reporting Radiographer who works in the NHS and private healthcare sectors. She has worked at Royal Cornwall Hospitals Trust since qualifying from Bristol in 1999, with a specialist interest in paediatrics. She is also a member of the European Society of Paediatric Radiology AI Taskforce. Other professional activities include forensic radiography, career coaching and guest lecturing on the MSc Reporting and Advanced Practice modules for Plymouth and Exeter Universities.

Brigitta Fazzini, BSc(Hons), PgDiP DTN, MSc (Crit Care and Adv Clin Practice), NMP(V300)
Brigitta is an Advanced Critical Care Practitioner in the Adult Critical Care Unit at the Royal London Hospital. She is an honorary research fellow with Queen Mary University of London. She is a clinical academic passionate about critical care and critical care outreach and applied clinical research. She is the deputy chair of the Intensive Care Society (ICS) Professional Advisory Group for Advanced Practice in Critical Care and part of the chair team of the Advanced Clinical Practitioners Academic Network (ACPAN) in the UK. Her highest hope is to proactively shape the future of intensive care speciality with an inclusive multidisciplinary approach promoting effective quality changes, education and research.

Helen Francis-Wenger
Helen began her nursing career in Essex and soon focused her work on emergency medicine (EM), holding roles within EM in secondary care. Now, focusing on higher education for postgraduates as a lecturer in advanced clinical practice at the University of Plymouth, she is a fellow of the Higher Education Academy. Helen remains clinically active as an ACP in emergency medicine in Cornwall's Royal Cornwall Hospitals Trust, and is member of the Royal College of Emergency Medicine as well as being a registered independent prescriber. Helen is a credentialled ANP and an active committee member of the Association of Advanced Practice Educators and RCN ANP committee.

Alexandra Gatehouse, BSc (Hons), MSc
Alex graduated from Nottingham University in 2000 with a BSc (Hons) in physiotherapy. Following junior rotations in the Newcastle Trust, she specialised in respiratory physiotherapy in adult critical care, also working in New Zealand. In 2012, she trained as an Advanced Critical Care Practitioner, completing a Master's in clinical practice in critical care and qualifying in 2014. Alex subsequently completed her non-medical prescribing qualification and continues to rotate within all the critical care units in Newcastle upon Tyne, also enjoying teaching on the regional transfer course. She is a co-founder of the Advanced Critical Care Practitioner Northern Region Group and a committee member of the North East Intensive Care Society. Alex has presented abstracts at the European Society of Intensive Care Medicine and the North East Intensive Care Society conferences.

Kirstin Geer, Advanced Critical Care Practitioner. North Cumbria Integrated Care.
Kirstin qualified as a nurse in 2005 and worked on an Emergency Admissions Unit before becoming a Critical Care Outreach. She began her Advanced Critical Care Practitioner training in 2014 and qualified in 2016.

Barry Hill, MSc, PGCAP, BSc (Hons,) Dip HE, OA Dip, RN, NMC, RNT/TCH, SFHEA
Barry is Associate Professor and Director of Employability, Northumbria University; Consultant Editor for the International Journal for Advancing Practice; Clinical Editor for the British Journal of Nursing. Barry is an experienced leader, academic, educator, researcher and clinical nurse. His current role is Associate Professor and Director of Employability for nursing, midwifery and health. He has a demonstrated history of working within academia in higher education. Barry is a senior fellow and an HEA mentor, a certified intensive care nurse, with an MSc in advanced practice (clinical); NMC registered nurse, NMC registered teacher and NMC registered independent and supplementary prescriber (V300). He is skilled in clinical research and clinical education, and is passionate about higher education, especially nursing science, advanced clinical practice, critical care, non-medical prescribing and pharmacology. Barry is a strongly education-focused professional who has published nine books, 60 book chapters and 100 peer-reviewed journal articles. He is the Consultant Editor for the International Journal of Advancing Practice and Clinical Editor for the 'At a glance' and 'Advanced clinical practice' series within the British Journal of Nursing.

Robin Hyde, MSc, BN, RN (Child) RNT, RNMP, PGCert TL, HE, FHEA
Robin is an Assistant Professor in children and young people's nursing at Northumbria University. He is an NMC registered children's nurse, nurse teacher, independent/supplementary prescriber, qualified advanced paediatric nurse practitioner and fellow of the Higher Education Academy. Robin has been a qualified nurse for over 18 years. He is an experienced clinician and academic, having held a range of roles across the NHS and HEI sectors in Scotland and England. Robin is currently in year three of a PhD research project, carrying out a realist evaluation of an advanced practice programme in the context of children and young people's healthcare.

Joanna Lavery, MSc Advanced Practice, NMP, PgDip, SCPDN, PGCert Teaching and Learning In Clinical Practice, BSc (Hons), Dip HE, RN, FHEA, Queen's Nurse
Joanna is a Senior Lecturer in adult nursing and programme lead specialist community practitioner in district nursing at Liverpool John Moores University. She qualified as a registered nurse in 1999. She worked in neurosurgery and critical care before embarking upon a role in the community as a district nurse. She held posts as District Nurse Care Manager and Community Matron. Joanna returned to secondary care to work as an advanced nurse practitioner in acute medicine and ambulatory emergency care in 2013. She has worked in higher education since 2019 teaching both undergraduate and postgraduate students.

Elizabeth Midwinter, RN, MSc, BSc (Hons)
Elizabeth is a Continuous Improvement Clinical Fellow at Lancashire Teaching Hospitals NHS Foundation Trust. She is a registered nurse and advanced clinical practitioner in emergency medicine, arriving here via the scenic route (theatres, ED, urgent care, primary care and ED again), before moving to education as a Lecturer at the University of Bolton and Matron for resuscitation and simulation. Whilst in the role, Elizabeth became involved in a number of projects and completed the Flow Coaching Academy, which sparked her passion for improvement and led her to her current role.

Stevie Park
Stevie is an Advanced Critical Care Practitioner at University Hospital Birmingham, Birmingham, UK.

Ollie Phipps

Ollie is a Course Director for non-medical prescribing and MSc advanced clinical practice (ACP) at Canterbury Christ Church University. He has a clinical background as a consultant nurse in acute medicine and he continues to work as an advanced clinical practitioner in an emergency department in Kent. Ollie has led the Health Education England and Royal College of Physicians ACP Credential Development for Acute Medicine and Respiratory Medicine. Previously, he was the credential lead for the Centre for Advancing Practice, the chair of the Royal College of Nursing's Advanced Nurse Practitioner (ANP) Forum, and the National Advanced Practice Steering Group. He is a published author on the subject of advanced practice within multiple texts and is an international keynote speaker on the subject. Ollie continues to be a national expert advisor for advanced practice. He also is an expert advisor for the National Institute for Health and Care Excellence (NICE) and the National Confidential Enquiry into Patient Outcome and Death (NCEPOD).

Jaclyn Proctor

Jaclyn is an Advanced Clinical Practitioner at Warrington and Halton Teaching Hospitals NHS Foundation Trust, Warrington, UK.

Sharon Riverol, MSc (dist) Advanced Practice, BSc (Hons), Dip HE Nursing Studies, Adult RN, PGCert, FHEA

Sharon is a Senior Lecturer in adult nursing and deputy programme lead for the Trainee Nursing Associate programme at Liverpool John Moores University. She qualified as a registered nurse in 2005. She started her nursing career in stroke rehabilitation before moving to coronary care and then acute medical care, and then moving into general practice. As a general practice nurse, Sharon was able to complete her V300, her nursing degree and then her Master's in advanced practice. Sharon's roles included nurse manager and advanced nurse practitioner before moving into higher education. She started in higher education in 2020, teaching undergraduates, postgraduates and apprentice students, and has now completed the PGCert and is a fellow of the Higher Education Academy.

Colin Roberts

Colin qualified as a GP in 1996 in Exeter. He has been involved in education since then, initially as a GP trainer and medical student educator, but increasingly focused on advanced practice. He now works as Associate Professor in advanced practice at Plymouth University. He remains clinically active as a GP, validating his academic role. Colin teaches advanced practice widely across the South West of England with a keen interest in developing a scientific foundation in advanced practitioners, underpinning clinical skills and diagnostics. He is a champion of the advanced practice role across all aspects of healthcare and works strategically in the region to enhance training routes and continuing professional development.

Vikki-Jo Scott, RN, MA Learning and Teaching, SFHEA, current PhD student

Vikki-Jo has a background in critical care nursing and returned to clinical practice to work in critical care during the initial peaks of the COVID-19 pandemic. Since working in academia, she has focused on continuing professional development for health and social care professionals. She teaches on many courses, including those focused on quality improvement and application of learning to practice as well as leading the Advanced Clinical Practice programmes. She is a senior fellow of the Higher Education Academy and up until 2020 was Dean of the School of Health and Social Care at the University of Essex, England. She is currently undertaking a PhD focused on advanced clinical practice and is a reviewer for the Centre for Advancing Practice accreditation processes.

Sara Stevenson-Baker, MSc, PGCE, BSc (Hons)

Sara is a Lecturer in nursing at King's College, London. She has worked in a variety of clinical and educational environments, including hospital and community within palliative care, oncology, general medicine and intensive care nursing and higher education. Sara has developed advanced clinical and educational skills by being committed to ensuring that her own practice, skills and knowledge are maintained. She has completed a BSc (Hons) degree in cancer nursing and an MSc in education for healthcare professionals. Sara successfully gained her Postgraduate Certificate in Education in 2012 and Advanced Assessment skills in 2011 at King's College University. She has also completed and delivered advanced communication training and Sage and Thyme Foundation communication training.

Vanessa Taylor, RGN, EdD, MSc Advanced Clinical Practice (Cancer Nursing), PGCE, BSc, DPSN

Vanessa is the Director of health and care partnerships/professor of cancer and palliative care at the School of Human and Health Sciences, University of Huddersfield, Huddersfield, UK. Following clinical roles in cancer and palliative care, Vanessa moved into higher education. Her activities and published work focus on cancer, palliative and end-of-life care and education, evaluation of education and its impact on workforce development and clinical practice. As chair of steering group/lead author for the RCN Career and Education Framework for Cancer Nursing and chair of steering group/lead author HEE (Yorkshire and the Humber) End of Life Care Learning Outcomes, Vanessa has published unique resources that distinguish levels of knowledge, skills and practice for the workforce in these fields. Most recently, Vanessa chaired the steering group developing the HEE ACP-Palliative and End of Life Care credential. She is a steering group member of the ACCEND project and chair of workstream 5 developing the 'Career pathway, core cancer capabilities in practice and education framework'. Vanessa is a member of the NHSE/I group developing a career pathway and education framework for palliative and end-of-life care. She was awarded a National Teaching Fellowship in 2020 and is chair of the Biosciences in Nursing Education Group.

John Wilkinson, MBBS, PGCert Med Ed

John is an Anaesthetics Registrar in the Northern School of Anaesthesia and Intensive Care Medicine, with a special interest in education and simulation. After studying medicine at Newcastle University and completing Foundation training in Newcastle Trust Hospitals, he trained in anaesthetic and critical care departments across the north of England, including as a clinical and education fellow in critical care. He has presented on the development of a novel educational resource at the annual meeting of the Society for Education in Anaesthesia. He has a particular interest in multidisciplinary team simulation training, including creating resources for sessions involving medical, nursing and midwifery students from Newcastle and Northumbria Universities.

Alison Wood, PhD, RGN

Alison is a Lecturer in non-medical prescribing in the Division of Nursing and Paramedic Science at Queen Margaret University, Edinburgh, Scotland. Alison's clinical nursing career has most recently focused on haemodialysis and renal medicine and this formed the focus of her PhD, exploring care in this clinical setting. Alison holds an honorary title within NHS Lothian as nurse consultant for non-medical prescribing and remains active in a clinical capacity alongside her full-time lecturing post. She is also a member of the Bioscience in Nurse Education (BiNE) group and engagement with science in pre- and postregistration healthcare education is a strong interest area, having led a project to develop a set of learning outcomes on physiology for pre-registration nurse education.

Joe Wood

Joe is an Advanced Critical Care Practitioner, physiotherapist and point-of-care ultrasound educator at the Medway NHS Foundation Trust, Kent, England.

Preface

The Advanced Practitioner: A Framework for Practice is the first of its kind. It provides a multiprofessional resource that uses the four pillars underpinning advanced practice as a framework: clinical practice, leadership and management, research and education. The text offers essential reading that is related to contemporary advanced clinical practice topics.

The Advanced Practitioner: A Framework for Practice has been written primarily for the trainee advanced practitioner. Advanced practitioners (APs) come from a range of professional backgrounds, including physiotherapy, pharmacy, paramedics, occupational therapy and nursing, practising across the age continuum and in a variety of spheres of practice, at the top of their licence. The focus of this text is on the adult person.

The advanced practitioner role offers the added value of an experienced clinician; it is a co-productive role that meets the needs of populations. Advanced practice offers a vision for the development of the workforce in a way that is consistent, ensuring safety, promoting quality and resulting in positive patient outcomes.

Advanced practice programmes have been developed to meet national and local policy drivers for workforce transformation through a Master's level programme. Using a level 7 taxonomy makes clear the expectation that practitioners working at this level are required to perform at Master's level. *The Advanced Practitioner: A Framework for Practice* is cognisant of this and the chapters in the text mirror this.

Readers will develop their knowledge, skills and behaviours required to act with a high level of autonomy, enhancing their skills in holistic and systematic assessment, complex decision making along with the provision of high-quality evidence-based interventions for patients and their families. This text will support the reader undertaking a programme of study to strengthen their learning through the application of theory related to their scope of practice in the workplace and the academic setting. The text will also be of value to those advanced practitioners who are seeking to update and review their knowledge and understanding of the various topics associated with advanced practice.

Throughout *The Advanced Practitioner: A Framework for Practice,* the service user is placed at the centre of all that is done, as is the case in practice. Key to education and training is understanding the importance of the time and experience required to build confidence in decision making and the management of risk. *The Advanced Practitioner: A Framework for Practice* facilitates individual and organisational development.

This is the 'go to' text for trainee advanced practitioners, with content written by experienced advanced practitioners and academics who are closely involved in the delivery of advanced practice programmes. A range of curricula have been assessed and wide consultation with key stakeholders has been undertaken to derive content for the chapters and format of the text.

Trainee advanced practitioners will undergo frequent assessment, using approaches such as consultation, observation tools, clinical portfolios and case-based discussion. Examination and procedural skills undertaken as part of the advanced practitioner role are assessed in practice. The trainee advanced practitioner is required to demonstrate competence, and there are a number of directly observed procedures that need to be undertaken along with the ability to 'see' the whole person and fuse biomedical science with the art of caring, providing health promotion advice, counselling, assessment, diagnosis, referral, treatment and discharge.

The Advanced Practitioner: A Framework for Practice focuses on regulatory body requirements such as those of the Health and Care Professions Council and Nursing and Midwifery Council. The text has been aligned to nationally established advanced practitioner curricula, including the Faculty of Intensive Care Medicine (FICM), the Royal College of Emergency Medicine (RCEM) and the Royal College of Nursing (RCN).

Created for the busy practising clinician, the 21 chapters in this text have been written by a variety of experts in the field, across a range of specialties, and the information provided is accessible and engaging. Each chapter has been written using an approach that will enable the reader to delve deeper into essential subject matter, encourage curiosity and offer safe and effective care to people.

High-quality colour illustrations, line drawings, tables, charts, graphs, and algorithms have been used in the comprehensive chapters to aid understanding as well as the retention of key facts. Pedagogical features are offered in such a way to support the trainee advanced practitioner to address the many curriculum requirements and to be successful when undertaking the various assessment challenges that they will face. These features aim to encourage the reader to delve deeper and challenge practice.

Containing numerous essential practical and theoretical components, *The Advanced Practitioner: A Framework for Practice* is the essential contemporary resource for all trainee advanced clinical practitioner as well as those healthcare students who are seeking to advance in this sphere of practice.

We sincerely hope you enjoy reading this text as much we have enjoyed editing it and providing you with a contemporary and useful resource as you make the transformation to advanced practitioner.

Ian Peate, London
Sadie Diamond-Fox, Newcastle
Barry Hill, Newcastle

Acknowledgements

We are grateful to the contributors of the text for their input as they worked and are working through the ongoing COVID pandemic. Ian would like to thank his partner Jussi for his continued support. Barry would like to thank his family and friends for their continued support and give a special thanks to the chapter contributors and co-editors Ian and Sadie. A big thank you to Wiley for this excellent opportunity. Sadie would like to thank her 'tribe'. This book is dedicated to her family (in particular Andy & Oscar), her friends and her contributor colleagues, without whom this would not have been possible.

CHAPTER 1

Advanced Clinical Practice

Sadie Diamond-Fox and Vikki-Jo Scott

Aim

The aim of this chapter is to provide the context in which this book is set and a background to the development of and current state of advanced practice in England. It sets out the framework within which advanced-level practice operates and how this has been utilised to structure this book to guide the reader through the fundamental aspects expected of advanced practitioners.

LEARNING OUTCOMES

After reading this chapter the reader will:

1. understand the context in which advanced clinical practice operates
2. know the current policy reference points for advanced clinical practice
3. be aware of the themes that shape implementation of advanced clinical practice
4. comprehend the shared definition of advanced clinical practice.

INTRODUCTION

Advanced-level practice began to emerge in the United States as far back as the 1960s (Dunn 1997). Examples of developing trained healthcare professionals to take on additional advanced tasks and skills or extended roles can now be found globally. Comparisons have been made between the UK trajectory and that in Europe and Australia, with recognition that different countries, and professions, specialties or particular healthcare services are at different stages of developing models of advanced practice (AP). The nomenclature surrounding this subject area is not universally applicable across the globe and can often

The Advanced Practitioner: A Framework for Practice, First Edition. Edited by Ian Peate, Sadie Diamond-Fox, and Barry Hill.
© 2024 John Wiley & Sons Ltd. Published 2024 by John Wiley & Sons Ltd.

TABLE 1.1 Definition of advanced clinical practice as defined by Health Education England.

Advanced clinical practice:

- is delivered by experienced, registered health and care practitioners
- is characterised by a high degree of autonomy and complex decision making
- is underpinned by a Master's level award or equivalent
- encompasses the four pillars of clinical practice, leadership and management, education and research
- demonstrates core capabilities and area-specific clinical competence
- embodies the ability to manage clinical care in partnership with individuals, families and carers
- includes the analysis and synthesis of complex problems across a range of settings, enabling innovative solutions to enhance people's experience and improve outcomes.

Source: Adapted from HEE (2017).

be confusing, therefore a detailed glossary of the application in the context of UK practice is included at the end of this chapter and Table 1.1 details the universally accepted definition of advanced clinical practice (ACP) within the UK.

This chapter will give the advanced practitioner the knowledge and understanding of the context of advanced clinical practice to provide a foundation which can be built upon in clinical practice in a supervised and independent manner.

Multi-Professional Framework for Advanced Clinical Practice (MPFfACP)

This chapter relates to the following areas of the MPFfACP:
1.2, 1.2, 2.2, 2.10, 2.11, 3.1, 3.2, 3.8, 4.6

(HEE 2017)

Accreditation Considerations

This chapter is applicable to the following specialist curricula:

- Acute Medicine (HEE 2022a)
- Critical Care (ACCP) (FICM 2015)
- Emergency Care – Adult & Child (RCEM 2022)
- Learning Disability and/or Autism (HEE 2020a)
- Mental Health (HEE 2022b)
- Older People (HEE 2022c)
- Primary Care (HEE 2020b)
- Surgical Care (HEE 2020c)

This is an ever evolving field and work continues to agree various competence and capability frameworks for advanced clinical practice in other clinical specialties, therefore the readers is encouraged to refer to https://advanced-practice.hee.nhs.uk/credentials

The Concept and History of Advanced-Level Practice

Initial development of AP roles is typified by a need to reconfigure services to address unmet need. Increasing life expectancy, complexity and disease burden, the European Working Time Directive and a subsequent shortage of medical personnel have often been cited as drivers for the implementation of advanced practice roles (Boulanger 2008; Evans et al. 2020; Torrens et al. 2020). However, caution is advised when rationalising their introduction and development to that of the medical substitution paradigm. Advanced practice roles complement existing medical models and are not designed to replace them. Since their inception, there has been great diversity in ACP roles and also some controversy surrounding them. Nevertheless, a colossal effort from professional bodies such as the Council of Deans of Health (CoDoH), the Association of Advanced Practice Educators (AAPE UK) and the royal colleges as well as HEE has led to a huge investment in workforce development in this area of service delivery, in order to meet patient needs in the future. Development in this area has also included the introduction of a multiprofessional definition of advanced clinical practice, the first of its kind, to provide clarity for employers, service leads, education providers, health professionals and ACPs themselves (HEE 2017) (Table 1.1).

Frameworks and Toolkits for Advanced Clinical Practice

Advanced practice has been evolving across the four UK countries over decades. Health Education England, NHS England, NHS Improvement and NHS Employers (2022) have developed the Advanced Practice Toolkit. This resource is aimed at practitioners, educators, employers, commissioners, those planning the workforce across systems and patients/service users. NHS Scotland (2018) have also developed an online repository of the national resources that pertain to all four nations.

A number of professional bodies have collaborated with Health Education England to create the 'Multi-Professional Framework for Advanced Clinical Practice in England' (MPfACP) (HEE 2017) (Figure 1.1). This framework sets out the definition of ACP, the scope of practice and practitioners this applies to, and the standards and capabilities that are expected in order to practise under this title. While this does not provide regulation of the title of 'advanced clinical practitioner', it has now provided a benchmark by which education and training providers can badge their products as leading to advanced clinical practice, employers can use to select individuals to work in ACP roles or undertake ACP-related tasks, and against which individuals can provide evidence to support their credentials as an ACP. Chapter 2 explores this subject in further detail.

Ensuring Quality and Governance in Advanced Practice

Since their inception, there has been great diversity in ACP roles and also some controversy surrounding them.

Before the release of the NHS Long-Term Plan (NHSE 2019), the CoDoH was commissioned by HEE, as part of the development and implementation of the Multi-professional Framework for ACP in England (HEE 2017), to revolutionise the interface between HEE and universities. Since the seminal CoDoH (2018) report, and in line with the Five Year Forward View (NHS England 2014, 2017), there have been several important developments for the ACP arena. As a result of significant investment and infrastructure, multiple initiatives are either well established or under way to strive for continued quality and governance and ultimately to promote patient safety.

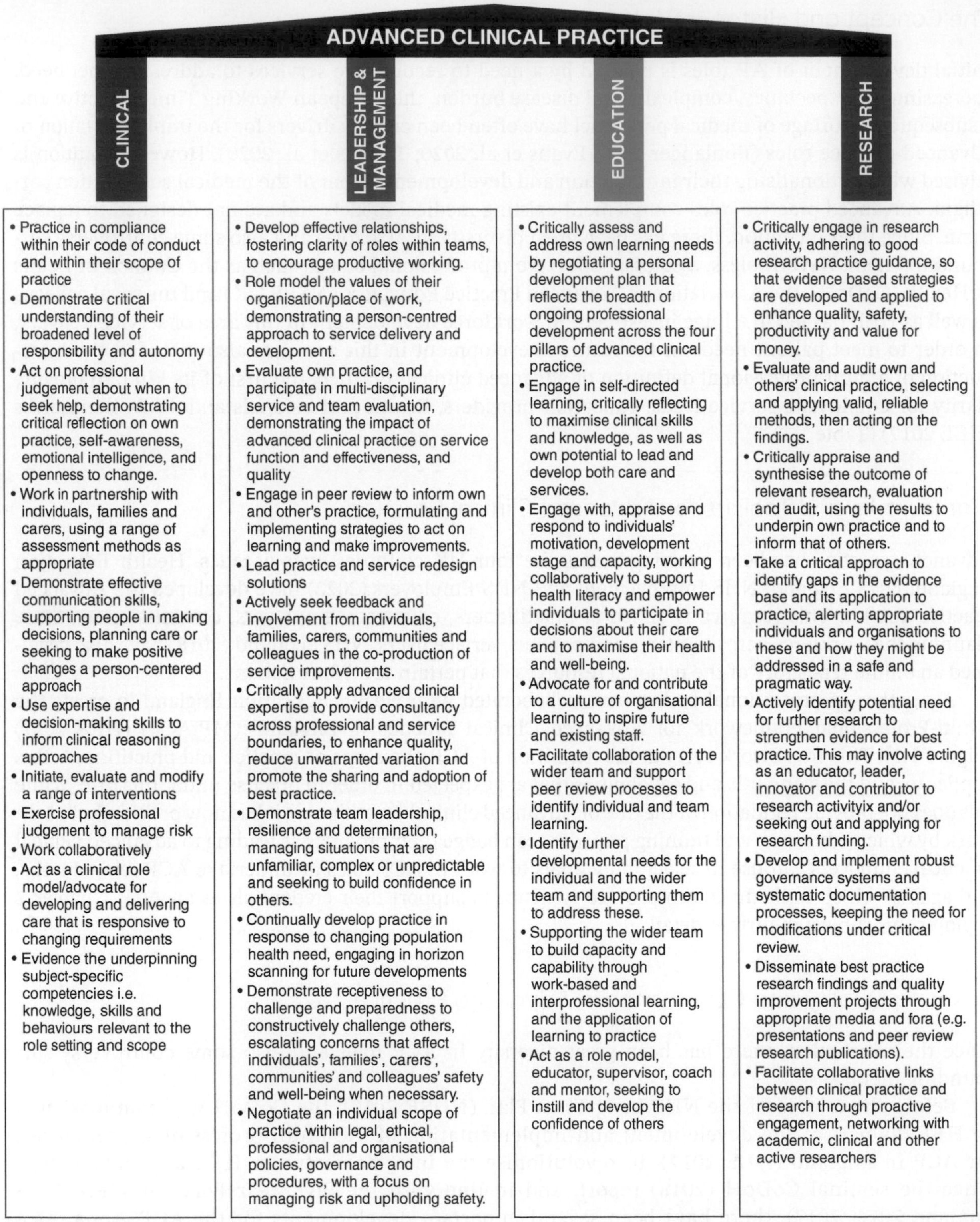

ADVANCED CLINICAL PRACTICE

CLINICAL

- Practice in compliance within their code of conduct and within their scope of practice
- Demonstrate critical understanding of their broadened level of responsibility and autonomy
- Act on professional judgement about when to seek help, demonstrating critical reflection on own practice, self-awareness, emotional intelligence, and openness to change.
- Work in partnership with individuals, families and carers, using a range of assessment methods as appropriate
- Demonstrate effective communication skills, supporting people in making decisions, planning care or seeking to make positive changes a person-centered approach
- Use expertise and decision-making skills to inform clinical reasoning approaches
- Initiate, evaluate and modify a range of interventions
- Exercise professional judgement to manage risk
- Work collaboratively
- Act as a clinical role model/advocate for developing and delivering care that is responsive to changing requirements
- Evidence the underpinning subject-specific competencies i.e. knowledge, skills and behaviours relevant to the role setting and scope

LEADERSHIP & MANAGEMENT

- Develop effective relationships, fostering clarity of roles within teams, to encourage productive working.
- Role model the values of their organisation/place of work, demonstrating a person-centred approach to service delivery and development.
- Evaluate own practice, and participate in multi-disciplinary service and team evaluation, demonstrating the impact of advanced clinical practice on service function and effectiveness, and quality
- Engage in peer review to inform own and other's practice, formulating and implementing strategies to act on learning and make improvements.
- Lead practice and service redesign solutions
- Actively seek feedback and involvement from individuals, families, carers, communities and colleagues in the co-production of service improvements.
- Critically apply advanced clinical expertise to provide consultancy across professional and service boundaries, to enhance quality, reduce unwarranted variation and promote the sharing and adoption of best practice.
- Demonstrate team leadership, resilience and determination, managing situations that are unfamiliar, complex or unpredictable and seeking to build confidence in others.
- Continually develop practice in response to changing population health need, engaging in horizon scanning for future developments
- Demonstrate receptiveness to challenge and preparedness to constructively challenge others, escalating concerns that affect individuals', families', carers', communities' and colleagues' safety and well-being when necessary.
- Negotiate an individual scope of practice within legal, ethical, professional and organisational policies, governance and procedures, with a focus on managing risk and upholding safety.

EDUCATION

- Critically assess and address own learning needs by negotiating a personal development plan that reflects the breadth of ongoing professional development across the four pillars of advanced clinical practice.
- Engage in self-directed learning, critically reflecting to maximise clinical skills and knowledge, as well as own potential to lead and develop both care and services.
- Engage with, appraise and respond to individuals' motivation, development stage and capacity, working collaboratively to support health literacy and empower individuals to participate in decisions about their care and to maximise their health and well-being.
- Advocate for and contribute to a culture of organisational learning to inspire future and existing staff.
- Facilitate collaboration of the wider team and support peer review processes to identify individual and team learning.
- Identify further developmental needs for the individual and the wider team and supporting them to address these.
- Supporting the wider team to build capacity and capability through work-based and interprofessional learning, and the application of learning to practice
- Act as a role model, educator, supervisor, coach and mentor, seeking to instill and develop the confidence of others

RESEARCH

- Critically engage in research activity, adhering to good research practice guidance, so that evidence based strategies are developed and applied to enhance quality, safety, productivity and value for money.
- Evaluate and audit own and others' clinical practice, selecting and applying valid, reliable methods, then acting on the findings.
- Critically appraise and synthesise the outcome of relevant research, evaluation and audit, using the results to underpin own practice and to inform that of others.
- Take a critical approach to identify gaps in the evidence base and its application to practice, alerting appropriate individuals and organisations to these and how they might be addressed in a safe and pragmatic way.
- Actively identify potential need for further research to strengthen evidence for best practice. This may involve acting as an educator, leader, innovator and contributor to research activityix and/or seeking out and applying for research funding.
- Develop and implement robust governance systems and systematic documentation processes, keeping the need for modifications under critical review.
- Disseminate best practice research findings and quality improvement projects through appropriate media and fora (e.g. presentations and peer review research publications).
- Facilitate collaborative links between clinical practice and research through proactive engagement, networking with academic, clinical and other active researchers

FIGURE 1.1   The four pillar of advanced clinical practice based upon the Health Education England Multi-professional Framework. *Source*: Hill B, Diamond-Fox S 2022/John Wiley & Sons.

Chapters 2 and 3 explore this area in further detail, but broadly these initiatives include the following.

- Development of the MPfACP (HEE 2017)
- Launch of the Centre for Advancing Practice to support education and training for advanced practitioners
- HEE accreditation of ACP university training programmes
- Area-specific workforce development interventions (HEE 2022c)
- ACP level 7 apprenticeships – incorporating skills development, technical knowledge and practical experience through a work-based training programme (NHS Employers 2022)
- Multiprofessional consultant-level practice capability and impact framework (HEE 2020b)
- Guidance for the supervision of ACPs (HEE 2020b,d)
- Signpost for Continuing Professional Development (HEE 2021)
- Advanced Practice Governance Maturity Matrix (HEE 2022f)
- ePortfolio (supported) route (HEE 2022g)

HOW TO USE THIS BOOK

This book provides a guide to the expected standards for the advanced clinical practitioner across a range of topic areas, field specialties and context through the application of a standard pedagogy which appears within boxes throughout this text (Table 1.2). Each chapter is designed to give the reader a point of reference for developing their knowledge and skills and to help them to seek out opportunities within their practice context to gain the experience needed to become a competent and confident advanced practitioner across all four pillars of advanced practice (Figure 1.1).

In this book, we have deliberately provided reference to a broad range of examples and potential applications to practice through in-text citations in each chapter and also within the further resources sections detailed in the end of each chapter. This reflects the burgeoning body of evidence that notes the incredible diversity of advanced-level practice operating in the healthcare context today and has developed in many ways, often at the forefront of innovation. We do not attempt to provide an exhaustive account of all the different types of advanced roles that are occurring; in fact, this is the antithesis of AP which is based on taking a ground-breaking approach to address service need and so will continue to develop in ways that cannot be captured by a book that has been written at one particular time.

CONCLUSION

Exciting times lie ahead for the development of new AP roles and the expansion of existing AP posts within the NHS. We still have a way to go when considering the long-term workforce development support for this group of clinicians, who, by nature of the career path they have chosen, are inherently driven to progress. The launch of the HEE Centre for Advancing Practice (https://advanced-practice.hee.nhs.uk/) has already proved to be the hub for such activity. Medical colleges and professional groups have representation from advanced practitioners on central committees and in clinical lead roles for key work streams, giving this workforce an important opportunity to shape the development of these specialties for the future. Other networks created to provide

TABLE 1.2   An explanation of the pedagogy used within this book (boxed).

Multi-professional Framework for Advanced Clinical Practice (MPFfACP)	Provides direct mapping of chapter content to the MPFfACP (HEE 2017)
Accreditation considerations	Provides direct mapping of chapter content to published ACP accreditation frameworks, e.g. Royal College of Emergency Medicine (RCEM 2022)
Clinical investigations	These provide a link to relevant clinical investigations that pertain to the content of the chapter
Examination scenarios	Encourage the application of diagnostic and management skills to a case scenario in the context of each chapter
Fields of practice – paediatrics	Considerations for ACPs working in the field of paediatrics
Fields of practice – mental health	Considerations for ACPs working in the field of mental health
Fields of practice – learning disabilities	Considerations for ACPs working in the field of learning disabilities
Learning events	Pertinent topics that encourage reflection
Pharmacological principles	Principles of pharmacology and prescribing in the context of the chapter content. This may include considerations of the scientific basis underlying the principles of drug therapy, or important considerations the practitioner should reflect upon when considering prescribing practices
Red flags	Pathological considerations in the context of the provision of health and care which relate to the chapter subject/content
Orange flags	Psychological considerations in the context of the provision of health and care which relate to the chapter subject/content
Green flags	Social considerations in the context of the provision of health and care which relate to the chapter subject/content
Case studies	These are related to chapter content. They will be challenging case studies and data led, encouraging the reader to analyse the data, make clinical decisions and apply the decisions to practice

Please note the pedagogy has been applied in the context of relevance to each chapter, therefore not all chapters will contain all the boxes detailed above.

education, support and research opportunities are now developing, building an important infrastructure to support this growing workforce.

> **Take Home Points**
> - Advanced practice is diverse and continues to develop, reflecting its position as a way to address service needs in innovative ways.
> - The Multi-Professional Framework for Advanced Clinical Practice provides the definition, scope and standards that advanced practitioners need to operate in England. This is the key reference point for the expected capabilities of advanced practitioners.
> - Key policy developments have placed an emphasis on advanced practice to address workforce needs that reflect the ambition to 'grow for the future'.

REFERENCES

Boulanger, C. (2008). The advanced critical care practitioner: trailblazing or selling out? *Journal of the Intensive Care Society* 9 (3): 216–217.

Council of Deans of Health. (2018). Advanced clinical practice education in England. `https://tinyurl.com/y2a7cnoa`

Dunn, L. (1997). A literature review of advanced clinical nursing practice in the United States. *Journal of Advanced Nursing* 25: 814–819.

Evans, C., Poku, B., Pearce, R. et al. (2020). Characterising the evidence base for advanced clinical practice in the UK: a scoping review protocol. *BMJ Open* 10: e036192.

Faculty of Intensive Care Medicine (2015). Curriculum Training for Advanced Critical Care Practitioners – Part 1 Handbook. `www.ficm.ac.uk/careersworkforceaccps/accp-curriculum`

Health Education England (2017) Multi-professional framework for advanced clinical practice in England. `www.hee.nhs.uk/sites/default/files/docuemtns/HEE%20ACP%Framework.pdf`

Health Education England (2020a). Advanced Clinical Practice: Capabilities framework when working with people who have a learning disability and/or autism. `www.skillsforhealth.org.uk/wp-content/uploads/2020/11/ACP-in-LDA-Framework.pdf`

Health Education England (2020b). Multiprofessional consultant-level practice capability and impact framework. It was accessed via `https://advanced-practice.hee.nhs.uk/reports-and-publications/`

Health Education England (2020c). Surgical Advanced Clinical Practitioner (SACP) Curriculum and Assessment Framework. `www.iscp.ac.uk/media/1141/sacp_curriculum_dec20_accessible-1.pdf`

Health Education England (2020d) Workplacc Supervision for Advanced Clinical Practice: An integrated multi-professional approach for practitioner development. `www.hee.nhs.uk/sites/default/files/documents/Workplace%20Supervision%20for%20ACPs.pdf`

Health Education England (2021). Advancing Practice: Signpost for continuing professional development. `www.hee.nhs.uk/sites/default/files/documents/Signposting%20for%20CPD.pdf`

Health Education England (2022a). Advanced Clinical Practice in Acute Medicine Curriculum Framework. `https://healtheducationengland.sharepoint.com/sites/APWC/Shared%20Documents/Forms/AllItems.aspx?id=%2Fsites%2FAPWC%2FShared%20Documents%2FCredentials%2FCredentials%20Endorsement%20Documents%2FAdvanced%20clinical%20practice%20in%20acute%20medicine%20curriculum%20framework%2Epdf&parent=%2Fsites%2FAPWC%2FShared%20Documents%2FCredentials%2FCredentials%20Endorsement%20Documents&p=true&ga=1`

Health Education England (2022b). Advanced Practice Mental Health Curriculum and Capabilities Framework. `https://healtheducationengland.sharepoint.com/sites/APWC/Shared%20Documents/Forms/AllItems.aspx?id=%2Fsites%2FAPWC%2FShared%20Documents%2FCredentials%2FCredentials%20Endorsement%20Documents%2FAdvanced%20practice%20in%20mental%20health%20curriculum%20and%20capabilities%20framework%2Epdf&parent=%2Fsites%2FAPWC%2FShared%20Documents%2FCredentials%2FCredentials%20Endorsement%20Documents&p=true&ga=1`

Health Education England (2022c). Different types of area-specific workforce development interventions within advanced-level practice. `https://tinyurl.com/3w9zhphj`

Health Education England (2022f). Advanced Practice Governance Maturity Matrix. `https://tinyurl.com/4xkw26yu`

Health Education England (2022g). ePortfolio (supported) Route. `https://advanced-practice.hee.nhs.uk/eportfolio-route/`

Health Education England, NHS England, NHS Improvement and NHS Employers (2022). The Advanced Practice Toolkit. www.e-lfh.org.uk/programmes/advanced-practice-toolkit/

NHS England (2014). The NHS Five Year Forward View. https://tinyurl.com/nyfwceu

NHS England (2017). Next Steps on the NHS Five Year Forward View. https://tinyurl.com/l6xt5lt

NHS England and NHS Improvement (2019). The NHS Long Term Plan. https://tinyurl.com/y65q8n6f

NHS Scotland (2018). Advanced Practice Toolkit. www.advancedpractice.scot.nhs.uk/uk-progress.aspx

Royal College of Emergency Medicine (2022). Emergency Medicine Advanced Clinical Practitioner Curriculum 2022 Adult. https://rcem.ac.uk/acp-curriculum/

Torrens, C., Campbell, P., Hoskins, G. et al. (2020). Barriers and facilitators to the implementation of the advanced nurse practitioner role in primary care settings: a scoping review. *International Journal of Nursing Studies* 104: 103443.

FURTHER READING

Centre for Advancing Practice Resources: https://advanced-practice.hee.nhs.uk/resources-news-and-events/

Hill, B. and Diamond-Fox, S. (2022). *Advanced Clinical Practice at a Glance*. Chichester: Wiley-Blackwell.

SELF-ASSESSMENT QUESTIONS

1. Define the context in which advanced clinical practice operates.
2. Recite the current policy reference points for advanced clinical practice.
3. Discuss the themes that shape implementation of advanced clinical practice.
4. Discuss the shared definition of advanced clinical practice.

GLOSSARY

Advanced-level practice Includes all practitioners who have progressed to an advanced level through further education and training (HEE 2017).

Advanced clinical practice A defined level of practice within clinical professions such as nursing, pharmacy, paramedics and occupational therapy. This level of practice is designed to transform and modernise pathways of care, enabling the safe and effective sharing of skills across traditional professional boundaries (HEE 2017).

Advanced clinical practitioner (ACP) ACPs come from a range of professional backgrounds such as nursing, pharmacy, paramedics and occupational therapy. They are healthcare professionals educated to Master's level and have developed the skills and knowledge to allow them to take on expanded roles and scope of practice in caring for patients (HEE 2017).

Capabilities Extent to which individuals can adapt to change, generate new knowledge and continue to improve their performance (HEE 2017).

Centre for Advancing Practice A health education initiative to oversee the workforce transformation of advanced-level practice, by establishing and monitoring standards for education and training, accrediting advanced-level programmes, supporting and recognising educational and training equivalence, and growing and embedding the advanced and consultant practice workforce.

Competencies   What individuals know or are able to do in terms of knowledge, skills and behaviour (HEE 2017).

Master's level award   This is an award that uses the relevant descriptors set at level 7 by the Framework for Higher Education Qualifications (FHEQ). See also: www.gov.uk/what-differentqualification-levels-mean/listof-qualification-levels

Multiprofessional   A term used to denote co-operation of health professionals from three or more different health professions.

Nomenclature   A system of names or terms, or the rules for forming these terms in a particular field of arts or sciences.

Practitioner   A non-medical clinical member of the workforce who may come from any professional background (HEE 2017).

CHAPTER 2

The Advanced Clinical Practice Curriculum

Rachael Daw and Ollie Phipps

Aim

The aim of this chapter is to explore the necessary requirements for practitioners, employers and higher educational institutions to ensure that practitioners are adequately trained with the correct knowledge, skills and behaviours to ensure competence, capability, safety, governance and quality assurance for service users, patients and the public.

LEARNING OUTCOMES

After reading this chapter the reader will:

1. understand the role and level of practice of the advanced clinical practitioner
2. appreciate the scope of learning required for advanced clinical practice
3. understand the requirement for practitioners to be clinically competent and embrace the four pillars of advanced practice within their speciality, sector and setting
4. understand the need for Level 7 academic study and how this relates to advanced clinical practice.

INTRODUCTION

With an ever changing and evolving healthcare system, the purpose of advanced practice and the role of advanced clinical practitioners (ACPs) are now recognised to be essential, and are expected to be relied upon to a greater extent for future workforce development (NHS Long Term Plan 2019). The NHS Multi-professional framework (MPF) for advanced practice in England (HEE 2017) describes the high level needed for a consistent approach to developing the role of ACPs to ensure quality, safety and governance are in place.

The Advanced Practitioner: A Framework for Practice, First Edition. Edited by Ian Peate,
Sadie Diamond-Fox, and Barry Hill.
© 2024 John Wiley & Sons Ltd. Published 2024 by John Wiley & Sons Ltd.

It is essential that those undertaking advanced roles are educationally prepared with the correct knowledge, skills and behaviours. The MPF (HEE 2017) sets out an agreed definition of advanced clinical practice in England for all health and care professionals and a clear set of standards which must be met and maintained. It articulates what it means for individuals to practise at an advanced level from that achieved on initial registration within their profession, and outlines the skills and knowledge that ACPs should develop to undertake clinical decision making in the context of complexity and uncertainty (HEE 2017).

Subsequent developments and guidance, including area-specific clinical competencies, the ACP Apprenticeship and the accreditation of higher education programmes and individual ACPs, have added further to the clarity of expectation for ACP education which will be further discussed within this chapter. However, in some sectors there remains a degree of misunderstanding of the scope and level of practice for ACP, which can only be improved by a more consistent approach to education, development and governance.

As understanding of the standards of practice for ACP increases, it should continue to be acknowledged that ACP is not a specific role but rather a level of practice that includes core competencies (aligned to the four pillars of ACP defined by the MPF), as well as area-specific knowledge and skills which will differ according to the demands of a specific role. Advanced practice roles can cover a spectrum ranging from those with a specialist emphasis but encompassing a breadth of supporting knowledge and skills to more generalist roles, covering a broader scope of practice. In both scenarios, the role may be closely aligned to the medical model or different, but complementary, to it (Figure 2.1).

This variability, coupled with the differences in foundation knowledge and skills of the multiple professions that might present for ACP training and education, means that every individual practitioner will present with a unique set of learning needs. It is essential therefore that the ACP curriculum offers flexibility to meet individual requirements, whilst also preserving the consistency and quality required to ensure governance and safety necessary for this level of practice. These complexities in ACP development consequently necessitate a collaborative approach to learning between higher education institutions (HEIs), individual trainees and their employing organisations, to ensure achievement of authentic, applicable skills through both academic and work-based learning and assessment.

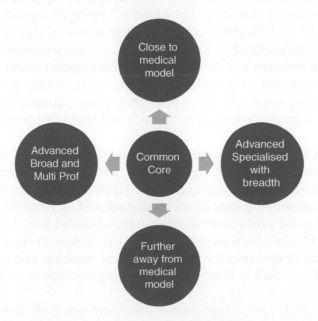

FIGURE 2.1 Advanced practice spectrum. *Source*: Adapted from HEE (2021).

Multi-professional Framework for Advanced Clinical Practice (MPFfACP)

This chapter relates to the following areas of the MPFfACP:
3.1–3.8

(HEE 2017)

Accreditation Considerations

This chapter relates to the following specialist curricula:

- Acute Medicine (HEE 2022a)
- Critical Care (ACCP) (FICM 2015)
- Emergency Care (RCEM 2022)
- Learning Disability and/or Autism (HEE 2020a)
- Mental Health (HEE 2022b)
- Older People (HEE 2022c)
- Primary Care (HEE 2020b)
- Surgical Care (HEE 2020c)

CURRICULUM DEVELOPMENT

The MPFfACP (HEE 2017) identifies the necessity for ACPs to be educated to Level 7, with their practice underpinned by 'a Master's level award or equivalent'; the curriculum for ACP development must therefore be appropriate to this level. The Quality Assurance Agency for Higher Education (2020) descriptor for Level 7 qualifications emphasises the nature of this level of study to develop and achieve systematic understanding of knowledge and critical awareness of current problems, ability to critically evaluate research and the skill to deal with complex issues systematically and creatively, making sound judgements in the absence of complete information. These attributes, along with self-direction in learning and autonomy in problem solving, planning and implementing tasks, are clearly commensurate with the core skills of the ACP and should be central to their learning and development.

Any curriculum for ACP, whether it is delivered by a HEI or negotiated between a clinician and their employer for development in practice, must ensure that the practitioner is able to achieve and demonstrate all the capabilities for ACP as outlined in the MPFfACP (HEE 2017). Historically, there has been a strong focus in practice and education on the clinical pillar of ACP, but the skills and knowledge of all four pillars are essential to the practitioner working at the advanced level defined by HEE. The capabilities described in the MPF have been mapped to Level 7 taxonomy to support the expectation that this will be the assured level of operation for the ACP. Critical thinking, ability to systematically solve problems and an analytical approach to competently managing complexity are therefore integral to the core capabilities.

The MPFfACP (HEE 2017) also acknowledges that there are three key elements consistently required in the workplace to support the education pathways and progression to achieve the capabilities: development of competence and capability, supervision and support, and assessment of competence and capability. For an individual working towards achieving advanced-level practice in a specific clinical setting, it may be necessary to complete generic education via a Master's level award, alongside completion of a specialty curriculum of capabilities in practice, to encompass all the required elements of their development. To facilitate achievement of role-specific ACP capability, it is suggested in the MPFfACP (HEE 2017) that trainee ACPs should engage in a programme of learning that includes specialist training, work-based units to ensure meaningful clinical exposure, interprofessional learning and support and workplace assessment.

Unlike pre-registration training and education, the curriculum of learning for ACP is not entirely predetermined by regulatory bodies and HEIs, for students to follow from start to finish to reach a specified endpoint. Instead, the learning pathway is negotiated and developed between the learner, their employer and the education provider, in order to achieve the educational goals which will ensure that the practitioner has the requisite skills, knowledge and behaviours to safely meet the needs of their individual advanced practice role. Most HEIs providing advanced practice education offer an MSc programme covering the core elements of the four pillars of ACP as well as modules tailored to fulfil specific areas of interest and capability requirements. Generic clinical skills, leadership and education, and research modules are commonly mandatory features of ACP programmes accounting for most of the required credits; these are then frequently complemented by specific optional modules selected to meet the trainee's individual learning needs. The choice of optional elements may be influenced by the employer, for whom there is a specific skill or knowledge requirement that must be fulfilled by the ACP to meet the requirements of their job description.

A relatively recent development in the ACP education landscape is the possibility of programme accreditation by Health Education England (HEE). It is hoped that through accreditation of ACP programmes, equality and standard of provision will be achieved, which will offer assurance to key stakeholders. To the benefit of practitioners and their employers, graduates of accredited programmes will automatically be accredited as ACPs. It will also be possible for ACPs to be accredited through a portfolio route; an individual's portfolio might reflect their own 'curriculum of learning' through a combination of work-based learning and formal educational modules. It will, however, need to be clearly mapped to the ACP capabilities and demonstrate that the practitioner has achieved appropriate Level 7 standards across the four pillars, as assessed by an educational assessor trained in the standardised assessment of the Framework.

The introduction of the ACP apprenticeship standard in England in 2018 has also influenced the evolution of the ACP curriculum. The apprenticeship route to ACP education enables employers, largely NHS Trusts, to utilise their 'apprenticeship levy' to support existing employee development and is rapidly becoming the routine approach for funding training and education. The ACP apprenticeship standard is aligned to the MPFfACP (HEE 2017) and requires apprentices (students) to provide evidence of achievement of the required knowledge, skills and behaviours, alongside their academic achievements. Like all English apprenticeship programmes, the ACP apprenticeship also requires apprentices to complete an 'endpoint assessment' to demonstrate their overall achievement of the standard and show their understanding of values and citizenship throughout.

Despite a move towards a more standardised curriculum for ACP in higher education, it is recognised that modes of delivery and pedagogical approaches may vary between HEIs. It is also understood that within the educational framework, and in clinical practice, there may be a degree of overlap between the pillars, meaning that some core elements of learning may be included in different sections of the curriculum, depending on the institution. Programme accreditation will, however, ensure that on completion an ACP will have demonstrated achievement of all the skills and knowledge required for the core capabilities.

Understanding the Context of ACP

Understanding the history and context of the development of advanced practice in the health and social care environment is important for the individual ACP's appreciation of their own role and responsibility, and where ACP fits into the current healthcare landscape. Teaching and learning regarding the context of advanced practice may be included in ACP programmes in standalone modules or incorporated into other areas of the curriculum. Topics covered might include national and global social and political drivers for ACP, including relevant policy and legislation, the ethical and legal implications of ACP, quality and governance, evidence-based practice and professional issues such as interprofessional working and regulation.

THE CLINICAL PRACTICE CURRICULUM

In HEIs, teaching and learning for ACP will usually focus on the core clinical skills required for clinical practice at an advanced level. To achieve the core capabilities outlined in the MPF (HEE 2017), the emphasis of learning will be on the processes of history taking and information gathering, physical examination, clinical decision making and diagnostic reasoning, and management planning, in the presence of complexity.

RED FLAGS – PATHOLOGICAL CONSIDERATIONS

The syllabus for learning is commonly aligned to key functional systems, an understanding of which will be valuable to all ACP roles. In this context the significance of recognising risks, red flags and the practitioner's own limitations and scope of practice is central to the knowledge and skills required for capability in practice.

The requisite knowledge and theory and the fundamental principles of clinical skills may be taught in the educational setting, facilitated by simulation of practice, but in order to be valid and applicable, much of the learning required for clinical capability must take place in the workplace. Nevertheless, when embedded within an accredited package of learning, there exists the additional attribute of academic assurance (Garrett et al. 2001).

The development of specialty-specific clinical capabilities is not always part of the core curriculum for ACP educational programmes, but may be included in optional modules or where HEIs offer a programme that supports a specific capability curriculum. Here, work-based learning is essential for the development of the practical skills and critical thinking necessary for attainment of capability that applies to real-world situations.

CLINICAL INVESTIGATIONS

Clinical capability 1.4 of the MPFfACP (HEE 2017) concerns clinical investigation/diagnostic test interpretation. Clinical decision support tools such as the BMJ Best Practice reference suite (see: https://bestpractice.bmj.com/info) can aid evidence-based decision making when deciding which tests to perform.

Pharmacology and Prescribing Principles

Clinical capability 1.7 of the MPFfACP (HEE 2017) concerns initiation, evaluation and modification of a range of interventions, including prescribing. Clinical decision support tools such as Medicines-Complete (see: https://about.medicinescomplete.com) can aid ACPs to make the best clinical decisions on the use and administration of drugs and medicines.

ORANGE FLAGS – PSYCHOLOGICAL CONSIDERATIONS

The National Institute for Health and Care Excellence mental health services guidance and quality standards repository (www.nice.org.uk/guidance/conditions-and-diseases/mental-health-and-behavioural-conditions/mental-health-services) may support ACPs when considering this area of their respective curricula.

GREEN FLAGS – SOCIAL CONSIDERATIONS

The National Institute for Health and Care Excellence social care guidance and quality standards repository (www.nice.org.uk/About/NICE-Communities/Social-care) may support ACPs when considering this area of their respective curricula.

THE LEADERSHIP AND MANAGEMENT CURRICULUM

The ACP curriculum for leadership and management will facilitate learners' development of knowledge, skills and behaviours, enabling them to understand the role of the ACP as a leader, and to embody and model the core leadership values of healthcare, including inclusive and compassionate leadership (West 2021; NHS Leadership Academy n.d.). The focus is usually on local, clinical leadership relevant to the individual's area of practice, starting with personal and professional development, and role transition. The syllabus may also include leadership theory and principles, and change management and quality improvement. The aims for learning, which may additionally incorporate risk management, human factors and handling demanding situations, would ultimately be to give the learner the confidence to apply knowledge and skills to practice, enabling them to successfully lead and develop teams and services to meet the needs of service users.

THE EDUCATION CURRICULUM

The ACP must understand educational principles and be competent in their application in relation to themselves, patients, service users and family and carers, and also, other professional and healthcare workers. To inform their own development, ACPs must be able to critically reflect on their own learning needs and formulate a suitable personal development plan to guide their professional development; they will also need to engage in peer review both as a reviewer and a reviewee. ACPs will also contribute to the identification of wider team development needs and support the development of capacity and capability within their clinical area. Regarding the education of patients and service users, one of the key roles of ACPs is to empower individuals to achieve personal autonomy in the management of their own health and well-being, so an understanding of health literacy and motivation is therefore essential for the role (Seedhouse 2017). The education curriculum for ACP will therefore include, in addition to general educational principles, appropriate theories and practice of such skills as coaching, mentoring and motivation.

THE RESEARCH CURRICULUM

In order to fulfil the research capabilities outlined in the MPFfACP (HEE 2017), it is essential for the ACP to understand the key principles of research, including ethics, governance and good practice in order to inform their own, and lead others', evidence-based clinical practice. The research curriculum will therefore include ethical principles, research methodologies and critical appraisal. Understanding of these principles and their application to clinical practice will enable ACPs to identify gaps in the evidence base, what methods of research or enquiry might be most appropriate, and how the findings of research can be disseminated, bridging the divide between academia and implementation. Research is often identified as the least understood and exercised pillar of ACP; it is therefore vital that the education process facilitates the development of skills and confidence in this domain for the future development of the role.

ASSESSMENT FOR ACP

Assessment is a fundamental function of education, providing a means to ensure standards and capability. When clearly linked to learning outcomes and focused on the learner's development and achievement of their educational aims, assessment will also drive learning. Assessment for ACP should be aligned to the MPFfACP (HEE 2017) and enable the learner to demonstrate competence and capability, relevant to their area of practice.

Due to the broad scope of the four pillars of practice and varying pedagogical approaches to ACP development, assessment can take numerous different forms, but all assessment at this level should aim to enable authentic demonstration of the individual's learning of appropriate knowledge and skills. Assessment throughout a programme of learning will provide evidence of that learning and facilitate the development of a portfolio, which may in itself be a summative assessment tool, such as in an apprenticeship programme.

In HEI environments, assessment of the leadership and management, education and research pillars may take an established approach involving written essays to demonstrate knowledge and understanding, and critical appraisal and thinking skills, in given topic areas. However, more recently, even in traditional research-intensive universities, there is a move towards authentic approaches to assessment that reflect the 'real-world' applications of the learning. It is therefore now possible that a learner's portfolio of assessments might include academic posters, presentations of practice development, critical reflections, personal development plans, quality improvement or leadership projects, amongst numerous other creative opportunities.

Assessment of clinical competence and capability for ACP presents a challenge to learners, HEIs and employers, but is essential to ACP development as outlined in the MPF. To ensure effective learning and development, it is first essential that all parties understand the requirements of competence and capability, how the learning will be achieved and how it will be assessed, as this will vary significantly between specific roles (Table 2.1) (HEE 2020d).

TABLE 2.1 The differences between competence and capability.

Competence	Capability
'The ability to consistently perform to defined standards in the workplace'	'The ability to be competent and beyond this work effectively in complex situations that require flexibility and creativity'
Stable environments with familiar problems	Dealing with complexity in unpredictable situations

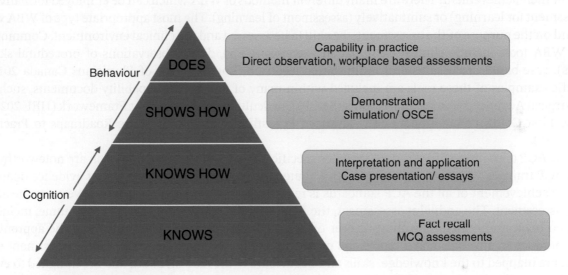

FIGURE 2.2 Miller's triangle. *Source*: Adapted from Miller GE (1990).

A process of triangulation, providing evidence of numerous methods and sources and thus increasing reliability, may be advocated for the assessment of clinical capability. Miller's triangle (Miller 1990) provides a model of how different elements of clinical skill and knowledge might be assessed to demonstrate competence and capability in practice (Figure 2.2).

As mentioned earlier, academic programmes may offer clinical skills education in the form of taught modules; assessment of these modules, which provide a basis for practice-based skill development, might include knowledge-based exams such as multiple-choice and short-answer formats. Further demonstration and interpretation of this knowledge might be assessed in the form of case presentations, and this may also be assessed in practice in the form of case-based discussions with clinical supervisors. In the education environment, observed structured clinical examinations (OSCEs) are frequently used to assess clinical competence, and despite concerns regarding the applicability of this form of assessment to clinical practice, due to their perceived validity and reliability, they continue to be a mainstream method for assessing clinical competence (Lavery 2022). Based on an extensive review of current literature, Lavery (2022) advocates for OSCEs to be used in collaboration with other work-based assessment (WBA) methods to enhance the experience and outcomes of advanced practitioners and to improve clinical practice.

Examination Scenario
As a trainee ACP, or a qualified ACP supporting a trainee ACP, how would you prepare for undertaking an OSCE?

Work-based assessment offers the opportunity for authentic evaluation of the practitioner's competency in the clinical environment, integrating and applying academic learning into practice. The close proximity of the assessment to the assessed skill offers validity which reassures both the learner and the educator of their achievement. There are many different methods of WBA which can be employed formatively (assessment for learning) or summatively (assessment of learning). The most appropriate type of WBA will depend on the purpose of the assessment, the skill to be assessed and the clinical environment. Commonly used WBA tools include clinical examination exercises (CEX), direct observations of procedural skills (DoPs), case-based discussions and multi-source feedback (Royal College of Physicians Canada 2014). Specific examples of these tools are included within many of the specific capability documents, such as the Surgical Advanced Clinical Practitioner (SACP) Curriculum and Assessment Framework (HEE 2020c) or the First Contact Practitioners and Advanced Practitioners in Primary Care Roadmaps to Practice (HEE n.d.).

The ACP apprenticeship standard includes specific elements of assessment, which are noteworthy as most ACP trainees will now be funded via this route. The completion of a portfolio of evidence demonstrating achievement of all the ACP standards is required before the apprentice can move on to the endpoint assessment. The endpoint assessment, the final essential requirement of the programme, includes an open book exam, including short-answer questions based on three case studies that the apprentice must produce in advance, and a report and presentation of a change in practice. These assessment elements are mapped to the knowledge, skills and behaviours of the ACP standard and are designed to evaluate the overall achievement of the apprentice across the programme.

SPECIALIST CURRICULUMS, CREDENTIALS AND CAPABILITY FRAMEWORKS

As advanced practice has evolved, several professional organisations, supported by HEE and other key stakeholders, have created specialty-specific curriculum and capability frameworks to provide a standardised national structure that assists employers in the training and appointment of regulated healthcare workers in ACP roles across England.

The purpose of these curriculum frameworks is to develop ACPs who have the correct knowledge, skills and behaviours (KSBs) and to acknowledge their scope of practice and level of competence. On successful completion, learners will be able to demonstrate to their employer that they can be trusted to undertake the role of ACP within the NHS and/or other health and social care settings (HEE 2022d).

The capabilities in practice (CiPs) within curriculum frameworks will be mapped to the MPF and will also outline specific capabilities required for specialist areas of practice. As part of the holistic development of responsible clinicians, these professional capabilities must be demonstrated at every stage of training (HEE 2022d).

The HEIs provide high-quality Master's level courses in advanced practice but these do not always include specialty-specific competences or nationally defined curricula. There is variation in the range of competences acquired, and no standardisation of the level of competence for a specific area of practice. Specific ACP credential resources provide an opportunity for standardisation and consistency in a specific clinical area.

First Contact Practitioners and Advanced Practitioners – Roadmaps to Practice

Highlighted in the NHS Long Term Plan (2019), the development of multiprofessional first contact practice (FCP) roles aims to alleviate pressures on medical services in primary care, by utilising nurses and allied health professionals (AHPs) trained to an advanced level to provide essential services. The FCP and Advanced Practitioners in Primary Care Roadmaps to Practice are supportive documents that provide a clear educational pathway to advanced practice for clinicians wishing to pursue a career in primary care. These capability frameworks clearly articulate capabilities and provide guidance on the expected supervision needed to support the roadmap to practice. By providing a standard of practice, there is a solid governance structure around FCP roles and advanced practice in primary care, ensuring gold standard care that puts patient safety first. To date, specific roadmaps have been launched for podiatry, paramedics, occupational therapy, dietitians and musculoskeletal practitioners (HEE n.d.).

SUPERVISION AND CPD STRATEGIES

The provision and delivery of high-quality workplace supervision for practitioners developing in ACP is crucial for both professional and patient safety (HEE 2017); it requires an integrated approach in which developing ACPs are supported by multiprofessional supervisors. The developing ACPs should have a nominated 'co-ordinating education supervisor' who supports the practitioner during the period of development, and access to a variety of 'associate workplace supervisors' who are matched to specified aspects of practitioner development, including specific clinical skills sets and across all the pillars of ACP (HEE 2020, 2022d). ACP supervisors should be appropriately qualified and experienced clinicians with an in-depth knowledge and understanding of the learner's role and learning requirements. It is recognised that in some areas, particularly those where there is not a well-established ACP workforce, it may be necessary for the supervisor to be from a different 'parent profession' to the trainee. This can present challenges in terms of understanding the trainee's base level of knowledge and experience, but can be overcome through training for the supervisor, which is essential for a successful supportive relationship.

The supervision process for the developing ACP should underpin their growth in confidence and capability by providing a context for their learning and facilitating the application of new academic knowledge to clinical practice, ultimately enabling them to function autonomously to provide safe and effective patient care. Regular supervision will allow opportunities for reflection on practice and reasoning for management choices, identification of skill gaps and learning opportunities, and also to recognise achievements and progression.

The supervision process for both trainee and qualified ACPs should function in tandem with, and identify areas of need for, the individual's continuing professional development (CPD). CPD is the systematic maintenance, improvement and continuous acquisition and reinforcement of lifelong knowledge, skills and competencies of health professionals, with the purpose of meeting patient, health service and individual professional learning needs (Executive Agency for Health Consumers 2013). As such, appropriately considered CPD enables employees and employers to ensure that the right person, with the right skills, is available at the right place and time.

The onus for CPD lies with the individual practitioner, but employers do have a responsibility to support individuals and ensure that they have opportunities to develop and maintain their capabilities to fulfil their role. ACP CPD should encompass all four pillars at an advanced level, taking a person-centred approach which is aligned to local and national strategies and facilitates an improvement-focused culture, promotes organisational values and supports the development of others, enabling the management of complexity and a positive patient experience (HEE 2021).

Fields of Practice – Paediatrics

At the time of writing, an ACP Paediatric curriculum is being developed. HEE and the Royal College of Paediatrics and Child Health (RCPCH) are creating a curricular framework that will consist of key capabilities and learning outcomes across 11 domains which map across five patient groups: non-hospital paediatrics, hospital paediatrics, neonatal, critical care and child with complex needs. The curricular framework encompasses the four pillars that underpin ACP practice (RCPCH 2022).

Fields of Practice – Mental Health

The Advanced Practice Mental Health Curriculum and Capabilities Framework (HEE 2022b) allows the advanced practitioner in mental health (AP-MH) to deliver high-quality, effective care for people experiencing mental health illnesses/conditions. It enables regulated healthcare professionals to develop theoretical knowledge and clinical skills to practise in the specialist areas of mental health. The framework enables practitioners to develop their knowledge, skills and professional behaviour to work autonomously in providing care to patients requiring complex assessment and treatment. Practitioners will also learn to develop their leadership and management skills, to support the wider mental health team and contribute to organisational learning. Finally, the curriculum is designed to promote and share evidence-based knowledge to enhance mental health services and person-centred care (HEE 2022b).

Fields of Practice – Learning Disabilities

In 2020 HEE launched the Advanced Clinical Practice: Capabilities framework for those working with people who have a learning disability and/or autism. This framework provides a definition of advanced clinical practice for AHPs and nursing staff in learning disabilities and autism services (HEE 2020a). In recent years, the learning disabilities and autism workforce has been the focus of much attention, not least because of the national Transforming Care Programme which aims to develop health and care services so that people with a learning disability and/or autism can live as independently as possible, with the right support and close to home. More recently, the Learning Disabilities Mortality Review (LeDeR) Programme has highlighted the persistence of preventable health inequalities and that people with a learning disability die, on average, 15–20 years sooner than people without a learning disability. The ACP framework sets out the capabilities (including knowledge, skills and behaviours) characterised by a high degree of autonomy, complex decision making and management of risks. The LeDeR programme has highlighted the need for:

- healthcare co-ordination for people with complex or multiple health conditions
- assurance that effective reasonable adjustments are being provided for people with a learning disability and their families
- mandatory learning disability awareness training for all staff supporting people with a learning disability (HEE 2020a).

Learning Events

1. Student A has completed a Level 7 Clinical Skills and Examination module, passing an MCQ exam and OSCE. How can they now develop and demonstrate their capability in practice?
2. On completion of their MSc ACP programme (accredited by HEE), practitioner B, now an accredited ACP, has moved into an ACP role in emergency care. What now are their considerations for future learning and development?

Case Study

Student A is newly appointed ACP trainee. They have several years of clinical experience in their area of specialty and as such have a depth of knowledge and skills related to the patient group. However, they have never been responsible for initial assessment of patients as they are admitted or for planning patient management.

The service for which student A works is undergoing a period of restructure and they have been asked to lead a review of educational support for new starters.

Supervisor B is student A's co-ordinating supervisor; they are an experienced ACP in the clinical area and in supervising trainees and students.

Tutor C is student A's academic advisor, an HEI lecturer in ACP, formerly an ACP in a different clinical specialty and parent profession.

1. What would be the first steps for student A to achieve the required capabilities in practice of the ACP role for which they are training?
2. What are the responsibilities of supervisor B, and how might they support student A to achieve the capabilities in practice?
3. What is the role of tutor C in facilitating student A to achieve the competencies for their ACP role?

CONCLUSION

The curriculum for the education of ACPs is continually evolving to meet the needs of healthcare services and the populations they serve. It is essential that ACPs are educated to the high level required to meet the capabilities set out in the MPF to ensure consistency and safety for the public. Developing the ACP curriculum is a complex process that requires robust assurances of standard, but also flexibility to accommodate different professional groups and areas of practice. It is therefore essential that contributions to ACP education are included from employers, educators, key stakeholders and professional organisations, as well as the training and qualified ACPS themselves.

Take Home Points

- Understand the role and level of practice of the ACP.
- Appreciate the scope of learning required for advanced clinical practice.
- Understand that practitioners need to be clinically competent and embrace the four pillars of advanced practice within their specialty, sector and setting.
- Understand the need for Level 7 academic study and how this relates to advanced clinical practice.

REFERENCES

Executive Agency for Health Consumers. (2013). Study concerning the review and mapping of continuous professional development and lifelong learning for health professionals in the European Union. European Union. http://ec.europa.eu/health//sites/health/files/workforce/docs/cpd_mapping_report_en.pdf

Faculty of Intensive Care Medicine (2015). Curriculum for Training for Advanced Critical Care Practitioners. www.ficm.ac.uk/sites/ficm/files/documents/2021-10/ACCP%20Curriculum%20Part%20I%20-%20Handbook%20v1.1%202019%20Revision.pdf Accessed 15th September 2022

Garrett, J., Comerford, A., and Webb, N. (2001). Working with partners to promote intellectual capital. In: *Work-Based Learning: A New Higher Education?* (ed. N. Solomon and D.J. Boud), 44–58. Buckingham: Society for Research into Higher Education & Open University press.

Health Education England (2017). Multi-professional Framework for Advanced Clinical Practice In England. www.hee.nhs.uk/sites/default/files/documents/multi-professional framework for advanced clinical practice in england.pdf

Health Education England (2020). Advanced Clinical Practice: Capabilities framework when working with people who have a learning disability and/or autism. www.skillsforhealth.org.uk/wp-content/uploads/2020/11/ACP-in-LDA-Framework.pdf

Health Education England (2020). Workplace Supervision for Advanced Clinical Practice: An integrated multi-professional approach for practitioner development. https://www.hee.nhs.uk/sites/default/files/documents/Workplace%20Supervision%20for%20ACPs.pdf

Health Education England (2020). Surgical Advanced Clinical Practitioner (SACP) Curriculum and Assessment Framework. www.iscp.ac.uk/media/1141/sacp_curriculum_dec20_accessible-1.pdf

Health Education England (2021). Advancing Practice: Signpost for Continuing CPD. https://www.hee.nhs.uk/sites/default/files/documents/Signposting%20for%20CPD.pdf

Health Education England (2022a). Advanced Clinical Practice in Acute Medicine Curriculum Framework. https://healtheducationengland.sharepoint.com/sites/APWC/Shared%20Documents/Forms/AllItems.aspx?id=%2Fsites%2FAPWC%2FShared%20Documents%2FCredentials%2FCredentials%20Endorsement%20Documents%2FAdvanced%20clinical%20practice%20in%20acute%20medicine%20curriculum%20framework%2Epdf&parent=%2Fsites%2FAPWC%2FShared%20Documents%2FCredentials%2FCredentials%20Endorsement%20Documents&p=true&ga=1

Health Education England (2022b). Advanced Practice Mental Health Curriculum and Capabilities Framework. https://healtheducationengland.sharepoint.com/sites/APWC/Shared%20Documents/Forms/AllItems.aspx?id=%2Fsites%2FAPWC%2FShared%20Documents%2FCredentials%2FCredentials%20Endorsement%20Documents%2FAdvanced%20practice%20in%20mental%20health%20curriculum%20and%20capabilities%20framework%2Epdf&parent=%2Fsites%2FAPWC%2FShared%20Documents%2FCredentials%2FCredentials%20Endorsement%20Documents&p=true&ga=1

Health Education England (2022c). Advanced Clinical Practice in Older People Curriculum Framework. https://healtheducationengland.sharepoint.com/sites/APWC/Shared%20Documents/Forms/AllItems.aspx?id=%2Fsites%2FAPWC%2FShared%20Documents%2FCredentials%2FCredentials%20Endorsement%20Documents%2FAdvanced%20clinical%20practice%20older%20people%20curriculum%20framework%20%20%2Epdf&parent=%2Fsites%2FAPWC%2FShared%20Documents%2FCredentials%2FCredentials%20Endorsement%20Documents&p=true&ga=1

Health Education England (2022d). The Centre for Advancing Practice. Advanced Practice Workplace Supervision. Minimum Standards for Supervision. `https://healtheducationengland.share-point.com/sites/APWC/Shared%20Documents/Forms/AllItems.aspx?ga=1&id=%2Fsites%2FAPWC%2FShared%20Documents%2FResources%20and%20News%2FAdvanced%20practice%20workplace%20supervision%2FAdvanced%20practice%20workplace%20supervision%2D%20Minimum%20standards%20for%20supervision%2Epdf&parent=%2Fsites%2FAPWC%2FShared%20Documents%2FResources%20and%20News%2FAdvanced%20practice%20workplace%20supervision`

Health Education England (n.d.) First Contact Practitioners & Advanced Practitioners - Roadmaps to Practice. `www.hee.nhs.uk/our-work/allied-health-professions/enable-workforce/ahp-roadmaps/first-contact-practitioners-advanced-practitioners-roadmaps-practice`

Health Education England, NHS England and Skills for Health (2020). Core Capabilities Framework for Advanced Clinical Practice (Nurses) Working in General Practice/Primary Care. `www.hee.nhs.uk/sites/default/files/documents/ACP%20Primary%20Care%20Nurse%20Fwk%202020.pdf`

Lavery, J. (2022). Observed structured clinical examination as a means of assessing clinical skills competencies of ANPs. *British Journal of Nursing* 31 (4): 214–220.

Miller, G.E. (1990). The assessment of clinical skills/competence/performance. *Academic Medicine* 65: S63–S67.

National Health Service (2019). The NHS Long Term Plan. `www.longtermplan.nhs.uk/wp-content/uploads/2019/08/nhs-long-term-plan-version-1.2.pdf`

NHS Leadership Academy (n.d.) The Nine Leadership Dimensions. `www.leadershipacademy.nhs.uk/resources/healthcare-leadership-model/nine-leadership-dimensions/`

Quality Assurance Agency for Higher Education (2020). Characteristics statement. Master's degree. `https://tinyurl.com/yygdaphz`

Royal College of Emergency Medicine (2022). Emergency Care Advanced Clinical Practitioner Curriculum – Adult. `https://rcem.ac.uk/wp-content/uploads/2022/09/ACP_Curriculum_Adult_Final_060922.pdf`

Royal College of Paediatrics and Child Health (2022). Advanced Clinical Practitioner (ACP) Paediatric Curricular Framework. `www.rcpch.ac.uk/education-careers/supporting-training/acp-curriculum`

Royal College of Physicians and Surgeons Canada (2014). Work-based Assessment: A Practical Guide. `www.surgeons.org/-/media/Project/RACS/surgeons-org/files/becoming-a-surgeon-trainees/work-based-assessment-a-practical-guide.pdf?rev=64c62242e777411eb43be8ac781dfa4a&hash=DCEE633AC11B7EE63975DF1A6948C99A`

Seedhouse, D. (2017). *Thoughtful Health Care. Ethical Awareness snd Reflective Practice.* Sage Publications `https://sk.sagepub.com/books/thoughtful-health-care.`

West, M. (2021). *Compassionate Leadership: Sustaining Wisdom, Humanity and Presence in Health and Social Care.* Swirling Leaf Press.

FURTHER READING

Advance Higher Education (2022). Inclusive curriculum design in higher education. `www.advance-he.ac.uk/knowledge-hub/inclusive-curriculum-design-higher-education`

Health Education England (2022). Credentials. `https://advanced-practice.hee.nhs.uk/credentials`

SELF-ASSESSMENT QUESTIONS

1. As a trainee ACP, what are your learning needs in relation to the MPF for ACP and any relevant capability curriculum?
2. How will you identify your need for CPD and supervision and what documents and guidance will support this?
3. How will you evaluate and assess your skills to prove your competency and capability in practice?
4. How can you ensure that you continue to fulfil all the domains of the MPF for ACP?

GLOSSARY

Advanced clinical practitioners apprenticeship   Delivered in partnership with employers, this flexible and innovative Level 7 apprenticeship will prepare experienced registered healthcare professionals to develop their professional careers as advanced clinical practitioners (ACPs).

Capabilities   Extent to which individuals can adapt to change, generate new knowledge and continue to improve their performance (HEE 2017).

Competencies   What individuals know or are able to do in terms of knowledge, skills and behaviour (HEE 2017).

Endpoint assessment (EPA)   The national ACP Level 7 apprenticeship pathway requires all students to complete an Endpoint Assessment module in Year 3. The ACP EPA provides independent synoptic assessment of the knowledge, skills and behaviours of the ACP apprenticeship standard. For further details of the national EPA assessment plan, please visit: https://haso.skillsforhealth.org.uk/wp-content/uploads/2018/03/2018.03.22-Advanced-Clinical-Practitioner-Assessment-Plan.pdf

Knowledge, skills and behaviours (KSBs)   The main assessment methods used in an Endpoint Assessment (EPA) for apprenticeship awards. See also EPA.

Leadership Academy   An NHS initiative that focuses on the development of health and care leadership. Its curriculum of programmes, resources and activities brings world-class learning and development to NHS people and partners. The Rosalind Franklin Programme has been identified by Health Education England as the preferred programme for ACP Leadership development. www.leadershipacademy.nhs.uk/programmes/rosalind-franklin-programme/

Master's level award   This is an award that uses the relevant descriptors set at Level 7 by the Framework for Higher Education Qualifications (FHEQ). See also: www.gov.uk/what-differentqualification-levels-mean/listof-qualification-levels

NHS Long-Term Plan   A 10-year plan focused on adapting the NHS to integrate new medical advances and the changing healthcare needs of society. It includes measures to prevent 150 000 heart attacks, strokes and dementia cases, and better access to mental health services for adults and children.

Pedagogy/pedagogical   Relating to the practice of teaching and its methods.

Stakeholder   An employee, investor, customer, etc. who is involved in or buys from a business and has an interest in its success. In healthcare, the main stakeholders are patients, providers (professionals and institutions), payers and policy makers (the 'four Ps').

CHAPTER 3

Scope of Practice and Management of Patient Care

Ollie Phipps

> **Aim**
> The aim of this chapter is to explore the legal, ethical and professional issues which affect advanced clinical practice (ACP) and to inform those working at an advanced level.

LEARNING OUTCOMES

After reading this chapter the reader will:

1. understand the legal and ethical considerations pertaining to the role and level of practice of advanced clinical practitioners (ACPs)
2. understand the ethical considerations pertaining to the role and level of practice of ACPs
3. be aware of their own scope of professional practice and how they should develop and grow it safely, within the law, supported by an appropriate governance framework
4. understand the need for practitioners to be clinically competent and to demonstrate this through capabilities in practice using the correct knowledge, skills and behaviours.

INTRODUCTION

The development of advanced practice within the UK has seen changes in traditional professional boundaries. Due to this, multiprofessional advanced practitioners must be aware of the professional, legal and ethical considerations that they may face. Advanced practitioners are a developing part of the

The Advanced Practitioner: A Framework for Practice, First Edition. Edited by Ian Peate,
Sadie Diamond-Fox, and Barry Hill.
© 2024 John Wiley & Sons Ltd. Published 2024 by John Wiley & Sons Ltd.

modern healthcare workforce (HEE 2021). They make a vital contribution to patient care (NHS 2020) and consist of registered practitioners from a variety of healthcare professional (HCP) backgrounds who have advanced-level capabilities which embrace the four pillars of practice, as set out in the Multiprofessional Framework for Advanced Clinical Practice in England (MPFfACP) (HEE 2017).

Multi-Professional Framework for Advanced Clinical Practice

This chapter relates to the following areas of the MPFfACP:
1.2, 1.2, 2.2, 2.10, 2.11, 3.1, 3.2, 3.8, 4.6

(HEE 2017)

Accreditation Considerations

This chapter is applicable to the following specialist curricula:

- Acute Medicine (HEE 2022a)
- Critical Care (ACCP) (FICM 2015)
- Emergency Care – Adult & Child (RCEM 2022a,b)
- Learning Disability and/or Autism (HEE 2020a)
- Mental Health (HEE 2022b)
- Older People (HEE 2022c)
- Primary Care (HEE 2020)
- Surgical Care (HEE 2020c)

This is an ever evolving field and work continues to agree various competence and capability frameworks for ACP in other clinical specialties; therefore the readers is encouraged to refer to https://advanced-practice.hee.nhs.uk/credentials

THE MULTI-PROFESSIONAL FRAMEWORK (MPFFACP)

The MPFfACP expands the definition of ACP in England (HEE 2017). The framework is designed to enable a consistent understanding of ACP, building on work carried out previously across England, Scotland, Wales and Northern Ireland. The core capabilities of ACP are articulated in this framework and these will apply across all ACP roles, regardless of the health and care professional's setting, subject area and job role (HEE 2017).

The MPFfACP requires that health and care professionals working at the level of ACP should have developed and can evidence the underpinning competencies (knowledge, skills and behaviours) applicable to the specialty or subject area (HEE 2017). It must be recognised that every practitioner is responsible and accountable for their actions and omissions. This is reflected within each HCP's code of conduct (NMC 2015; HCPC 2016). It must also be remembered that every person is responsible for upholding the law of the land.

Governance

Many titles exist for people working at an 'advanced level', such as 'advanced clinical practitioner', 'advanced nurse practitioner', 'advanced paramedic' and 'advanced practice therapeutic radiographer'. It is essential to note that some professionals have adopted or been given the term 'advanced' but may not have the correct credentials or simply are not working at an 'advanced' level for many reasons (HEE 2017).

With the development of advanced practice across the UK, the four nations have taken a different approach to its implementation. It is essential that clear local governance structures exist to support the development, implementation and ongoing strategy for both the employer and advanced practice employee (HEE 2017). There should be policies highlighting the clear difference between base registration, enhanced practice and advanced practice which explore the agreed scope of practice and freedom to act (HEE 2017).

Employers may need to review their workforce to ensure there is no misunderstanding for colleagues and, more importantly, the public. Appropriate governance meetings of an advanced practice assurance group, or similar, should exist with a reporting route to the Trust board or similar. An executive should be identified to hold the portfolio of advanced practice and an advanced practice lead should be appointed, where possible, to steer the development of advanced practice within an organisation. To embed advanced practice and ensure that it is fit for purpose, it is essential that governance is in place and should consider the following.

- Practice governance and service user safety requirements
- Adherence to legal and regulatory frameworks
- Support systems and infrastructure for delegated roles (e.g. requesting diagnostic tests, administering medicines)
- Professional and managerial pathways of accountability
- Continued assessment against, and progression through, the capabilities identified within this framework
- Location of ACP within a career framework that supports recruitment and retention, and succession planning to support workforce development
- Regular constructive clinical supervision that enables reflective practice together with robust annual appraisal.

(HEE 2017)

The above considerations are embedded within the Health Education England Centre for Advanced Practice Governance Maturity Matrix (HEE 2022c).

Legal Issues

Advanced practice will often involve exploring new ways of working and touching upon roles that were traditionally performed by other professional groups, for example medical staff. Therefore, it is essential that any legal implications are fully explored to ensure that new areas of practice are appropriate for the obligations of current legislation and statutes. It must be noted that ignorance of the law is not an appropriate or sufficient defence.

The law relates to rules that govern and oversee our society, with the purpose of maintaining justice, upholding social order and preventing harm to both individuals and property. The UK Parliament can implement laws across the four countries (England, Wales, Scotland, Northern Ireland). However, the devolved nations all have powers and judicial systems to implement laws that affect an individual country on devolved issues, and health is one.

Regulation Statements of Standards and Code of Conducts

Each HCP is responsible for upholding their individual professional code of conduct and professional standards. This is even more important when working as an advanced practitioner, given the higher level decision making, undertaking procedures with potential risks and making possible discharge decisions. Each professional code must be understood.

Nursing and Midwifery Council (NMC)

'The Code presents the professional standards that nurses, midwives and nursing associates must uphold in order to be registered to practise in the UK. It is structured around four themes – prioritise people, practise effectively, preserve safety and promote professionalism and trust. Each section contains a series of statements that taken together signify what good nursing and midwifery practice looks like' (NMC 2015).

Health and Care Professions Council (HCPC)

'The role of the standard of conduct, performance and ethics set out how we expect registrants to behave and outline what the public should spect from their health and care professional. They help us make decisions about the character of professionals who apply to our Register and we use them if someone raises a concern about a registrant's practice. Our registrants work in a range of different settings, which include direct practice, management, education, research and roles in industry. They also work with a variety of different people, including patients, clients, carers, and other professionals' (HCPC 2016).

General Pharmaceutical Council (GPhC)

'The standards apply to all pharmacists and pharmacy technicians in Great Britain. There are nine standards that every pharmacy professional is accountable for meeting. The standards for pharmacy professionals describe how safe and effective care is delivered. They are a statement of what people expect from pharmacy professionals, and also reflect what pharmacy professionals have told us they expect of themselves and their colleagues' (GPhC 2017).

Scope and Capability

Defining Scope of Practice

For HCPs, acknowledging one's scope of professional practice is important, as it defines the limit of knowledge, skills and experience. This scope is supported by the professional activities undertaken in one's working role and essential boundaries must be identified, acknowledged and maintained. It is acknowledged that a professional's scope will change over time as their knowledge, skills and experience develop.

With the evolution of advanced practice and the expansion of entrustable professional activities, traditional professional boundaries have significantly changed, and this is demonstrated as the multiprofessional workforce comes together at an advanced level.

The provision of healthcare has evolved and is incorporated into many healthcare settings, from primary care to secondary care, from a generalist stance or within specialties. This variability and breadth have meant that advanced practice has become immersed in attempts to define and provide structure.

As this level of practice is unique to the work setting, it is acknowledged that no one profession can encompass all the expertise needed to treat and care for patients. For all, it must include the four fundamental strands of advanced practice: a clinical element, research element, educational element and management/leadership element. Technological and clinical advances across all sectors have brought about changes to practice and have contributed to the level and quantity of postqualification education required to advance.

Often contentious is the definition of what advanced practice is. No one definition will fit perfectly for all advanced practitioners or indeed some work environments. Advanced practice is occasionally described as a blurring of the boundaries of traditional roles or registered HCPs. Yet this 'blurring' of boundaries implies assuming aspects of a variety of roles and is needed to provide better, more holistic care to all which can be seen as a positive evolution of healthcare.

Competency vs Capability

Competency and capability are two terms that pertain to human ability. Capability describes the quality of being capable. Does the individual have the ability to learn the knowledge and skills required and is it within their capacity? Capability can also be used to describe a person's implied abilities, or abilities that are not yet developed. With experience, time and practice, a person's capabilities can develop into competence. Capabilities serve as the starting point of being able to do something and gradually becoming more adept in performing the task.

Competence describes the quality of an individual's work. Competence can also be applied to the improvement or development of one's abilities and skills. Once competence has been met, it can result in an increased quality of work and/or performance. Competence can include a combination of knowledge, skills, abilities, behaviours and attitude.

Knowledge, Skills and Behaviours

Employers, higher education institutions, capability frameworks and curriculums must set out the knowledge, skills and behaviours required to be competent.

- *Knowledge* – the information, technical detail and 'know-how' that someone needs to have to successfully carry out the required duties. Some knowledge will be more specific, whereas some may be more generic.
- *Skills* – the practical application of knowledge needed to successfully undertake the duties. They are learnt through on- and/or off-the-job training or experience.
- *Behaviours* – mindsets, attitudes or approaches needed for competence and working as a professional. Whilst these can be innate or instinctive, they can also be learnt. Behaviours tend to be very transferable. They may be more similar across occupations than knowledge and skills – for example, team worker, adaptable and professional.

Competence

Each advanced practitioner must possess the correct knowledge, skills and behaviour to undertake their role and to demonstrate competence, professionally and educationally. Although embracing the four pillars of advanced practice, as experts, advanced practitioners must be professionally mature and have significant experience of practice. They must always work within their scope of professional practice and acknowledge their professional limitations and restrictions.

Multiprofessional Registrations and Scope of Practice

Advanced clinical practice is multiprofessional, which differentiates it from other health and care provision by registered professionals (HEE 2021). Developing ACP will be complex as each practitioner will have different professional starting points reflecting different professional registrations, prior practice and previous supervision and assessment experience. It must therefore be acknowledged that there is no single underpinning, pre-registration professional training for professionals developing to work at an advanced level of practice. The scope of practice for different registered professions varies, and not all professional registrations extend to independent or supplementary prescribing (HEE 2021).

RED FLAGS – PATHOLOGICAL CONSIDERATIONS

Clinical capability 1.6 of the MPFfACP (HEE 2017) concerns clinical reasoning approaches. Clinical decision support tools such as the BMJ Best Practice reference suite (see: https://bestpractice.bmj.com/info) can aid the ACP in consideration of red flag diagnoses that may present within their scope of practice.

ORANGE FLAGS – PSYCHOLOGICAL CONSIDERATIONS

The National Institute for Health and Care Excellence mental health services guidance and quality standards repository (www.nice.org.uk/guidance/conditions-and-diseases/mental-health-and-behavioural-conditions/mental-health-services) may support ACPs when considering their scope of practice.

GREEN FLAGS – SOCIAL CONSIDERATIONS

The National Institute for Health and Care Excellence social care guidance and quality standards repository (www.nice.org.uk/About/NICE-Communities/Social-care) may support ACPs when considering their scope of practice.

Expanding Scope and Scope Creep

Those training, and those working, at an advanced level must be aware of their competence and capability. With various curriculums and capability frameworks being developed and implemented, advanced practitioners have guidance on where their knowledge, skills and professional behaviour must sit. However, someone beginning their advanced practitioner journey must acknowledge that it will take years to acquire the knowledge, skills and experience to work at an advanced level.

For some, advanced practice touches on the knowledge and skills which were traditionally associated with medicine, but with the development of the multiprofessional workforce, bringing a different set of knowledge and skills, the advanced practitioner is seen as being 'value added' rather than a role substitute.

Responsibility and Accountability

All healthcare practitioners working either at their base registration or at an advanced level must understand that they are both responsible and accountable for the decisions they make.

Expanding one's scope of practice should be done following the correct preparation, education and experience.

The concepts of accountability and responsibility are closely linked and are at the centre of the codes of conduct for those professionally regulated by the Nursing and Midwifery Council (NMC 2015) and the Health and Care Professions Council (HCPC 2016). Advanced practitioners have an obligation to undertake their role, and associated tasks, using sound professional judgement. As their level of practice expands, they should realise that this will increase the level of responsibility. Regulated HCPs are responsible for maintaining their competence in practice. They are answerable for decisions made within their professional practice, and the consequences of those decisions. Advanced practitioners should be able to justify their decision making and understand the associated legislation, ethical principles, professional standards and guidelines, including evidence-based practice.

Dunning–Kruger Effect

The Dunning–Kruger effect is pertinent in advanced practice. Here, incompetence and metacognitive defects can lead to an individual overestimating their abilities and performance. People in this group find it a challenge to recognise genuine levels of competence when applied to themselves or (objectively) in more competent peers. Gaining insight into one's own limitations and inadequacies is also a challenge by social comparison demonstrating an inability to 'see' their own deficits in relation to their peer's performance. The presence and prevalence of this effect in advanced practice must be recognised and challenged to counterbalance the effect of imposter syndrome, thus creating a balanced, objective practitioner.

Imposter Syndrome

Imposter syndrome is common phenomenon amongst advanced practitioners and can be interpreted both positively and negatively. Here, the practitioner doubts their credentials and ability to function, and is often plagued by a fear of being exposed as inadequate. This phenomenon is driven by anxiety and self-doubt, or because of attempted perfection. Often, it is associated with high-pressure environments, especially in healthcare, and comparing oneself to another colleague. Imposter syndrome is the sense that someone else is better than you, although competent HCPs possess the same skills, knowledge and experience.

Professional Issues

Advanced practitioners are pioneers of a new style of practice which challenges the traditions associated with professional roles. With the development of the advanced practitioner role, which is undertaken by members of the multiprofessional workforce, working within professional silos has significantly changed. Within areas such as acute and emergency care, nurses, physiotherapists and paramedics, for example, despite keeping their own professional identity, will work together undertaking the same role and the same procedures, working alongside one another. Each profession brings its own dimension of expertise to the patient, while embracing its own scope of practice. This is seen as being 'value added' for both the patient and the healthcare team. However, each professional group has its restrictions, often associated with legislation or its professional regulator, i.e. independent prescribing.

CLINICAL INVESTIGATIONS

Radiology (IRMER)

The Ionising Radiation (Medical Exposures) Regulations 2017 (IR[ME]R) lay down basic measures for the protection of patients from unnecessary or excessive exposure to medical X-rays. They also have specific guidance for employers, practitioners, operators and referrers in their responsibilities as duty holders.

The employer is responsible for putting into place a system of policies, protocols and procedures which will govern referrals and ensure that justification of exposures takes place, and that a clinical evaluation of all radiographs is recorded. The aim is to ensure that radiation doses to patients are kept as low as is reasonably practicable. The employer is responsible for ensuring that the diagnostic findings and clinical evaluation of each medical exposure are recorded in the patient's notes. If it is known before an exposure that no clinical evaluation will occur, then the exposure cannot legally be justified and therefore should not take place. The Medical Exposures Directive requires that each request for a medical X-ray must be justified by a practitioner or authorised by a radiographer (Reg.6.(1).(a)) prior to exposure being made.

Practitioners and operators are responsible for justifying and authorising individual medical exposures based upon assessment information supplied by the referrer. The practitioners and operators must consider:

- the specific objectives of the exposure and the characteristics of the patient involved
- the total potential or therapeutic benefits, including direct health benefits to the individual and society
- any potential detriment to the individual
- the efficacy, benefits and risks of available alternative techniques.

The practitioner must pay special attention to:

- the necessity of the exposure
- exposures on medical-legal grounds
- exposures that have no direct health benefit for the individual
- the urgency of the exposure in cases involving an individual where pregnancy cannot be excluded, in particular if the abdominal and pelvic regions are exposed; this also applies to those who were female at birth but may be transgender or non-binary. If the practitioner or operator considers the request not to be compliant with IR(ME)R, they are legally bound to refuse the imaging request.

Responsibilities of referrer

- *The form*: the radiology request form is a legal document and must be filled in accordingly. It is essential that correct patient identification details are recorded as well as giving sufficient clinical and medical data and a provisional diagnosis. Referrers must provide a legible signature uniquely identifying the referrer and a contact number for any queries.

Informing the patient of the risk and benefit of radiation exposure is important. Under IR(ME)R (2017) 'wherever practicable, and prior to an exposure taking place, the patient or their representative is provided with adequate information relating to the benefits and risks associated with the radiation dose from exposure'. In the first instance, this discussion should be had with the patient by the referrer prior to referral for X-ray. This should include how the imaging will allow them to be able to make a diagnosis or monitor the progress of the patient's treatment, and how the benefits from having the X-ray, and making the right diagnosis or providing the correct treatment, outweigh the very low risk involved with the X-ray itself.

Over recent years, advanced practitioners have been prevented from ordering investigations primarily due to a misunderstanding of their role. Therefore, in 2021, the Royal College of Emergency Medicine created a protocol entitled 'Radiology Requesting Protocol for Extended and Advanced Clinical Practitioners in the Emergency Department' (RCEM 2021) to set out the clear standards which were supported by the Clinical Radiology Faculty of the Royal College of Radiologists.

CLINICAL INVESTIGATIONS

Blood Tests

Clinicians requesting blood investigations must acknowledge that the responsibility for ensuring that results are acted upon rests with the person requesting the test. That responsibility can only be given to someone else if they accept by prior agreement; this includes discharging patients before results are back and forwarding to primary care colleagues (BMA 2020).

Patients should be kept informed in a sensitive and appropriate manner of the findings of investigation results, the actions taken as a result, and in a manner that is in keeping with the principles of the duty of candour (RCEM 2020).

Indemnity

Legal accountability involves advanced practitioners ensuring that they have professional indemnity insurance in case there is a substantiated claim of professional negligence. Regulators need to ensure that registrants have this indemnity arrangement in place, and it is now a condition of their registration. The indemnity insurance must be appropriate for their level of practice. If you are employed, your employer has vicarious liability for your actions and omissions while in its employment and is responsible for your actions. However, the practitioner must have been working within their level of competence and following their organisation's policies, procedures and guidelines.

Indemnity Insurance

Healthcare professionals, by law, must have in place an appropriate indemnity arrangement in order to practise and provide care in the UK. It is your responsibility as a registered HCP to ensure that appropriate cover is in place for your whole scope of practice. The requirement for professional indemnity is to make sure that if someone has suffered harm through the negligent action of a practitioner, they will be able to claim any compensation to which they are entitled. Regulators know that the professionals on their registers take this obligation very seriously. Professionals do not need to hold an arrangement, but it is your responsibility as a professional to ensure that appropriate cover is in place for your whole scope of practice. If you practise without an appropriate indemnity arrangement in place, you may be removed from your professional body's register and will be unable to practise until appropriate indemnity cover is in place. If you are an employee in the NHS or independent sector, your employer will normally have indemnity arrangements that will cover your work.

Appropriate cover is an indemnity arrangement which is appropriate to your role and scope of practice. It must take into account the nature and extent of the risks of practising in your role. The cover must have enough financial resources to meet an award of damages for a range of situations if a successful claim is made against you, including the costs of a large claim or several smaller claims. If your indemnity provider does not have enough resources to meet the cost of a claim, then you will have to secure alternative indemnity cover to meet the indemnity requirement.

To help you to decide whether you have appropriate cover, you should think about what your job involves and where you work; who you provide care to and the level of care you provide; the risks involved with your practice; and the possible size of any claim for damages. You could seek advice from your professional body, trade union or insurer to inform your decision. As noted above, if you are an employee in the NHS or independent sector, your employer will normally have indemnity arrangements that will cover your work but it is your responsibility to check. If you work for the NHS, you will already have an appropriate indemnity arrangement. The NHS insures its employees for work carried out on its behalf, which means you will be covered if a successful claim is made against you in that employment. Outside the NHS, many employers are likely to have professional indemnity arrangements that will provide appropriate cover for all the relevant risks related to your job and scope of practice. Arrangements may vary between employers and it is your responsibility to check with them.

In 2019, NHS Resolution created a new state-backed indemnity scheme for general practice in England called the Clinical Negligence Scheme for General Practice (CNSGP). It covers clinical negligence liabilities in general practice for incidents that occur on or after 1st April 2019 and provides a fully comprehensive indemnity for all claims within its scope. All providers of NHS primary medical services will be eligible for cover under the CNSGP, including out-of-hours providers. Therefore, if you are working in general practice and are carrying out activities in connection with the delivery of primary medical services, it is likely you will be covered by the scheme.

Negligence

Duty of Care

Duty of care consists of three primary elements of tort (duty of care, breach and causation). Whilst there are many situations in which an individual might have acted carelessly, unless they have a duty of care to the person harmed by their carelessness, then no claim will arise. However, the term 'duty of care' covers the responsibility of an individual to not harm others through carelessness.

Breach of Duty

Breach of duty of care is concerned with the standard of care that ought to have been applied in the situation. Therefore, if the conduct of the individual or organisation fell below the standard that a reasonable person would have expected, they will have been negligent in their duty.

Causation

Causation within medical negligence cases occurs after proving that negligence through a breached duty of care caused injury. Proving this is known as 'establishing causation'.

Examination Scenario

As an advanced practitioner, with a base registration as a registered nurse, you are asked to review a pregnant woman with an excessively high blood pressure. Professionally and legally, are you able to manage this patient or do restrictions exist?

Fields of Practice – Paediatrics

Those working and treating children must ensure that they are competent to undertake such a role. The person must possess the correct knowledge and have the right skills and professional behaviours. Those working with children must ensure that they have the correct indemnity and insurances to cover paediatric practice.

Fields of Practice – Mental Health

The field of mental health is a specialist area. HEE have created a curriculum to support the training of advanced practitioners working in the speciality of mental health (2022b). This curriculum allows the advanced practitioner in mental health (AP-MH) to deliver high-quality, effective care for people experiencing mental health illnesses/conditions. It enables regulated HCPs to develop theoretical knowledge and clinical skills to practise in the specialist areas of mental health. The framework enables practitioners to develop their knowledge, skills and professional behaviour to work autonomously in providing care to patients requiring complex assessment and treatment. Practitioners will also learn to develop their leadership and management skills to support the wider mental health team and contribute to organisational learning. Finally, the curriculum is designed to promote and share evidence-based knowledge to enhance mental health services and person-centred care.

MENTAL HEALTH ACT 1983 AND SECTIONS

The Mental Health Act is the main piece of legislation that covers the assessment, treatment and rights of people with a mental health disorder. In most cases, it covers when people are treated in hospital or another mental health facility, how they have agreed or volunteered to be there. However, there are cases when a person can be detained under the Mental Health Act, which is known as sectioning or being sectioned under the Mental Health Act (1983). People detained under the Mental Health Act need urgent treatment for a mental health disorder and are at risk of harm to themselves or others.

- Section 2 – Admission for Assessment and Treatment (2 doctors, one approved for 28 days)
- Section 3 – Admission for Treatment (2 doctors, one approved for 6 months)
- Section 4 – Emergency Admission (any doctor for 72 hours)
- Section 136 – Removal to a Place of Safety (by a police officer for 72 hours)
- Section 5(2) - Detention of Inpatient (doctor in charge or deputy for 72 hours)
- Section 5(4) - Detention of Inpatient (qualified nurse for 6 hours)

Fields of Practice – Learning Disabilities

Those working with and treating people with learning disabilities and autism must ensure that they are competent to undertake such a role. The person must possess the correct knowledge and have the right skills and professional behaviours. Those working with people with learning disabilities and autism must ensure that they have the correct indemnity and insurances to cover this type of practice.

Mental Capacity Act

The Mental Capacity Act (MCA) 2005 is designed to protect and empower people who may lack the mental capacity to make their own decisions about their care and treatment for those aged 16 and over. It covers day-to-day decisions such as what to wear or what to buy, but also serious life-changing decisions like whether to move into a care home or have major surgery.

It must be acknowledged that someone can lack capacity to make some decisions (for example, to decide on complex financial issues) but still have the capacity to make other decisions (for example, to decide what items to buy at the local shop). The MCA also allows people to express their preferences for care and treatment, and to appoint a trusted person to make a decision on their behalf should they lack capacity in the future.

Learning Events

- An advanced practitioner has completed a MSc in ACP. Some concerns have been raised about their clinical practice and there is a possibility that they are working outside their scope of practice – seeing patients independently and starting treatments without any discussion with a senior clinician. How should this be handled? How should the practitioner and their manager develop their scope of practice and demonstrate their capability in practice?

- A patient presents with shortness of breath. An advanced practitioner reviews the patient's chest X-ray and notes it as 'unremarkable – nothing abnormal detected'. Four hours later the patient collapses, has a cardiac arrest and dies. The coroner asks for the advanced practitioner to demonstrate their capability in the management of the patient's initial presentation and to state how they are competent to interpret a chest X-ray. How would you respond in this situation?

Pharmacology and Prescribing Principles

Prescribing Capability

To support all prescribers in prescribing safely and effectively, a single prescribing competency framework was published by the Royal Pharmaceutical Society (RPS) in 2016. It agreed to revise and update the framework in collaboration with the other prescribing professions and members of the public. Going forward, the RPS will continue to maintain and publish this framework for all regulators, professional bodies, education providers, prescribing professions and patients/carers to use (RPS 2021).

Patient Group Direction Practice – Short Overview

For those who are unable to legally prescribe medications, a Patient Group Direction (PGD) is an alternative, although this does not replace independent prescribing. PGDs are written instructions for the supply or administration of medicines to groups of patients. PGDs provide a legal framework that allows the supply and/or administration of a specified medicine(s) to a predefined group of patients needing prophylaxis or treatment for a condition described in the PGD, without the need for a prescription or an instruction from a prescriber. Using a PGD is not a form of prescribing. PGDs need to include the name of the authorised, registered health professional using them. PGDs can only be used by those HCPs listed in the legislation. Organisations should have policies and processes in place to consider all options before a service is designed or commissioned using PGDs. Before a PGD is developed, the organisation must ensure that PGDs are appropriate, legal and that relevant governance arrangements are in place (RCN 2022).

Multiprofessional Prescribing

Each individual profession needs to acknowledge the differences associated with the legalities of prescribing within the Human Medicines Regulations 2012. Some professions are limited to individual cohorts of patients, while others are limited on schedule drug prescribing, and others have minimal restrictions. Please refer to your regulator's information on independent and supplementary prescribing.

Ethics

Advanced practitioners should be prepared to make appropriate ethically informed judgements to support their practice. However, it is not easy, as professionals have struggled with understanding ethics and ethical dilemmas for centuries. Ethics is supported by principles which consist of rules, standards and guidelines which come from theoretical positions regarding what is good for humans. For advanced practitioners to practise in an ethically sound way, they must balance ethical considerations with professional values and relevant legislation.

An individual, usually a patient, will sit at the heart of ethical decision making. The advanced practitioner should seek advice in complex situations where legal, ethical and professional issues need to be considered. On occasions, the advanced practitioner will be expected to discuss the ethical problem with the individual/patient, to see how their needs can be compassionately met while addressing the challenges of clinical practice. On other occasions, if the individual is unable to discuss their needs, the advanced practitioner will need to weigh up the ethical considerations and, if necessary, consider the individual's best interests. Four key aspects must be considered: autonomy, non-maleficence, beneficence and justice.

Autonomy

Health professionals must respect a patient's decision to accept or refuse care. Advanced practitioners should be the patient's advocate, to ensure that patients receive all the necessary information to make a well-informed decision. This information must include potential risks, benefits and complications. Care should be discussed and planned with the patient, putting their wishes at the centre of what is done. Many influences will affect a patient's decision, including culture, age, social system, previous experience, general health and awareness of other patients' experiences.

Non-maleficence

The main principle of 'non-maleficence' within medical ethics is – 'do no harm'. The advanced practitioner should select interventions that will cause the least amount of harm to achieve a beneficial outcome (benefit versus risk). The patient is at the centre of the decision. Non-maleficence has many implications for advanced practitioners. An example of this is when treating the terminally ill and withdrawing treatment, etc.

Beneficence

The principle of beneficence ensures that the advanced practitioner takes positive actions to help others. This can be as simple as consoling an upset patient, through to administering analgesia to someone in pain. Beneficence is at the centre of all professional actions while engaging with patients. On occasions, beneficence may clash with a patient's autonomy.

Justice

Care is provided on a fair and equal basis, no matter what the patient's financial or social status.

THE RIGHT TO LIFE AND THE RIGHT TO DIGNITY

The Universal Declaration of Human Rights (UDHR) is a historic document, drafted by representatives with different legal and cultural backgrounds from all regions of the world. The Declaration was proclaimed by the United Nations General Assembly in Paris on 10 December 1948 as a common standard of achievement for all people and all nations (United Nations 1948).

Human rights most recently discussed within the context of medicine are:

- the right to life
- the right to health
- the right to autonomy
- the right to dignity
- the right to privacy
- the right to equality
- the right not to be tortured or subjected to cruel or inhuman treatment.

Three key concepts to understand are as follows.

- The Right to Life is for many a key human right, which can cause disagreements within medical ethics as well as legal systems across the world. The meaning of life and right to life has implications in the context of medicine particularly in the context of euthanasia and abortion. Article 2 of the European Convention on Human Rights (ECHR) protects the right to life to every person.
- The Right to Autonomy is protected by Article 8 of the ECHR and the right to choose and decide what medical treatment an individual receives.
- The Right to Dignity is covered in Article 3 and emphasises the right to die with dignity and the right to be protected from treatment, or a lack of treatment which may result in someone's death.

Consent

The principle of consent is associated with international human rights law and is a key aspect of the principle of autonomy. It allows an individual, where capacity exists, to make their own decision. Consent is essential; failure to obtain it could constitute 'trespass against the person' and if a patient is touched without consent, this may constitute a crime of battery in English law or assault in Scottish law. All practitioners have a responsibility to ensure that they gain consent before proceeding with care or treatment.

Gillick Competence

Children are legally defined as being under the age of 18. Like children aged 16 to 18, children under the age of 16 can consent to their own treatment if they are believed to have enough intelligence, competence and understanding to fully appreciate what is involved in their treatment, which is known as Gillick Competence (NSPCC 2022).

Case Study

- An advanced practitioner assesses an 85-year-old woman who is acutely unwell with decompensated heart failure. The AP examines the woman and reviews her investigations. It is noted she has a severe acute kidney injury but is also significantly overloaded with fluid. She is diagnosed with cardiorenal syndrome.
  1. What are the key points that should be evaluated and discussed in terms of treatment escalation, resuscitation status and necessary treatment plan?
  2. Can an ACP make these decisions?
  3. Where should this be documented?

- An ACP has recently been signed off as competent to insert a Seldinger intercostal chest drain. The procedure is undertaken on a 50-year-old man, who suddenly becomes breathless, with chest pain and is acutely unwell. The procedure is taken over by a colleague.
  1. What should be required to deem someone capable and competent to undertake a procedure?
  2. Who should be able to assess this?
  3. What governance framework should be in place?

Confidentiality

Healthcare professionals have a professional and legal responsibility to respect and protect the confidentiality of service users at all times (HCPC 2016). As a HCP, you are not expected to be an expert on the law, but you must keep up to date with and meet your legal responsibilities.

DEVELOPMENT AND REGULATION

As this alternative 'arm' to provide healthcare in the UK continues to evolve, mechanisms of governance have been difficult to hone due to the variability in roles and environments where advanced practice can be found. In 2008, calls to have new parts added to the NMC and HCPC registers were not authorised as the Council for Healthcare Regulatory Excellence (CHRE) deemed that regulators should ensure that their codes of conduct should adequately reflect the requirement for health professionals to stay up to date and operate safely within their areas of competence.

In addition, organisations are encouraged to develop local governance frameworks, policies and procedures to support and regulate advanced practice, taking support and guidance from the relevant advisory groups for the disciplines involved.

All these factors play a pivotal role in the continued expansion and prevalence of advanced practice roles and all professionals involved in these roles. There is a need to ensure awareness and the ability to address them all. Encompassing the four fundamental strands of advanced practice is essential but interpersonal skills and insight are equally important in ensuring that advanced practice is a sustainable development in the future workforce planning and longevity of the NHS.

CONCLUSION

The development of advanced practice within the UK has seen changes in traditional professional boundaries. Due to this, multiprofessional advanced practitioners must be aware of the professional, legal and ethical considerations that they may face. Each advanced practitioner and advanced practice lead must understand the complexities associated with practice development and implementation.

Take Home Points
- To practise effectively and within your professional registration, you must possess the correct knowledge, skills and professional behaviours to undertake your role. This includes working within your role as a newly qualified registrant, as a specialist practitioner and as an advanced practitioner.
- Advanced practitioners must be able to demonstrate a critical understanding of their broadened level of responsibility and autonomy. They must acknowledge the limits of their own competence and professional scope of practice, including when working with complexity, risk, uncertainty and incomplete information.
- Advanced practitioners must be aware of the legalities and ethical complexities associated with their practice.

REFERENCES

British Medical Association (2020). Duty of care when test results and drugs are ordered by secondary care. www.bma.org.uk/advice-and-support/gp-practices/communication-with-patients/duty-of-care-when-test-results-and-drugs-are-ordered-by-secondary-care

Faculty of Intensive Care Medicine (2015). Curriculum for Training for Advanced Critical Care Practitioners. www.ficm.ac.uk/sites/ficm/files/documents/2021-10/ACCP%20Curriculum%20Part%20I%20-%20Handbook%20v1.1%202019%20Revision.pdf

General Pharmaceutical Council (2017). Standards for Pharmacy Professionals. www.pharmacyregulation.org/sites/default/files/standards_for_pharmacy_professionals_may_2017_0.pdf

Health and Care Professions Council (2016). Standards of Conduct and Ethics. www.hcpc-uk.org/standards/standards-of-conduct-performance-and-ethics

Health Education England (2017). Multi-professional Framework for Advanced Clinical Practice in England. www.hee.nhs.uk/sites/default/files/docuemtns/HEE%20ACP%Framework.pdf

Health Education England (2020a). Advanced Clinical Practice: Capabilities framework when working with people who have a learning disability and/or autism. www.skillsforhealth.org.uk/wp-content/uploads/2020/11/ACP-in-LDA-Framework.pdf

Health Education England (2020b). Workplace Supervision for Advanced Clinical Practice: An integrated multi-professional approach for practitioner development. www.hee.nhs.uk/sites/default/files/documents/Workplace%20Supervision%20for%20ACPs.pdf

Health Education England (2020c). Surgical Advanced Clinical Practitioner (SACP) Curriculum and Assessment Framework. www.iscp.ac.uk/media/1141/sacp_curriculum_dec20_accessible-1.pdf

Health Education England (2021). Advancing Practice: Signpost for continuing CPD. www.hee.nhs.uk/sites/default/files/documents/Signposting%20for%20CPD.pdf

Health Education England (2022a). Advanced Clinical Practice in Acute Medicine Curriculum Framework. https://healtheducationengland.sharepoint.com/sites/APWC/Shared%20Documents/Forms/AllItems.aspx?id=%2Fsites%2FAPWC%2FShared%20Documents%2FCredentials%2FCredentials%20Endorsement%20Documents%2FAdvanced%20clinical%20practice%20in%20acute%20medicine%20curriculum%20framework%2Epdf&parent=%2Fsites%2FAPWC%2FShared%20Documents%2FCredentials%2FCredentials%20Endorsement%20Documents&p=true&ga=1

Health Education England (2022b). Advanced Practice Mental Health Curriculum and Capabilities Framework. https://healtheducationengland.sharepoint.com/sites/APWC/Shared%20Documents/Forms/AllItems.aspx?id=%2Fsites%2FAPWC%2FShared%20Documents%2FCredentials%2FCredentials%20Endorsement%20Documents%2FAdvanced%20practice%20in%20mental%20health%20curriculum%20and%20capabilities%20framework%2Epdf&parent=%2Fsites%2FAPWC%2FShared%20Documents%2FCredentials%2FCredentials%20Endorsement%20Documents&p=true&ga=1

Health Education England (2022c). Governance of Advanced Practice in Health and Care Provider Organisations. https://advanced-practice.hee.nhs.uk/resources-news-and-events/governance-of-advanced-practice-in-health-and-care-provider-organisations/

Health Education England, NHS England and Skills for Health (2020). Core Capabilities Framework for Advanced Clinical Practice (Nurses) Working in General Practice/Primary Care. www.hee.nhs.uk/sites/default/files/documents/ACP%20Primary%20Care%20Nurse%20Fwk%202020.pdf

National Society for the Prevention of Cruelty to Children (2022). Gillick competency and Fraser guidelines. https://learning.nspcc.org.uk/child-protection-system/gillick-competence-fraser-guidelines

NHS (2020). We are the NHS: People Plan 2020/21 – action for us all. www.england.nhs.uk/wp-content/uploads/2020/07/We-Are-The-NHS-Action-For-All-Of-Us-FINAL-March-21.pdf

Nursing and Midwifery Council (2015). The Code. www.nmc.org.uk/globalassets/sitedocuments/nmc-publications/nmc-code.pdf

Royal College of Emergency Medicine (2020). Management of Investigation Results in the Emergency Department. https://rcem.ac.uk/wp-content/uploads/2021/10/RCEM_BPC_InvestigationResults_200520.pdf

Royal College of Emergency Medicine (2021). Radiology Requesting Protocol for Extended and Advanced Clinical Practitioners in the Emergency Department. https://res.cloudinary.com/studio-republic/images/v1636645964/Radiology_Requesting_Protocol_for_Extended_and_-ACPs_-in_the_ED/Radiology_Requesting_Protocol_for_Extended_and_-ACPs_-in_the_ED.pdf?_i=AA

Royal College of Emergency Medicine (2022a). Emergency Medicine Advanced Clinical Practitioner Curriculum (Adult). https://res.cloudinary.com/studio-republic/images/v1662469600/ACP_Curriculum_Adult_Final_060922/ACP_Curriculum_Adult_Final_060922.pdf?_i=AA

Royal College of Emergency Medicine (2022b). Emergency Medicine Advanced Clinical Practitioner Curriculum (Child). https://res.cloudinary.com/studio-republic/images/v1662477148/ACP_Curriculum_Children_Final_060922_1108919893/ACP_Curriculum_Children_Final_060922_1108919893.pdf?_i=AA

Royal College of Nursing (2022). Patient Specific Directions (PSDs) and Patient Group Directions (PGDs). www.rcn.org.uk/clinical-topics/medicines-management/patient-specific-directions-and-patient-group-directions

Royal Pharmaceutical Society (2021). Prescribing Competency Framework. https://www.rpharms.com/portals/0/rps%20document%20library/open%20access/professional%20standards/prescribing%20competency%20framework/prescribing-competency-framework.pdf

The Ionising Radiation (Medical Exposure) Regulations (2017). www.legislation.gov.uk/uksi/2017/1322/contents/made

United Nations (1948). Universal Declaration of Human Rights. www.un.org/en/about-us/universal-declaration-of-human-rights

FURTHER READING

Leslie, K., Moore, J., Robertson, C. et al. (2021). Regulating health professional scopes of practice: comparing institutional arrangements and approaches in the US, Canada, Australia and the UK. *Human Resources for Health* 19: 15.

Science Direct Topics (2022). Scope Practice. www.sciencedirect.com/topics/nursing-and-health-professions/scope-of-practice

SELF-ASSESSMENT QUESTIONS

1. As an advanced practitioner assessing a pregnant woman, when would you need to refer to a midwife or medical practitioner?
2. How do you deem yourself competent with the correct knowledge, skills and behaviours to assess and treat an individual?
3. Do you understand what your duty of care is and what constitutes a breach of your duty of care?
4. What requirements should be in place to protect you from litigation?

GLOSSARY

Advanced paramedic practitioners (APPs)   APPs offer a high level of clinical skills and leadership. They co-ordinate and provide clinical advice for some of the more complex incidents they attend, whilst also being responsible for a team of senior paramedics.

Advanced Practice Governance Maturity Matrix   The Matrix is designed to be a developmental activity for health and care provider organisations and can also be used to foster discussion within their own organisation and with the relevant regional Faculty for Advancing Practice.

Advanced practice therapeutic radiographer   The College of Radiographers uses the term advanced practice in the education and career framework for the radiography workforce: www.sor.org/learning-advice/professional-body-guidance-and-publications/documents-and-publications/policy-guidance-document-library/education-and-career-framework-for-the-radiography

Council for Healthcare Regulatory Excellence   The Council for Healthcare Regulatory Excellence (CHRE) was a UK health regulatory body set up under the National Health Service Reform and Health Care Professions Act 2002. CHRE has now changed its name to the Professional Standards Authority for Health and Social Care (the Authority) under the Health and Social Care Act 2012, section 222.

Governance framework   A recommended framework for the development of advanced clinical practitioners (ACPs). It aims to provide employers with guidance on issues which should be addressed within their own governance policy or processes, from identifying the need for an ACP to postqualification support. The aim is to provide a set of standards and support mechanisms to enable employers to embed and grow ACPs within their organisations.

Scope creep   A term commonly used in project management. It refers to changes, continuous or uncontrolled growth in a project's scope, at any point after the project begins.

Scope of practice   Describes the procedures, actions and processes that a healthcare practitioner is permitted to undertake in keeping with the terms of their professional licence.

Service user   A broad phrase to refer to those who use or are affected by healthcare services.

CHAPTER 4

Principles of Physiology for Advanced Practice

Colin Chandler, Alison Wood, and Robin Hyde

Aim

The aim of this chapter is to explore physiological concepts that will equip trainee APs to develop their future practice. This chapter assumes that a level of physiology knowledge has already been achieved. These concepts will help trainees to develop their understanding of relevant physiology in their own areas and understand future advances.

LEARNING OUTCOMES

After reading this chapter the reader will:

1. have an understanding of the interaction between activity, context and individuals as related to physiology (to facilitate person-centred assessment)
2. be able to explain how the body adapts its function to changing internal and external demands
3. understand the importance and influence of lifestyle on bodily functions throughout different stages of life
4. understand how interactions between cells of the body and the microbiome environment can lead to changes in function at the membrane and cellular levels.

The Advanced Practitioner: A Framework for Practice, First Edition. Edited by Ian Peate, Sadie Diamond-Fox, and Barry Hill.

INTRODUCTION

Our understanding of the body's physiology is partial; this will develop over the advanced practitioner's (APs) careers as new knowledge is found and the physiological concepts we draw upon are applied to patient care and advanced practice. This chapter builds on the qualified practitioner's existing level of physiology education (BINE 2016; Wood et al. 2020) and is considered against the backdrop of the advanced practice frameworks and curricula which indicate varying degrees of physiology knowledge, mostly 'hinting towards' physiology requiring to be understood (Table 4.1).

The rationale for a conceptual approach at this advanced level is that concepts are the big ideas which provide structure for understanding in an area, they are transferable to sub areas, they are useful tools for problem solving and to aid future understanding (Michael et al 2017).

We are in an information age where it is easy to search for and find material; this may be good information, misinformation or even disinformation. The skill is first to know what to look for and where; second, in assessing its value; and third, putting it together to address the question you started with. This is where a conceptual understanding can provide structure to fit information, current and future, into the individual contexts of a physiological or practice situation. It can provide a scaffold for future learning of physiology and in particular its application into the practice context.

TABLE 4.1 Frameworks and curriculum for ACP which mention physiology as a requirement.

Multi-professional Framework for Advanced Clinical Practice (HEE 2017) www.hee.nhs.uk/sites/default/files/docuemtns/HEE%20ACP%Framework.pdf	1.6 Use expertise and decision-making skills to inform clinical reasoning approaches when dealing with differentiated and undifferentiated individual presentations and complex situations, synthesising information from multiple sources to make appropriate, evidence-based judgements and/or diagnoses
Faculty of Intensive Care Medicine (2019) Curriculum for Training for Advanced Critical Care Practitioners: Syllabus. www.ficm.ac.uk/sites/ficm/files/documents/2021-10/accp_curriculum_part_iii_-_syllabus_v1.1_2019_revision.pdf	Highlight core knowledge of basic science: • Cellular physiology • Homeostasis • Systems anatomy, physiology, and pathophysiology: Respiratory; Cardiovascular; Neurological; Gastrointestinal and hepatic; Renal; Musculoskeletal; Endocrine; Immunity; Blood and coagulation
Royal College of Emergency Medicine (2019) Advanced Clinical Practitioner Curriculum and Assessment [Adult and Paediatric]. www.ficm.ac.uk/sites/ficm/files/documents/2021-10/accp_curriculum_part_iii_-_syllabus_v1.1_2019_revision.pdf	Some outcomes and skills which identify physiology specifically: • Identify physiological perturbations causing anaphylactic shock • Recognise significance of major physiological perturbations • Recalls the relevant physiology and pharmacology [including toxicity of local anaesthetic agents, its symptoms, signs and management, including the use of lipid rescue]

(Continued)

TABLE 4.1   (Continued)

Royal College of Emergency Medicine (2019) Advanced Clinical Practitioner Curriculum and Assessment [Paediatric Only]. `https://rcem.ac.uk/wp-content/uploads/2021/10/EC_ACP_Curriculum_2017_Paediatric_Only-for-publication-last_edit_14-03-2019.pdf`	Some outcomes and skills which identify specifics of physiology A few examples: • Understand the psychological and physiological and socioeconomic effect of alcohol misuse and illicit drug use – opioids, amphetamines, ecstasy, cocaine, GHB • Know the neuroanatomy and physiology relevant to balance, coordination, and movement • Know the basic anatomy and physiology of the eye and visual pathways
Scottish Government (2021) Transforming Nursing Roles: Advanced Nursing Practice - Phase II: Paper 7. `www.gov.scot/binaries/content/documents/govscot/publications/advice-and-guidance/2021/04/transforming-nursing-roles-advanced-nursing-practice-phase-ii/documents/transforming-nursing-roles-advanced-nursing-practice-phase-ii/transforming-nursing-roles-advanced-nursing-practice-phase-ii/govscot%3Adocument/transforming-nursing-roles-advanced-nursing-practice-phase-ii.pdf`	No outcome related but evidence of learning required including: ▪ Anatomy and physiology
Royal College of General Practitioners (2015) General Practice Advanced Nurse Practitioner Competencies. London: RCGP	1.2 Accurately assesses, diagnoses, monitors, co-ordinates and manages health/illness state of individuals during acute or enduring episodes 7.5 Distinguishes between normal and abnormal development and age-related physiological and behavioural changes in complex, acute, critical and chronic illness

In this chapter, we will look at five areas which draw on multiple physiological concepts and relate these to current practice situations. Use these in the future to add or challenge new ideas and information and their fit or relevance to clinical practice (Michael et al. 2017).

Multi-Professional Framework for Advanced Clinical Practice (MPFfACP)

This chapter relates to the following areas of the MPFfACP:
1.6

(HEE 2017)

Accreditation Considerations

This chapter is applicable to the following specialist curricula:

- Acute Medicine (HEE 2022a)
- Critical Care (ACCP) (FICM 2015)
- Emergency Care – Adult and Child (RCEM 2022)
- Learning Disability and/or Autism (HEE 2020a)
- Mental Health (HEE 2022b)
- Older People (HEE 2022c)
- Primary Care (HEE 2020b)
- Surgical Care (HEE 2020c)

HOW THE BODY ADAPTS TO DIFFERENT SITUATIONS

Life is not a static event; we are constantly moving from one activity to another and in consequence placing different demands on our bodies with these shifting contexts of life. An example would be the change from a sedentary activity (rest, sleep, working at a desk) to one involving exercise (moving within a home, walking to a shop or taking part in a marathon). This change will present the body with the need to ensure sufficient energy supply to the muscles involved and manage any waste products whilst maintaining as near optimum balance within the internal environment. The core concepts here involve transport, usually passive down gradients, and energy supply. Within the body, these gradients may be due to pressure, concentration and volume and will have a tendency to move down the gradient from high to low. Often, these gradients will exist across barriers such as cell membranes which will be permeable to some substances but not others. Transport across cell membranes can involve transporters, gap junctions, voltage-gated sodium channels and receptor-gated non-selective cation channels (Figure 4.1). Proteins, which will be explored in more detail in a later section, provide the means to cross these barriers and in some cases transport against a concentration gradient which requires the use of energy (active transport).

Energy supply is paramount but needs to be in the right amount and place. In the cell, energy is stored, transported and released by the making and breaking of a chemical bond, the most common of which is the addition of an extra phosphate to adenosine diphosphate (ADP) to produce adenosine triphosphate (ATP). The energy stored in this bond is released when the reaction is reversed (ATP to ADP) and powers molecular-level activity within the cell. The pathways to transform our food intake to this level of cellular energy currency are complex, involving many chemical reactions and transport across membranes, distribution throughout the body and metabolic pathways within the cell requiring sufficient oxygen supply. This, combined with the management of waste products (CO_2 and metabolites), can challenge the control of the internal environment (homeostasis) and is better described as a homeodynamic mechanism where some factors may vary widely within safe limits (heart rate [HR], blood pressure [BP], O_2 saturation, pH) whilst others are tightly controlled ($[K^+]$, $[Ca^{++}]$).

In anticipation and during exercise, HR, cardiac output, respiratory rate and volume will increase dramatically with a moderate increase in blood pressure as the demand for perfusion of active muscle increases. Some elements of this will be under neural or endocrine control, others a local response to the prevailing conditions within the tissue. These changes will tend to reverse after exercise, but at varying timescales. This provides the context for clinical interpretation of blood results. Other conditions will

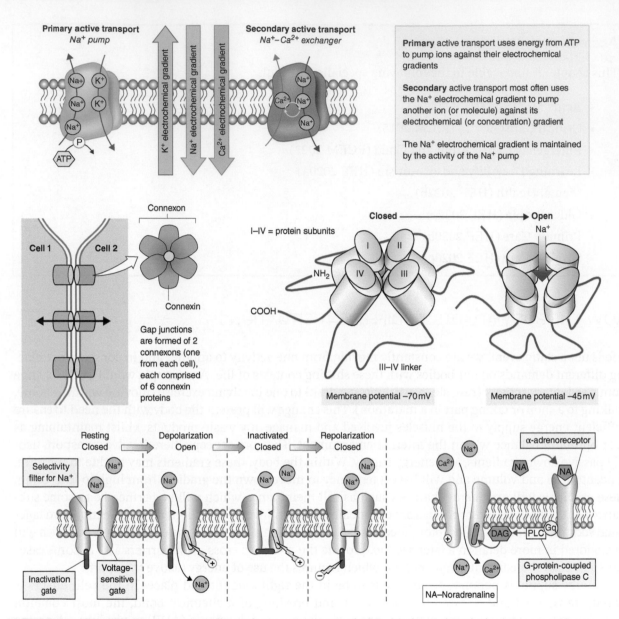

FIGURE 4.1 Transport routes across cell membranes. *Source*: Ward J.P.T., Linden R. (2017) Physiology at a Glance. Chichester: John Wiley & Sons.

also play into this homeodynamic mix, such as altitude, heat or cold, pressure changes, ageing and a variety of pathologies (Hawley et al. 2017). When walking at altitude, multiple integrated responses are required to cope with the challenges to whole body homeostasis posed by such exercise. The muscle-centric approach sees cardiovascular and respiratory responses becoming "service functions". This is a salutary warning that in many of the bodies activities both in health and disease, the interaction between systems is complex and often competing or conflicting in the pursuit of the activity whilst maintaining stability in the body. When exercising at altitude (3000 – 5000m), a conscious adaptation is required to balance oxygen demand with reduced supply to avoid the unwanted consequences of hyperventilation, i.e. slow the walk down and control breathing to find a sustainable slow pace. This illustration shows that we need to apply bioscience knowledge to facilitate the whole person, in the context of their desired activities and participation in society.

Pharmacological Principles – Antipyretics

Body temperature control is a major component of normal homeostatic control. Paracetamol is a common agent used for control of pyrexia (high temperature). Paracetamol's antipyretic properties have remained obscure for centuries, but it is hypothesised that they may result from several mechanisms, including inhibition of two specific enzymes implicated in temperature homeostasis: cyclo-oxygenase and transient receptor potential ankyrin 1 (TRPA1) (Mirrasekhian et al. 2018).

RED FLAGS – PATHOLOGICAL CONSIDERATIONS

It is not uncommon to analyse an arterial blood gas (ABG) sample to explore the cause of an acute deterioration in health state, i.e. increasing respiratory distress, decreasing level of consciousness, cardiac dysfunction. Such an analysis draws on chemical and physical principles that explain how substances dissolve and ionise in aqueous solution and the relationship between hydrogen ion concentration and acidity or alkalinity.

The body's internal environment contains many salts and weak acids in aqueous solution (Figure 4.2). When a weak acid dissolves in water, some of it will dissociate into its ionic components and some will remain in the undissociated state. For example, carbonic acid H_2CO_3 will partially dissociate into hydrogen ions (H^+) and bicarbonate ions (HCO_3^-). There will also be a range of salts dissolved in the aqueous solution,

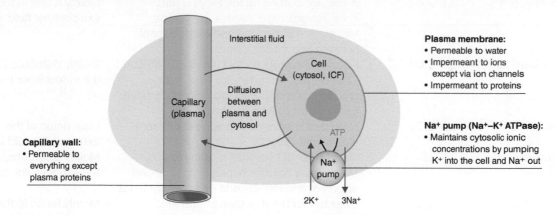

Constituents of physiological fluids (approximate values, intracellular varies between tissues)		Plasma	Interstitial	Intracellular	Unit
Water:	% total body water	13%	22%	65%	%
	(volume in a **70 kg** person)	(3.5)	(9.5)	(27)	L
Osmolality		290	290	290	mosmol/kg H₂O
Cations:	Na⁺	140	140	10	mmol/L
	K⁺	4	4	140	mmol/L
	Ca²⁺ (free)	1	1	0.0001	mmol/L
Anions:	Cl⁻	108	129	3–30	mmol/L
	HCO₃⁻	26	26	9	mmol/L
	Proteins⁻	10	1	50	mmol/L
	Other anions (mainly PO₄³⁻, SO₄³⁻)	3	0	60–88	mmol/L

Notes: Ca²⁺ (and Mg²⁺) tend to bind to plasma proteins, and their free concentrations are about 50% of the total. Ionic concentrations are sometimes given in mEq/L to reflect the amount of charge, where an equivalent (Eq) is 1 mole of charge. So 1 Eq of a monovalent ion such as Na⁺ = 1 mole, but 1 Eq of Ca²⁺ = 0.5 mole

FIGURE 4.2 Physiological fluid compartments. *Source*: Ward J.P.T., Linden R. (2017) Physiology at a Glance. Chichester: John Wiley & Sons.

e.g. sodium chloride (NaCl) which will dissociate into sodium ions (Na^+) and chloride ions (Cl^-). Together, these provide a chemical buffer solution which can maintain an almost constant pH when small amounts of acid or base are added. If extra hydrogen ions are added, some will combine with the bicarbonate ions and form undissociated carbonic acid so that the ratio between the ionic and undissociated forms of the weak acid is maintained. In effect, it is absorbing some of the excess hydrogen ions. If a base is added, e.g. further bicarbonate ions, then these will combine with hydrogen ions or other positively charged ions to maintain the dynamic ratios of dissociation of weak acids and salts. In this way, the effect of adding strong acid or base is minimised by the buffering effect of the weak acids and salts within the solution.

CLINICAL INVESTIGATIONS – SERUM ELECTROLYTES

Electrolytes	Normal Values in Extrasellar Fluid (Mmol/l)	Function	Main Distribution
Sodium (Na)	135–145	Important cation in generation of action potentials. Plays an important role in fluid and electrolyte balance	Main cation of the extracellular fluid
Potassium (K^+)	3.5–5	Important cation in establishing resting membrane potential. Regulates pH balance. Maintains intracellular fluid volume	Main cation of the intracellular fluid
Calcium (Ca^{2+})	2.1–2.6	Important clotting factor. Plays a part in neurotransmitter release in neurons. Maintains muscle tone and excitability of nervous and muscle tissue	Mainly found in the extracellular fluid
Magnesium (Mg^{2+})	0.5–1.0	Helps to maintain normal nerve and muscle function; maintains regular heart rate, regulates blood glucose and blood pressure. Essential for protein synthesis	Mainly distributed in the intracellular fluid
Chloride (Cl)	98–117	Maintains a balance of anions in different fluid compartments	Main anion of the extracellular fluid
Hydrocarbons (HCO_3^-)	24–31	Main buffer of hydrogen ions in plasma. Maintains a balance between cations and anions of intracellular and extracellular fluids	Mainly distributed in the extracellular fluid
Phosphate– organic (HPO_4^-)	0.8–1.1	Essential for the digestion of proteins, carbohydrates and fats and absorption of calcium. Essential for bone formation	Mainly found in the intracellular fluid
Sulphate (SO_4^{2-})	0.5	Involved in detoxification of phenols, alcohols and amines	Mainly found in the intracellular fluid

Source: Peate I (ed.). Fundamentals of Applied Pathophysiology: An Essential Guide for Nursing and Healthcare Students. Chichester: John Wiley & Sons, Incorporated, 2017.

During exercise, the muscles require energy; to provide this, they need a substrate, oxygen and produce carbon dioxide as a waste product. This carbon dioxide is transported from the muscle to the blood and via the circulation to the lungs where it is exhaled. Increases in cardiac output and respiratory rate facilitate this during exercise. Seventy percent of the carbon dioxide is transported in combination with water to form carbonic acid which then dissociates as described above. The hydrogen ions are buffered within the red blood cell by haemoglobin. Bicarbonate and hydrogen ions move out into the plasma down their concentration gradient and have the potential to lower the pH, but will be buffered within the plasma (Figure 4.3a).

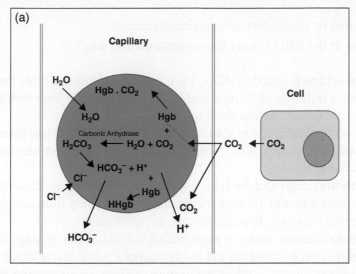

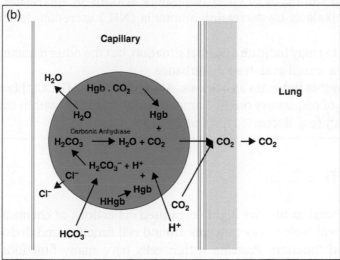

FIGURE 4.3 Transport of carbon dioxide (a) from cells to blood, (b) from blood to alveoli. *Source*: Ward J.P.T., Linden R. (2017) Physiology at a Glance. Chichester: John Wiley & Sons.

At the lungs, this process is reversed, and carbon dioxide moves down its concentration gradient into the air-filled spaces of the alveoli where it is breathed out (Figure 4.3b).

Case Study and Clinical Investigations

Reflect on this aspect of respiratory physiology in connection with interpreting ABG results in a clinical situation.

- Are they normal?
- Is there an acidosis? If so, is this of respiratory or metabolic origin?
- Is there an alkalosis? If so, is this of respiratory or metabolic origin?

- Is this compensated by respiratory or renal mechanisms?
- What parameters in the ABG answer these questions and why?

If the pH is low (an acidosis) and the $[HCO_3^-]$ is normal then this indicates that the acidosis is of metabolic origin, namely a build-up of H^+ ions within the body possibly from another non-respiratory source (e.g. infection, renal failure, ketoacidosis).

If the pH is high then this indicates an alkalosis, and if the $[HCO_3^-]$ is low then this alkalosis is of respiratory origin, namely a low level of CO_2 within the body possibly from respiratory hyperventilation (e.g. stress, panic attack, sepsis).

If the pH is high (an alkalosis) and the $[HCO_3^-]$ is normal then this indicates that the alkalosis is of metabolic origin, namely a loss of H^+ ions within the body possibly from another non-respiratory source (e.g. vomiting, renal diuretics, hypercalcaemia, hypokalaemia).

Respiratory compensation can occur to renormalise the pH either through hyperventilation to raise the pH or hypoventilation to lower the pH in the case of a metabolic acidosis or alkalosis.

Renal compensation can occur to offset respiratory acidosis by increasing HCO_3^- retention to buffer excess acid, or alkalosis by decreasing ammonia (NH_3) excretion, leading to a decrease in plasma HCO_3^-.

Normal pH (7.35–7.45) may indicate a normal situation, but the other parameters should be examined as it can also show a mixed acid–base disturbance.

If the pH is low then this indicates an acidosis. Alongside this, if $[HCO_3^-]$ is raised then this indicates that the acidosis is of respiratory origin, namely a build-up of CO_2 within the body possibly from a respiratory insufficiency (e.g. decreased respiratory drive, drowning).

KEY CONCEPTS OF THE CELL

Cells, which are fundamental to life, are highly organised collections of chemicals contained within a membrane. This section will look at key concepts around cell function and division, DNA and protein production, structure and function. Proteins within cells have many functions providing structural support, catalysing and controlling metabolic reactions, transporting molecules, acting as recognition markers and receptor sites. They form the main building blocks from which the cell is assembled, and can occur in the cell's aqueous environment or embedded within membranes.

The structure of the protein is fundamental to its function. Alterations to the structure, either by changing the sequence of amino acids or the way it is folded, can inactivate or change its action, in some cases leading to a toxic build-up within the cell or failure to control a metabolic process. All nucleated cells within the human body contain an identical sequence of DNA.

The DNA is a double helix of pairs of bases arranged on sugar-phosphate strands (Figure 4.4). Each human cell has around 3 billion base pairs in its genome; less than 2% of these, around 21 000 genes, are used to code for proteins. The remaining DNA is involved in controlling which genes are switched on to produce proteins within a specific cell, or may be 'junk DNA' acting either as spacer material within the sequence or with some other, as yet unknown, function.

The production of proteins is a multistage process. First, one of the strands of DNA is transcribed into a single strand of mRNA (messenger RNA), which provides the template for the sequence of amino acids that will be assembled in the translation phase. Following this, a variety of modifications may happen, including folding to establish its three-dimensional shape, binding to further chemicals (co-factors),

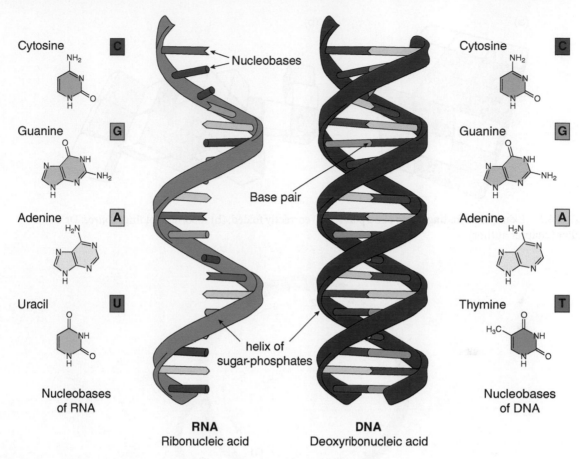

FIGURE 4.4 DNA and RNA structure. *Source*: Ward J.P.T., Linden R. (2017) Physiology at a Glance. Chichester: John Wiley & Sons.

binding to phosphate groups or sugars (phosphorylation, glycosylation), linking to other protein subunits, activation by removing some amino acids from the sequence or some other modification. Such a complex manufacturing process leaves plenty of scope for errors; most commonly, these would be errors in replicating the DNA sequences during cell division, resulting in missing out an amino acid, adding an extra or different one. Also, errors in the way the sequence is folded and bound to co-factors or other molecules can lead to misshapen proteins (imagine the puzzle of a string of 27 small cubes which can be folded into one large cube – getting the sequence of moves wrong leads to some very odd shapes – see Figure 4.5).

Fields of Practice – Learning Disabilities

Those working within a learning disabilities context should engage with the underlying physiological and biochemical changes which occur at the cellular level for those in this population. A recent study has speculated that gene E2 Rad6 is associated with one type of severe learning disability in humans. It has also been found to play a vital role in the cellular response to oxidative stress (Simões et al. 2022).

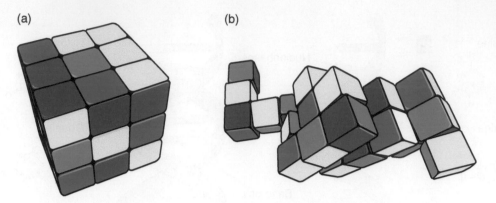

FIGURE 4.5   Example of folding using cube puzzle, (a) correctly folded, (b) incorrect folding. *Source*: Dr Colin Chandler (chapter author).

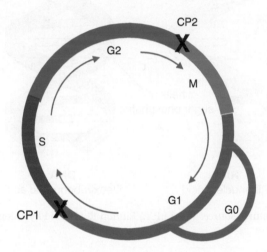

FIGURE 4.6   Cell cycle illustrating the sequence of phases during cell division. The phases are S (synthesis), M (mitosis) and G (gap G0, G1 and G2). Control of the cycle is achieved through checkpoints (CP1 and CP2).

Fortunately, cells have a range of quality control measures which weed out or correct most errors in protein production; some get through but are then usually caught by the immune system. Most mutations which could lead to altered cell function in cancer cells are destroyed by the immune system, but some do escape. Identifying the specific changes that occur in the genome, the transcription of the DNA or the protein produced is the basis of 'omics' (genomics, transcriptomics and proteomics), which are opening routes to personalised and more targeted interventions in the future (Marshall et al. 2022).

A fundamental property of cells is their ability to divide and produce more cells of the same type. This is described as the cell cycle which is an ordered sequence of phases leading to division into two identical daughter cells. Cell division consists of S (synthesis), M (mitosis) and G (gap G0, G1, and G2) phases (Figure 4.6).

In the adult, most cells remain in a quiescent state outside the cycle in the holding phase, termed G0. Progress through the cycle is regulated at checkpoints (CP1 and CP2) and any DNA damage stops the cycle at a checkpoint to allow repair. Where these checkpoints fail, genetic instability occurs, a feature of cancers. The main day job of the immune system is to detect and destroy cells which have genetic instability. Immunosurveillance removes thousands of incorrectly divided or damaged cells each day.

Occasionally, our immune system will encounter a foreign body such as a virus or bacterium and will then divert to destroy them. Immunotherapy and checkpoint inhibitors are exciting developments in the treatment of many cancers and will no doubt provide an extended range of cancer therapy in the future.

The development of personalised medicine is not new but as clinicians and researchers, we can use our knowledge on the genome to affect the way we diagnose and treat conditions and patients. Patterns are now being identified that help determine risks of disease and can establish the most effective treatments and interventions. As this progresses, the AP will be required to update their knowledge and practice in line with these new discoveries.

CONTROL – HOW THE BODY ALLOWS US TO ACHIEVE ACTION AND PARTICIPATION IN SOCIETY

Life is about living, not just existing, and our bodies enable us to engage with the world in which we exist – a mix of social, physical, psychological, emotional and spiritual environments. This is supported by our body's abilities to move, think, reason, communicate, learn and solve problems. The key physiological concepts that underpin these abilities are communication, adaptability or learning, and control of the interdependent organisational systems within the body.

Fields of Practice – Paediatrics

It is fascinating to watch a young child explore their environment. At first, this involves the challenges of developing control of movement and interacting with others. There are clear physical and emotional aspects to this early learning, and recognition of parents and other individuals is evident as well as toys and objects involved in play. In these early stages, the development of connections in the nervous system reflects the increasing levels of control and learning in movement and activity. Adaptation in the nervous system continues throughout life with the reinforcing, making and breaking of connections within the central nervous system (CNS). Such neuroplasticity underpins learning, recovery and functional change throughout life. Where loss of neuronal function occurs through cellular damage or pathology, within limits the nervous system will adapt over time to reduce this loss. This may be through establishing alternative pathways of control, with surviving neurons branching and forming new synapses or the regrowth of damaged axons within peripheral nerves to re-establish connection.

Fields of Practice – Mental Health

Physiology does have a strong connection with those who are under mental health services care or diagnoses. Taquet et al. (2021) have found a 'pattern of structural brain connectivity in children which robustly encodes a genetic vulnerability to psychiatric illness which crosses diagnostic boundaries'.

Much of the control of the body's internal environment is managed by the endocrine system; the timescales of this control can be immediate, within seconds, to longer term, over days, months or years. Intervention or change within such control is likely to follow a similar timeframe. Communication in both neural and endocrine systems is via chemical messengers, neurotransmitters and hormones.

These are released by the cells that produce them and travel through an aqueous environment to activate the target cells, usually through receptor proteins, though some may diffuse across the cell membrane and have a direct effect on intracellular mechanisms. Many of these chemical messengers are proteins which will match shape with their receptor site, resulting in an effect. This effect could be switching on, off or moderating a metabolic process, the transport of a substance across a membrane, the release of a further chemical substance and an alteration in the electrical potential across a membrane, to name but a few actions. Key to this will be the shape recognition between the transmitter substance and receptor site. If either of these is altered, then the response may not occur. This could be through changes in structure or numbers of transmitters or receptors. In the nervous system, this may be represented as a loss of neurons either from an area (as in stroke) or of a particular type (as the loss of dopaminergic cells in Parkinson disease), leading to a loss of function.

In diabetes mellitus (DM), the different types are characterised by different losses. In type 1 DM, there is a loss of insulin-producing beta cells in the pancreas, resulting in reduced production and hence the inability to respond to increases in blood sugar concentrations. In type 2 DM, there is a combination of impaired insulin secretion and insulin resistance. Impaired insulin resistance appears to be a dysfunction of the pancreatic beta cells which have a reduced response to raised plasma glucose levels. Insulin resistance seems to be related to age and weight, hence modifiable lifestyle factors such as diet and obesity are factors. It appears that obesity can lead to an increased resistance to the uptake of glucose into muscle, heart and fat cells. This may be due to an inflammatory response with reduced insulin-mediated activation of GLUT4, the transporter protein involved in the uptake of glucose into muscle, heart and fat cells, but the mechanism of this process is unclear at present.

Another aspect of control involves the processes dealing with cellular damage or degeneration. It is becoming clearer that disorders of cellular proteins, and in particular the way they are folded into the functional shape, are important. If these shapes are changed then the proteins may not be recognised and dealt with; they may thus accumulate and become toxic, disrupting cell function.

Autophagy is the normal housekeeping function of the cells in order to maintain their function; it includes processes that eliminate waste, protect against variations in nutrient availability, promote cellular remodelling and defend against invading pathogens. It acts to recycle proteins, lipids and nucleic acids through lysosomes, which are membrane-bound organelles containing an array of hydrolytic enzymes that deal with a range of substrates transported into the lysosomes by invagination or across the membrane. A further pathway in autophagy involves proteasomes, another form of membrane-bound organelle, which are responsible for most protein turnover.

Should these housekeeping functions in cells become disordered or unbalanced in some way then toxic substrates can accumulate. Oxidative stress arising from reactive oxygen species (ROS), which are hydrogen peroxide (H_2O_2), hydroxyl ions (OH^-) and superoxide ions (O_2^-), can lead to oxidative damage within cells. These ROS are normal products of mitochondrial energy production but are usually produced at low levels. However, if the mitochondria develop any defects, then their production can increase, leading to denaturation of cellular proteins. This denaturation will either be repaired or recycled as already described. But if the repair misfolds the protein then a toxic element may be produced which can collect within the cells, impairing function.

The cellular mechanism for the orderly destruction of cells is called apoptosis. This process is triggered within the cell and starts off a proteolytic cascade of reactions which dismantle the cell contents, leading to cell shrinkage. As the cell is disassembled it becomes a target for phagocytosis by macrophages. The process of necrosis involves overt damage to the cells, including rupture and the release of chemoactive substances. These initiate an inflammatory response and lead to an aggressive clean-up by the immune system which may have unintended consequences such as triggering autoimmune disorders.

CHANGES TO PHYSIOLOGY THROUGH THE LIFE COURSE

An indicator of change in physiology and pathology over the life course can be seen in the number and pattern of deaths for different age groups. The Global Burden of Diseases, Injuries and Risk Factors study 2019 provides a tool that can estimate mortality, incidence, prevalence, life expectancy and other data on a large range of diseases worldwide. It draws on a very large number of data sources. Figure 4.7 illustrates an extract of predicted mortality data for the UK in 2019 associated with major disease and injury categories.

The most obvious feature is that the majority of deaths are in the 80-plus age group – around 54% of all deaths. For children, those under one year of age are more vulnerable, but the death rates for children and adolescents are very low. There is a slight rise in numbers for young adults but again these numbers are small and only start to rise to any great extent above the age of 40. At 50–54 this is only just over 2% of

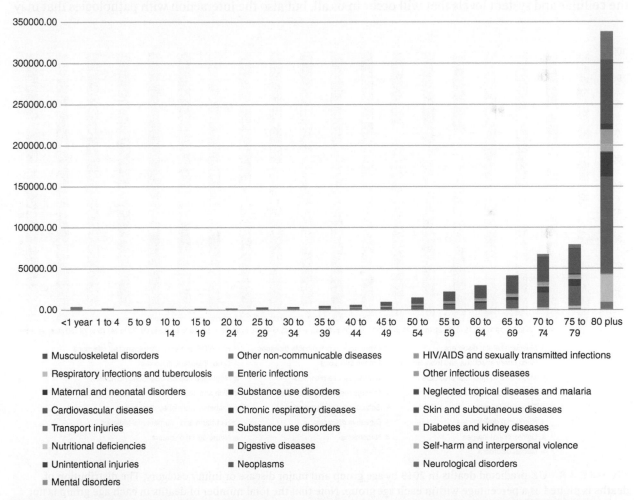

FIGURE 4.7   UK predicted deaths in 2019 by age group and major disease or injury category. Age group is shown on the horizontal axis and the height of the stacked bars represents the total deaths in that age group. The distribution of conditions leading to death is shown by the different colours in the stacked bars and within the diagram legend. *Source*: Data extracted from the Global Burden of Disease Collaborative Network. Global Burden of Disease Study 2019 Results. Seattle: Institute for Health Metrics and Evaluation, 2020. http://ghdx.healthdata.org/gbd-results-tool

the total deaths for the year. What is evident is that two main causes of deaths over 50 are neoplasms or cancer (red) and cardiovascular diseases (brown).

The causes of death in each age group are shown in Figure 4.8 as a percentage of total deaths in the age group. Whilst the risk of death is low in the younger age groups, it is interesting to see what the main risks are.

In the very young, under one year old, maternal and neonatal disorders are the most common cause of death (dark blue) followed by other non-communicable diseases (orange). Through childhood and adolescence, neoplasms or cancers feature as a cause (red). Self-harm and interpersonal violence (green) show up in the late teens to 50s. The impact of cancers increases from the 30s, peaking in the 60s at around 49%, then cardiovascular diseases (brown) which include cerebrovascular disorders increase in the elderly. Transport injuries (mid blue) are greatest in the 15–19 age group (22%).

Underlying these mortality statistics are a range of morbidities, many of which are related to ageing of cells and body tissues. As we consider ageing, we should think about the normal processes of ageing at the cellular and system levels that will occur in us all, but also the interaction with pathologies that may

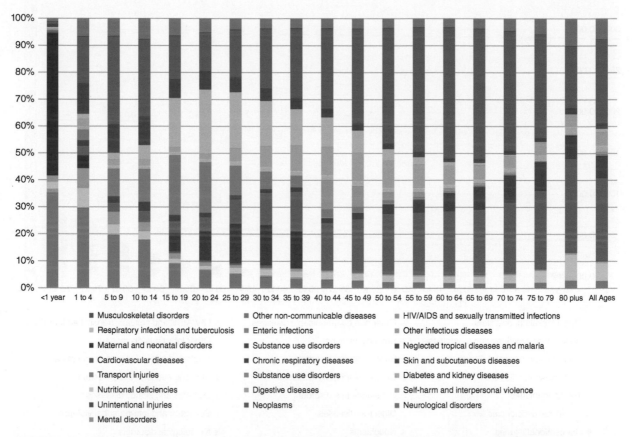

FIGURE 4.8   UK predicted deaths in 2019 by age group and major disease or injury category. The distribution of deaths is plotted as a percentage within each age group. Note that the total number of deaths in each age group is not shown but is very small in the age groups under 50 (each age group representing less than 2% of the total deaths). The distribution of conditions leading to death is shown by the different colours in the stacked bars and the legend is below. *Source*: Data extracted from the Global Burden of Disease Collaborative Network. Global Burden of Disease Study 2019 Results. Seattle: Institute for Health Metrics and Evaluation, 2020. http://ghdx.healthdata.org/gbd-results-tool

occur within the individual. All of these must be considered in the context of the person's life goals and how they may change and be reimagined.

ORANGE FLAGS – PSYCHOLOGICAL CONSIDERATIONS

The physiology of ageing can be viewed at many levels and may impact on an individuals psychological state. At the cellular level, we see changes in the way cells respond in terms of division and repair at different stages of the life course. At the tissue level, we can see growth, maturation, repair and decline of function with age. At the whole-body level, we see a complex interaction between the physical, psychological and social aspects of life with the possibility of interruption in one or more due to major pathology (e.g. cancer, dementia, cardiovascular disease, neurological conditions, arthritis, endocrine or gut conditions) affecting our healthy ageing trajectory. We can think of ageing as a long-term condition that will affect us all.

Ageing is a complex activity and the changes that constitute and influence it are complex biologically and not well understood. One view is that we see a gradual accumulation of molecular and cellular damage over time. This damage can lead to a decrease in physiological function and increased risk of many diseases. A general decline in the capacity of the individual ultimately will lead to death but these changes are very variable between individuals and not necessarily related to age. Many 70 year olds enjoy good physical and mental functioning, whilst others may be very frail and require significant support just to meet their basic needs.

GREEN FLAGS – SOCIAL CONSIDERATIONS

Beyond the biological side of older age, other significant changes occur which include changes in role, changes in social position and dealing with the loss of close relationships. As we progress through life, life goals and activities change, perhaps to select more meaningful goals and activities and so optimise existing abilities. In recent years we have seen a massive development of understanding of new technology across the whole age spectrum.

At the cellular level, there is a range of molecular damage, phenomena and processes that together make up the progressive dysfunction and eventual death of cells. This has been put into a conceptual framework called the nine hallmarks of ageing (López-Otín et al. 2013).

1. *Genomic instability*: the accumulation of genetic damage throughout life. This may be due to replication errors, damage from metabolic stressors within the cell leading to changes in the genetic material, or the addition of genetic material of viral origin. These changes will alter the genetic control of cellular function.
2. *Telomere attrition*: telomeres are located at the ends of chromosomes and protect them during replication. They are progressively shortened with each replicative cycle and once lost, further replication of the cell is not possible.
3. *Epigenetics* refers to the way genes are expressed; alterations in this affect the enzymatic systems within the cells and so change the way the cells work.
4. Loss of *proteostasis* is an impairment of protein homeostasis within the cell, disrupting structure and function. In response to stressors, there may be an unfolding and refolding of proteins, leading to damaged proteins which may collect within the cells or be degraded.

5. Deregulated *nutrient sensing* within the cells represents a reduction in control of nutrient use within the cell. Ageing in the cell appears to link to excess activity in anabolic processes, whereas decreased activity is related to longevity.

6. *Mitochondrial dysfunction*: mitochondria produce highly reactive oxygen species via their normal function. Over time, these lead to oxidative damage within the organelles, reducing their efficiency.

7. *Cellular senescence* is a halting of the cell cycle at a stable point, resulting in cells no longer being able to divide. Over time, a tissue will accumulate senescent cells leading to a reduction in its function.

8. *Stem cell exhaustion* limits the regenerative potential of tissues, in particular the production of immune cells.

9. *Altered intercellular communication*: whether this is endocrine, neural or a combination of the two, it reduces the body's ability to respond to damage and stimuli. This is of particular importance in the area of immunosurveillance against pathogens and premalignant cells. It also contributes to the increase in inflammatory activity with age – 'inflammaging'.

The first four of these hallmarks are causes of damage; the next three are responses to that damage; and the final two are consequences that ensue in ageing.

The complexity of ageing is summed up at the individual level in this quote from the Physiological Society:

The most important system in the body related to ageing is the one that fails first for the individual as this leads to a domino effect and ultimately multimorbidity.

(Physiology Society 2019, pp. 17, 19)

Healthy ageing appears to be very much about maintaining activity, particularly exercise. The failure of a system can lead to a reduction in the ability to exercise, causing subtle changes in lifestyle with consequent knock-on effects on other systems in the body, reducing their capacity and function.

The World Health Organization defines healthy ageing as the process of developing and maintaining the functional ability that enables well-being in older age. Functional ability is having the capabilities that enable people to be and do what they have reason to value. This includes a person's ability to meet their basic needs, to learn, grow, make decisions, to be mobile, to build and maintain relationships, and to contribute to society. Functional ability is within the intrinsic capacity of the individual but also relies on the relevant characteristics of their environment.

In old age, one can distinguish between healthy ageing, where there is some functional decline but not so much that it affects activity and participation in society, and years spent in poor health. This can be seen as the difference between healthy life expectancy and life expectancy and may be in the range of 15–20 years of poor health in the final years of life (Public Health England 2017). Related to this, Scott Murray (2017) developed the concept of well-being trajectories at the end of life, which map physical, social, psychological and spiritual well-being. Three trajectories are described.

1. *Rapid functional decline*, where physical and social well-being decline rapidly in parallel towards the end of life. Psychological and spiritual dimensions show a fluctuating pattern. This trajectory is typical for an individual with late-stage cancer.

2. *Intermittent decline*, typical of individuals with a life-limiting long-term condition. There is a general trend of decline with dips in the physical, social and psychological well-being with recovery towards the trend line.

3. *Gradual decline*, with a reducing level of physical well-being. The other dimensions are often well maintained, but show a rapid decline towards the end, with social followed by psychological and finally spiritual falling off. This trajectory is typical of frailty, dementia and long-term neurological conditions.

A further situation exists of sudden death often caused by trauma or an unexpected pathological event.

MICROBIOME/MICROBIOTA AND INTERACTIONS WITH THE MICROBIOLOGICAL ENVIRONMENT

Our bodies are made up of around 10^{13} cells which work together to enable us to carry out all the things we do, from the background tasks of digesting food, transporting blood around the body to distribute nutrients and oxygen and collect carbon dioxide for removal, right through to our brain cells working to sort out complex problems. But we are not alone – each of us carries a large number of micro-organisms in and on our bodies. This population of organisms, our *microbiota*, usually helps us to maintain our health, though on occasion it can get out of balance or in the wrong place and cause disease. There are around 10^{14} organisms in this microbiota, so each of us carries around 10 times as many micro-organisms as there are cells in our own bodies. Most of these are in our gut, a lot on our skin, and on our other body surfaces, with only a few in our internal environment, and those that do get there are usually dealt with quickly.

Every cell in our body with a nucleus contains an identical copy of our genetic material; this is a blueprint or plan of our body and is used to construct, develop and control the function of our cells. Each micro-organism will also have its own genetic material. The combined pool of this material is referred to as the *microbiome* and, with the advances in our understanding of genes, can be sequenced and analysed. The combined genomes of the microbiota amount to some 5 million genes, that is 100 times greater than the number of genes in each cell of our bodies.

In our bodies, we have many sites in which diverse microbial ecosystems are established. As soon as we are born, a process of colonisation by foreign (not us) micro-organisms starts. They inhabit most of our body surfaces that are exposed to the surrounding environment – skin, mouth, gut, cornea, and urogenital structures including, urethra and vagina.

Immediately after we are born, the microbiome that can be detected on and in us is influenced by the route of delivery; if vaginal delivery then we are covered with microbes from the vagina, if caesarean then skin microbes will predominate. Whilst the microbiome is established early in life, mainly over our first two years, over time it can alter due to changes in diet, lifestyle, environment, use of antibiotics and age. In the gut, a range of microbial metabolites can interact with host cell receptors, altering their metabolic balance, and may result in metabolic disease. Such microbial metabolites can be identified and related to a variety of conditions, for example irritable bowel disease or heart failure. Most of us for most of the time will live in harmony with our microbiotas and benefit from their contribution to our homeostasis. Only in acute infection or situations such as compromise of the immune system will the body's physiology become unbalanced which in the extreme case may lead to sepsis and death. The overuse of antibiotics, for even minor infections, has led to a situation where antimicrobial resistance genes within the microbiome are selectively preserved, with the result that the range of effective antibiotics is reducing.

Our understanding of the relationship between different organisms has evolved as our knowledge of their genetic make-up has increased. We now describe them in three groups, two of which are made up of the prokaryotic organisms Bacteria and Archaea. The third is the Eukarya which contains the eukaryotic organisms, many of which are unicellular but also include fungi, plants and animals. Genome analysis has provided a more direct way to show evolutionary relationships. A comparison of the complete DNA sequence of organisms shows how similar they are. This led to the identification of the three groups, but all have some similarities, suggesting a common ancestor. There are 63 genes in common to all three groups which are mainly involved in managing genetic material, while a further 264 genes are highly conserved and common to two of the groups.

In addition to these organisms that are capable of independent life there are the viruses which consist of genetic material, DNA or RNA, contained within a protein or glycoprotein shell. They commandeer host cells to reproduce. Some kill the host cell outright while others may insert themselves into the host DNA by reversing the transcription process of DNA to RNA. Their genome may then lie dormant in the host cells leading eventually to changes in function. Antiretroviral drugs target reverse transcriptase and have been successful in delaying or preventing the progression of HIV infection to AIDS (Alberts 2019).

The microbiota inhabiting the different surfaces of the body consist of bacteria, archea, viruses and some simple eukaryotes. In the gut, the microbiome has been linked to metabolic and other systemic disorders. Some pathogenic infections have been successfully treated with faecal transplant from a healthy gut microbiota. In health, the gut microbiota maintains a friendly relationship with the host most of the time, but where this commensal relationship changes, disease or damage may ensue. Links have been made between gut bacteria and obesity, type 1 diabetes, bowel disorders and a range of cancers. Further links have been made with brain function, involving an interplay of the nervous, digestive and immune systems which has been named the brain–gut–microbiome axis. The gut microbiota can produce a range of neurotransmitter substances that will normally contribute to the local control of gut function, sensation and peristalsis, but may also have a wider effect on unconscious behaviour and emotion mediated through serotonergic pathways in the brain. This raises interesting questions about the roles of our microbiomes which can be influenced by our lifestyle and behaviours (Shehata et al. 2022).

CONCLUSION

A solid understanding of physiology is key for healthcare practice and for the provision of safe patient care. Despite physiology being an implicit part of advanced practice standards, which often do not mention physiology directly (see Table 4.1), having this understanding, both of the body at 'rest' and 'extremes', provides the backdrop for the AP to support their clinical decisions and treatment plans as well as a person-centred approach to care planning and management.

We have presented here five areas which draw on multiple physiological concepts and begin to relate these to current healthcare practice. This baseline, we believe, supports both the practice challenges for the developing AP and systems approach to assessment and treatment which is considered in subsequent chapters within this text. We have provided a scaffold for future learning of physiology, presented in a way to support practitioners to engage with these concepts, to allow further development of knowledge in this area related to their role and to patient care.

Take Home Points
- Regardless of clinical specialty or field of practice, physiology underpins advanced practice and clinical assessment and decision making.
- Advanced practice frameworks require knowledge of physiology, and this underpins understanding of concepts related to pathophysiology.
- A concepts approach can provide an AP with a format to expand their knowledge base on physiology as they progress in this role.

REFERENCES

Alberts, B.(2019). *Essential Cell Biology,* 5e. New York: W.W. Norton.

Bioscience in Nurse Education (BiNE) (2016). Quality Assurance Framework for Biosciences Education in Nursing.https://s3.eu-west-2.amazonaws.com/assets.creode.advancehe-document-manager/documents/hea/private/bine_biosciences_qa_framework_b-qaf_july_16_1568037218.pdf

Faculty of Intensive Care Medicine (2015). Curriculum for Training for Advanced Critical Care Practitioners. www.ficm.ac.uk/sites/ficm/files/documents/2021-10/ACCP%20Curriculum%20Part%20I%20-%20Handbook%20v1.1%202019%20Revision.pdf

Hawley, J.A., Hargreaves, M., Joyner, M. et al. (2014). Integrative biology of exercise. Cell 159 (4): 738–749.

Health Education England (2017). Multi-professional Framework For Advanced Clinical Practice in England. www.hee.nhs.uk/sites/default/files/docuemtns/HEE%20ACP%Framework.pdf

Health Education England (2020a). Advanced Clinical Practice: Capabilities framework when working with people who have a learning disability and/or autism. www.skillsforhealth.org.uk/wp-content/uploads/2020/11/ACP-in-LDA-Framework.pdf

Health Education England (2020b). Surgical Advanced Clinical Practitioner (SACP) Curriculum and Assessment Framework. www.iscp.ac.uk/media/1141/sacp_curriculum_dec20_accessible-1.pdf

Health Education England (2020c). Workplace Supervision for Advanced Clinical Practice: An integrated multi-professional approach for practitioner development. www.hee.nhs.uk/sites/default/files/documents/Workplace%20Supervision%20for%20ACPs.pdf

Health Education England (2022a). Advanced Clinical Practice in Acute Medicine Curriculum Framework. https://healtheducationengland.sharepoint.com/sites/APWC/Shared%20Documents/Forms/AllItems.aspx?id=%2Fsites%2FAPWC%2FShared%20Documents%2FCredentials%2FCredentials%20Endorsement%20Documents%2FAdvanced%20clinical%20practice%20in%20acute%-20medicine%20curriculum%20framework%2Epdf&parent=%2Fsites%2FAPWC%2FShared%20Documents%2FCredentials%2FCredentials%20Endorsement%20Documents&p=true&ga=1

Health Education England (2022b). Advanced Practice Mental Health Curriculum and Capabilities Framework. https://healtheducationengland.sharepoint.com/sites/APWC/Shared%20Documents/Forms/AllItems.aspx?id=%2Fsites%2FAPWC%2FShared%20Documents%2FCredentials%2FCredentials%20Endorsement%20Documents%2FAdvanced%20practice%20in%20mental%20health%2-0curriculum%20and%20capabilities%20framework%2Epdf&parent=%2Fsites%2FAPWC%2FShared%20Documents%2FCredentials%2FCredentials%20Endorsement%20Documents&p=true&ga=1

Health Education England (2022c). Advanced Clinical Practice in Older People Curriculum Framework. https://healtheducationengland.sharepoint.com/sites/APWC/Shared%20Documents/Forms/AllItems.aspx?id=%2Fsites%2FAPWC%2FShared%20Documents%2FCredentials%2FCredentials%20Endorsement%20Documents%2FAdvanced%20clinical%20practice%20older%20people%20curriculum%20framework%20%20%2Epdf&parent=%2Fsites%2FAPWC%2FShared%20Documents%2FCredentials%2FCredentials%20Endorsement%20Documents&p=true&ga=1

López-Otín, C., Blasco, M., Partridge, L. et al. (2013). The hallmarks of aging. *Cell* 153 (6): 1194–1217.

Marshall, J.L., Peshkin, B.N., Yoshino, T. et al. (2022). The essentials of multiomics. *Oncologist* 27 (4): 272–284.

Michael J., W. Cliff, J. McFarland, H. Modell, A. Wright (2017) *The Core Concepts of Physiology.* New York: Springer Nature.

Mirrasekhian, E., Nilsson, J.L.Å., Shionoya, K. et al. (2018). The antipyretic effect of paracetamol occurs independent of transient receptor potential ankyrin 1-mediated hypothermia and is associated with prostaglandin inhibition in the brain. *FASEB Journal* 32 (10): 5751–5759.

Murray, S.A., Kendall, M., Mitchell, G. et al. (2017). Palliative care from diagnosis to death. *BMJ* 356: j878.

Physiological Society (2019). *Growing Older, Better*. London.: Physiological Society.

Public Health England (2017). Chapter 1: life expectancy and healthy life expectancy. www.gov.uk/government/publications/health-profile-for-england/chapter-1-life-expectancy-and-healthy-life-expectancy

Royal College of Emergency Medicine (2022). Emergency Care Advanced Clinical Practitioner Curriculum – Adult. https://rcem.ac.uk/wp-content/uploads/2022/09/ACP_Curriculum_Adult_Final_060922.pdf

Shehata, E., Parker, A., Suzuki, T. et al. (2022). Microbiomes in physiology: insights into 21st-century global medical challenges. *Experimental Physiology* 107 (4): 257–264.

Simões, V., Cizubu, B., Harley, L. et al. (2022). Redox-sensitive E2 Rad6 controls cellular response to oxidative stress via K63-linked ubiquitination of ribosomes. *Cell Reports* 39: 110860.

Taquet, M., Smith, S.M., Prohl, A.K. et al. (2021). A structural brain network of genetic vulnerability to psychiatric illness. *Molecular Psychiatry* 26: 2089–2100.

Wood, A., Chandler, C., Connolly, S. et al. (2020). Designing and developing core physiology learning outcomes for pre-registration nursing education curriculum. *Advances in Physiology Education* 44 (3): 464–474.

FURTHER READING

Alberts, B. (2019). *Essential Cell Biology*, 5e. New York: W.W. Norton.

Grumezescu, A.M. and Holban, A.M. (2018). *Diet, Microbiome and Health*. London: Elsevier.

Hawley, J.A., Hargreaves, M., Joyner, M. et al. (2014). Integrative biology of exercise. *Cell* 159 (4): 738–749.

Murray, S.A., Kendall, M., Mitchell, G. et al. (2017). Palliative care from diagnosis to death. *BMJ* 356: j878.

SELF-ASSESSMENT QUESTIONS

1. In the context of your clinical specialty, what would you consider to be the extremes of physiological changes you need to be familiar with (or encounter)?

2. Consider the relevant advanced practice frameworks to your role (see Table 4.1 for some examples). How does physiology support your clinical knowledge and skills detailed within the frameworks?

3. Within your role and area of practice:
   - How can exercise affect an individual's 'normal' physiology?
   - How do sedentary lifestyle factors, including raised body mass index (BMI)/overweight, affect an individual's 'normal' physiology?

GLOSSARY

Acidosis   Condition concerning the serum pH in which there is too much acid.

Adenosine diphosphate (ADP)   A biological molecule consisting of adenine, a sugar and two phosphate groups.

Adenosine triphosphate (ATP) ATP acts as an energy store by adding a further phosphate group to ADP. This is the main source of energy for use and storage at the cellular level.

Alkalosis Condition concerning the serum pH in which there is too much alkali.

Cell The basic unit from which a living organism is made; consisting of an aqueous solution of organic molecules enclosed by a membrane. This fundamental unit of life takes nutrients from its environment to provide energy or substrates to carry out specialised functions.

DNA (deoxyribonucleic acid) DNA is the genetic material in humans, consisting of the chemical building block called nucleotides. These are made of three parts: a phosphate group, a sugar group and one of four nitrogen bases. This forms a double helix.

Homeodynamic A dynamic balance between interrelated body systems maintaining an overall equilibrium, i.e. cardiovascular function, such as cardiac output in different activities.

Homeostasis Stable equilibrium between interdependent elements which is maintained by physiological processes.

Microbiome The combined genomes of a collection of micro-organisms such as bacteria, viruses or fungi that exist in a particular environment, i.e. gut or other body surfaces.

Microbiota Microscopic organisms of a particular environment, i.e. gut microbiota.

CHAPTER 5

Principles of Pathophysiology

Sarah Ashelford and Vanessa Taylor

Aim

The aim of this chapter is to examine the principles of pathophysiology and apply these to the top five major health conditions identified in the NHS Long Term Plan: cancer, cardiovascular disease, stroke, diabetes and respiratory disease (NHS 2019). By examining the underpinning pathophysiological principles, you will learn about several important disease mechanisms which can be applied to other conditions in your area of advanced practice. Throughout this chapter, knowledge from genomics and genetic information is included.

LEARNING OUTCOMES

After reading this chapter the reader will:

1. identify the main pathophysiological mechanisms that underpin most diseases and conditions
2. apply these pathophysiological mechanisms to the top five major conditions identified in the NHS Long Term Plan: cancer, cardiovascular disease, stroke, diabetes and respiratory disease
3. appreciate how developments in genomics enhance understanding of disease risk, prognosis and a personalised therapeutic plan
4. recognise how an understanding of disease mechanisms informs understanding of disease presentation, investigation, possible complications and the use of pharmacological treatments.

The Advanced Practitioner: A Framework for Practice, First Edition. Edited by Ian Peate, Sadie Diamond-Fox, and Barry Hill.
© 2024 John Wiley & Sons Ltd. Published 2024 by John Wiley & Sons Ltd.

Multi-Professional Framework for Advanced Clinical Practice (MPFfACP) (HEE 2017)

This chapter relates to the following areas of the MPFfACP:
1.6, 1.7, 3.1, 3.2

Accreditation Considerations

This chapter is applicable to the following specialist curricula:

- Acute Medicine (HEE 2022a)
- Critical Care (ACCP) (FICM 2015)
- Emergency Care – Adult and Child (RCEM 2022a,b)
- Learning Disability and/or Autism (HEE 2020a)
- Mental Health (HEE 2022b)
- Older People (HEE 2022c)
- Primary Care (HEE 2020b)
- Surgical Care (HEE 2020c)

This is an ever evolving field and work continues to agree various competence and capability frameworks for advanced clinical practice in other clinical specialties, therefore the reader is encouraged to refer to https://advanced-practice.hee.nhs.uk/credentials

INTRODUCTION

Pathophysiology can be defined as the study of how a disease disrupts normal biological function. With progress in molecular and cell biology, genomics and immunology, we now have considerable knowledge of how disruptions to normal function occur at the levels of the cell and molecular pathways within the cell (Kumar et al. 2017). Examining disruption of function at the cellular and molecular levels has enabled the illumination of general 'disease mechanisms' that underpin a wide range of diseases. These disease mechanisms are identified as neoplasia, inflammation, immunopathology (hypersensitivity and autoimmunity), infection and genetic (Kumar et al. 2017; Banasik and Copstead 2018).

We start this chapter by reviewing these general disease mechanisms. This focus will enable you to gain an in-depth understanding of the most fundamental mechanisms that underlie these conditions. This has applicability for understanding signs and symptoms and the rationale of many diagnostic and/ or screening tests used in clinical practice, including the use of tumour markers in cancer screening, the use of HbA1c in diagnosing and monitoring of diabetes, and the use of cardiac biomarkers for evidence of cardiac cell damage. Furthermore, knowledge of a disease or condition at the cell and molecular level is important for understanding pharmacodynamics – the study of a drug's molecular, biochemical and physiological effects or actions.

The Main Disease Mechanisms

Table 5.1 provides a summary of the main disease mechanisms identified above: neoplasia, inflammation, immunopathology, infection and genetic. In the subsequent sections of the chapter, we elaborate on these mechanisms and apply these to the top five conditions identified in the NHS Long Term Plan: cancer, cardiovascular disease, stroke, diabetes and respiratory disease (NHS 2019).

Fields of Practice – Learning Disability

Chromosomal disorders such as Down syndrome and Turner syndrome involve an alteration in chromosome number or structure. They most often arise 'out of the blue', rather than being due to an inherited mutation.

Fields of Practice – Mental Health

Schizophrenia and major depressive disorder have been classified as complex, multifactorial conditions which have a potential genetic link.

TABLE 5.1   Summary of the main disease mechanisms.

Disease Mechanism	Description	Common Examples
Neoplasia	The process by which a normal cell acquires new and unregulated growth properties, leading to the production of benign or malignant tumour. Neoplasia is a genetic disease of unregulated cell growth. A cancer is a malignant neoplasm which has the potential to invade neighbouring tissue and/or spread to a distant site in the body (metastasis). A benign tumour is one which does not have the ability to spread and metastasise. Neoplasia involves the accumulation of many genetic mutations in genes called oncogenes and tumour suppressor genes	Cancer is currently the second most common cause of death in the UK. Common cancers include breast, lung, colorectal and prostate cancer, leukaemias and lymphomas
Inflammation	Inflammation is a protective response to infection and/or injury, and part of the body's innate immune response. It involves a vascular (blood vessel) response leading to redness, swelling and heat and a cellular response involving infiltration of white blood cells into the tissues to remove the injurious agent. In its acute form, inflammation is protective, leading to removal of the injurious stimulus and the initiation of tissue repair. In its chronic form, it is a harmful disease mechanism, causing ongoing tissue damage, tissue remodelling and fibrosis	Atherosclerosis, COPD, inflammatory bowel disease, arthritis

TABLE 5.1   (Continued)

Disease Mechanism	Description	Common Examples
Immunopathology	*Hypersensitivity*: these are harmful immune reactions, often in response to innocuous chemicals from the environment (allergens). Hypersensitivity reactions involve components of the innate and adaptive immune response. There are four classes of hypersensitivity which each have a different underlying immune mechanism (Kumar et al. 2017). Type 1 hypersensitivity, for example, involves IgE antibodies binding to mast cells (covered in detail in the section on asthma)	Allergies, anaphylaxis, allergic asthma, toxic shock syndrome, organ transplant reactions
	Autoimmunity: involves breakdown in self-tolerance in which the immune system targets components of the body tissues (self-antigens) leading to cell, tissue and/or organ damage	Autoimmune thyroiditis, multiple sclerosis, rheumatoid arthritis, systemic lupus erythematosus (SLE), type 1 diabetes, myasthenia gravis
Infection	Injury results from invasion and tissue damage by a pathogenic agent. The main pathogenic agents in humans are viruses, bacteria, fungi and protists. Tissue injury arises through a complex interplay between the infecting agent and the host immune response. Pathogens, especially bacteria, may carry virulence factors, rendering them more harmful (or pathogenic)	Common infectious agents include SARS-CoV-2, influenza A and B, chlamydia, *Staphylococcus aureus*, *Escherichia coli* and *Candida albicans*
Genetic	Genetic mechanisms include alterations (mutations) in single genes, multiple genes and changes in chromosome structure and number. Complex (polygenic) disorders are the most common type of genetic disorder. With complex genetic disorders there is an interplay between many genes of small effect and environmental factors. By this definition, complex (polygenic) disorders tend to cluster in families but do not show the clear inheritance patterns of single-gene disorders.	Single-gene disorders: cystic fibrosis, sickle cell anaemia, Huntington disease. These are caused by mutation in single genes and show defined inheritance patterns
		Chromosomal disorders
	Genetics plays an important part in furthering our understanding of the basis of disease, from revealing biological pathways involved in pathogenesis to improving knowledge of the relative contributions of various genetic and environmental factors	Complex (polygenic disorders): heart disease, obesity, type 2 diabetes, hypertension, cancer
		Mental health conditions

In the next sections, we apply these principles to explain cancer, cardiovascular disease and stroke, diabetes and respiratory disease. With respiratory disease, we examine asthma and COPD.

CANCER

Cancer is a genetic disease of unregulated cell growth. There are over 200 types of cancers reflecting the diverse cell and tissue types from which cancers may originate. The different types of cancer have different aetiologies, patterns of growth and sites of metastases. Currently, in the UK, the most common cancers are breast, lung, colorectal and prostate (CRUK 2022).

Aetiology and Pathogenesis of Cancer

Cancers arise through a stepwise series of mutational events called carcinogenesis (Figure 5.1). The exact cause and sequence of mutational events will be unique for each individual cancer, but there are common risk factors for cancers (Figure 5.1).

Each primary tumour has a clonal origin, which means that the cancer originated from a single normal body cell. This cell, and its daughter cell population comprising the tumour, is subject to a series of mutational events – alterations in the genetic material – which initiate and confer a series of changes in its growth properties. Mutational events are permanent changes to the DNA and/or chromosome number

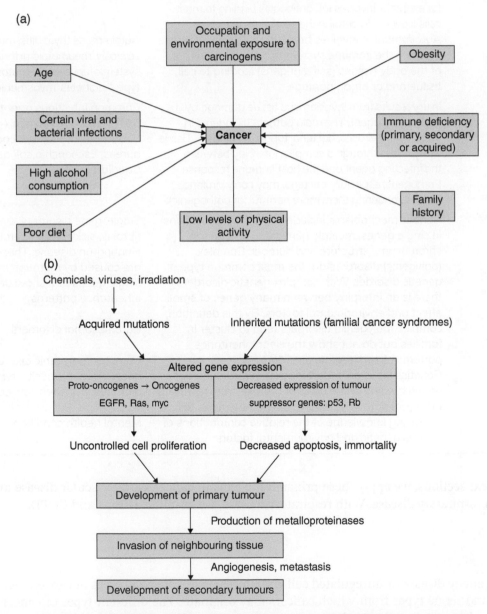

FIGURE 5.1   (a) Common risk factors for the development of cancer. (b) The process of carcinogenesis.

and/or structure, and are therefore passed on to the daughter cells during cell division (replication). As the daughter cells replicate, they acquire further mutations in their DNA and further alterations in replicative ability. With multiple rounds of replication, a mass of cells (or tumour) is produced that has acquired the properties of a cancer. These acquired capabilities include unlimited replicative ability (immortality), altered cell metabolism, the ability to evade the immune system and the ability to invade and spread to other sites (metastasis). The capabilities acquired by tumours through the sequential accumulation of mutations are known as the hallmarks of cancer (Hanahan and Weinberg 2011; Hanahan 2022), which are given in Table 5.2.

It is important to appreciate the multistep nature of carcinogenesis. Mutations arise sequentially, leading to the acquisition of the hallmarks of cancer, which is known as tumour progression. This, in part, highlights the importance of early detection and treatment of cancer.

The genes which acquire mutations in cancer fall into two main classes.

- *Proto-oncogenes*: these are growth-promoting genes. The normal function of proto-oncogenes is to promote and regulate normal cell growth and replication. Many proto-oncogenes are growth factor receptors or form key components of growth factor signal transduction pathways within the cell. Proto-oncogenes that have acquired mutations are called *oncogenes*. Gain-of-function mutations result in cells which can replicate in the absence of the normal growth factor control signals. Common examples of oncogenes include EGFR (epidermal growth factor receptor, or Her); Ras – a GTP binding protein involved in growth factor signal transduction pathways; and

TABLE 5.2 Eight hallmarks of cancer.

Hallmark	Description
1. Sustaining proliferative signalling	Normal cells depend on external growth signals for proliferation; cancer cells can generate their own growth signals
2. Evading growth suppressors	Multiple antiproliferative signals maintain homeostasis in normal tissues; cancer cells subvert the mechanisms that control cell cycle progression
3. Resisting cell death	Apoptosis, or programmed cell death, is a major mechanism in normal cells to prevent unregulated cell growth. Cancer cells develop mechanisms to evade apoptosis and continue replicating even in the presence of genetic damage
4. Enabling replicative immortality	Cancer cells acquire the ability to replicate indefinitely. This is achieved through the reactivation of the telomerase enzyme, leading to lengthening of the telomeres on the ends of chromosomes
5. Inducing or accessing vasculature	The growing tumour can trigger the formation of new vasculature (blood supply) to maintain its expansion
6. Tissue invasion and metastasis	Cancer cells acquire the ability to invade neighbouring tissue and spread throughout the body to form metastases
7. Avoiding immune destruction	Cancer cells acquire the ability to evade normal immune mechanisms which would lead to their destruction
8. Reprogramming energy metabolism	Cancer cells can switch to anaerobic respiration (the Warburg effect) (Liberti and Locasale 2016). The advantage of this for the cancer cells has not yet been resolved. One proposal is that it enables increased access to glucose and ATP production when glucose is in short supply

Source: Adapted from Hanahan and Weinberg (2011); Hanahan (2022).

VEGF (vascular endothelial growth factor) which promotes angiogenesis or the growth of a blood supply to the tumour.

- Oncogenes are important targets for recently developed targeted biological therapies, including monoclonal antibodies (MAB) such as trastuzumab (Herceptin®).
- *Tumour suppressor genes*: tumour suppressor genes normally function to form a network of checkpoints that prevent uncontrolled growth. In tumour progression, mutation and/or chromosome loss leads to loss of function of tumour suppressor genes. Common tumour suppressor genes include p53 and Rb. Other important genes involved in carcinogenesis include the DNA repair enzymes BRCA1 and BRCA2.

Clinical Investigations

Tumour markers may be used as part of diagnosis, in monitoring treatments, and assessing follow-up. They may also be used in the diagnosis, prognosis and screening of cancer.

A tumour marker is any substance, usually a protein, that can be related to the presence or absence of a tumour (Murphy et al. 2019). Tumour markers are not necessarily unique products of malignant tumours – they can also be raised in non-malignant conditions. In cancer, tumour markers may be expressed by the tumour in greater amounts than by normal cells, often in the blood, urine or body tissues. Examples include CA125 for ovarian cancer (NICE 2011), PSA for prostate cancer (NICE 2019) and AFP and hCG in tumours of possible germ cell origin, used in the diagnosis of metastatic malignant disease of unknown primary origin (NICE 2010).

The Genome UK: the future of healthcare (2020) strategy places the molecular characterisation of cancer at the forefront of targeted screening and personalised medicine for cancer.

Learning Events

1. Using the references, further reading and your own reading, explore further the use of tumour markers PSA, CA125 and CEA in the initial investigation and screening for cancer.
2. Explore the common sites of metastases for breast, lung, colorectal and prostate cancer.

Clinical Effects of Cancer

Local growth of tumours may cause obstruction of blood vessels and ducts and invade surrounding organs and tissues. However, most deaths arise from the metastatic spread of tumours (Hallmark 6), where tumours may cause widespread damage to distant glands and organs.

Paraneoplastic syndromes may cause widespread systemic effects. Paraneoplastic syndromes are caused by the tumour cell secreting hormones, or hormone-like substances, inappropriately. This is known as ectopic hormone production. Examples of paraneoplastic syndromes include syndrome of inappropriate antidiuretic hormone production (SIADH) and hypercalcaemia.

Learning Event

Choose one of the paraneoplastic syndromes to explore further. Consider which types of cancer the syndrome is most commonly associated with, and the main clinical consequences of the secretion of the hormone or hormone-like substance.

CARDIOVASCULAR DISEASE AND STROKE

In this section, we examine atherosclerosis which is the main cause of cardiovascular disease and stroke. Atherosclerosis is an example of a disease arising through a chronic inflammatory mechanism (Table 5.1). It is a progressive disease of large and medium-sized arteries, characterised by the build-up of fatty plaques, *atheromata* (singular: atheroma), within the walls of the arteries. The complications of atherosclerosis include coronary artery disease, peripheral artery disease, stroke, renal artery disease and aortic aneurysm (Lilly 2021).

Investigations

With the goal of primary and secondary prevention, risk assessment for cardiovascular disease should be carried out for all patients identified to be at risk (NICE 2023).

QRISK3 is a risk assessment tool for assessing CVD risk for primary prevention of CVD. It incorporates the risk factors for atherosclerosis and relevant co-morbidities to produce a percentage 10-year risk (Hippisley-Cox et al. 2017). Risk factors include age, gender, ethnicity, systolic blood pressure, body mass index, total cholesterol:high-density lipoprotein cholesterol ratio, smoking, family history of coronary heart disease in a first-degree relative aged less than 60 years, diabetes and hypertension.

Pathogenesis of Atherosclerosis

The development of an atheroma begins in late childhood or adolescence with the first appearance of a lesion called a fatty streak. The fatty streak comprises a collection of lipids (largely cholesterol) within the inner lining of the artery. Over many years, a fatty streak can progress to an atheromatous plaque (Figure 5.2). Plaque progression is driven by chronic inflammatory processes in the presence of widely recognised risk factors (including high levels of serum cholesterol). The initial lesion – the fatty streak – renders the wall of the artery permeable to the influx and build- up of low-density lipoprotein (LDL) particles within the intima (inner layer) of the arterial wall. Leucocytes are recruited into the vessel wall to 'scavenge' and sequester the potentially damaging LDL particles. Efflux of LDL-containing leucocytes is impaired, and these accumulate within the plaque as highly pathogenic 'foam cells'. Foam cells along with activated endothelial cells are the source of cytokines and other growth factors which set in motion the migration of smooth muscle cells from the media, or middle layer, of the vessel wall. The smooth muscle cells secrete fibrin and other molecules which lead to the formation of a protective fibrous cap underneath a core of lipid.

With disease progression, increase in size of the atheroma can lead to gradual narrowing of the lumen and arterial stenosis. The reduction in blood flow from arterial stenosis can lead to ischaemia and ischaemic injury of downstream tissues. More acutely, a complicated, unstable atheromatous plaque can rupture, leading to vessel thrombosis. Thrombosis often results in complete vessel obstruction and necrosis of the tissue. Atheromatous plaques cause weakening of the arterial wall, leading to aneurysm and potential rupture of the vessel (Figure 5.3).

In its mature or advanced stage, a fibrous plaque can be described as stable or unstable. A stable plaque has a small lipid core and a thick fibrous cap. Unstable, or vulnerable, plaques have a larger lipid core and a thin fibrous cap. An unstable plaque is more likely to rupture and cause thrombosis. The surface of a stable plaque can be subject to erosion and accumulate platelets and lead to thrombus formation. Unstable plaques tend to rupture and spill out the highly thrombogenic lipid core. The main clinical complications of atherosclerosis are detailed in Table 5.3.

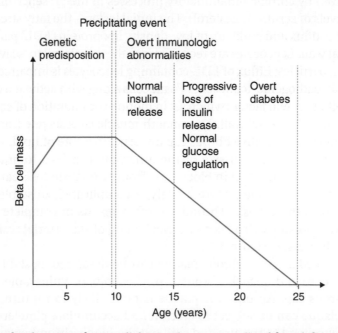

(a) Atherosclerosis progression

Normal artery → Fatty streaks → Fibrous plaque → Atherosclerotic plaque → Complicated lesions

(b)

Collagen
Cholesterol efflux
ABCA1
ABCG1
VSMC
Platelet
Thrombus
LDL
LOX-1
Monocyte
ox-LDL
IL-6
MMP
TNF-α
M1
MPO
Apoptotic macrophage
MCP-1
VCAM-1
SR-A
Cholesterol crystal
αvβ3
RBC
ICAM-1
OPN
SMC derived Foam cell
EC
Leukocyte
Monocyte
Macrophage
Foam cell
Neovascularization

FIGURE 5.2 (a,b) Pathophysiology of atherosclerosis and subsequent plaque rupture. *Source*: Zhang et al. 2022/John Wiley & Sons.

Precipitating event

Genetic predisposition

Overt immunologic abnormalities

Normal insulin release

Progressive loss of insulin release
Normal glucose regulation

Overt diabetes

Beta cell mass

5   10   15   20   25

Age (years)

FIGURE 5.3 Stages in the development of type 1 diabetes. The stages are listed from left to right: genetic predisposition, a precipitating event, overt immunological abnormalities, progressive loss of insulin release and overt diabetes. *Source*: Adapted from Eisenbarth GS, Jeffrey J (2008).

TABLE 5.3 The main clinical complications of atherosclerosis.

Complication	Description
Ischaemic heart disease: • Stable angina • Silent angina	Ischaemic heart disease is most often caused by atherosclerotic disease of the coronary arteries. Ischaemic heart disease arises when the myocardial oxygen supply is insufficient to meet myocardial oxygen demand. This results in myocardial hypoxia and the accumulation of waste metabolites (including lactate, serotonin and adenosine). Stable chronic angina usually manifests as a pattern of predictable, transient chest discomfort during exertion or emotional stress. It is generally caused by a fixed stenosis (narrowing) of a coronary artery due to an atherosclerotic plaque. Hypoxia will occur when an increased oxygen demand occurs with exertion or emotional stress but is not met because of reduced delivery due to the coronary artery stenosis. Asymptomatic episodes of myocardial ischaemia also occur that are clinically silent but can be detected by ECG or other laboratory techniques (Lilly 2021)
Acute coronary syndromes: • Unstable angina • Myocardial infarction (NSTEMI, STEMI)	Life-threating conditions forming a continuum that ranges from unstable angina to a large, acute myocardial infarction. Most acute coronary syndromes result from disruption of atherosclerotic coronary plaques with subsequent platelet aggregation and thrombus formation within the coronary artery (Lilly 2021). Unstable angina and non-ST segment elevated myocardial infarction (NSTEMI) are due to the formation of a partially occlusive thrombus. NSTEMI is distinguished from unstable angina by the presence of necrosis. A more severe ischaemia and a larger amount of necrosis manifest an ST segment elevated myocardial infarction (STEMI). This is the result of a thrombus which completely occludes the coronary artery
Aortic aneurysm	An aortic aneurysm forms at the site of atherosclerotic plaque formation. The fibrous plaque subjects the underlying media to increased pressure, which may provoke atrophy and loss of elastic tissue
Stroke: • Thrombotic • Embolic	Rupture or erosion of an atherosclerotic plaque within a carotid artery followed by thrombus formation. Thrombosis can occlude the vessel and result in cerebral infraction. With embolic stroke, fragments of the disrupted atherosclerotic plaque can embolise and block a downstream vessel
Peripheral artery disease	A term used to describe narrowing or occlusion of the peripheral arteries, affecting the blood supply to the lower limbs. This results in a reduction in blood flow to the affected limb. The narrowing or occlusion is most often due to arterial atherosclerotic disease. Peripheral artery disease affects around 13% of the Western population who are over 50 years old. Most patients are asymptomatic but many experience intermittent claudication (pain on walking). Critical limb ischaemia occurs when reduction in blood flow is so severe that it causes pain on rest or tissue loss (ulceration or gangrene) (Morley et al. 2018)
Renal artery stenosis	Narrowing of one or both renal arteries. It is the main cause of renovascular hypertension. One of the main causes of renal artery disease is renal artery stenosis following atherosclerotic renal artery disease. Hypertension results from activation of the renin–angiotensin system causing increased systemic vascular resistance and sodium retention (Dobrek 2021)

Pharmacological Principles

One of the key pharmacological treatments for primary prevention of cardiovascular disease is lipid-lowing therapy. This can help to reduce cardiovascular clinical events in patients with coronary artery disease, and in those at risk of developing CVD.

Statins are hydroxymethylglutaryl-CoA (HMG-CoA) inhibitors. HMG-CoA is an enzyme that catalyses the rate-limiting step in cholesterol synthesis in the liver. Statins are widely used to reduce blood cholesterol level.

Investigations

Cardiac-specific biomarkers can be used in the investigation of myocardial necrosis.

Troponin T and I are regulatory proteins, specific to cardiac myocytes that are involved with interactions between actin and myosin contractile proteins (Lilly 2021). Serum levels of troponin T and I rise within hours of onset of symptoms of myocardial infarction and remain elevated for 1–2 weeks. Between two and six hours, there is a steep increase in cardiac troponin representing myocardial necrosis, allowing for accurate detection of myocardial injury (McDonaugh and Whyte 2020).

Examination Scenario
A 76-year-old patient who identifies as male presents with central chest pain and shortness of breath. There are three classic components in the evaluation of the MI. 1. Clinical features 2. ECG findings 3. Cardiac biomarkers List the common features of each of the above.

DIABETES

Diabetes mellitus is a group of metabolic conditions that share the common underlying feature of hyperglycaemia (Kumar et al. 2017). In this section, we describe the aetiology and pathogenesis of type 1 diabetes to illustrate the development of an autoimmune disease, a type of immunopathology (Table 5.1).

Clinical Presentation

Polyuria (excessive or abnormally large production or passage of urine), polydipsia (excessive thirst or excess drinking) and polyphagia (excessive eating or appetite) are the classic triad of diabetes, and frequently occur in the initial presentation of those with type 1 diabetes. Initial presentation in those with type 1 diabetes can have progressed to metabolic ketoacidosis (as in the case study below). The acute biochemical disturbances that occur are a consequence of a deficiency of insulin and contribute to the presenting signs and symptoms of diabetes shown in Figure 5.5. These will be discussed further under 'Acute complications'.

The onset of type 2 diabetes is more insidious, and can include unexplained tiredness, repeated infections and slow wound healing. It is often picked up on routine blood tests in asymptomatic people. With type 2 diabetes, patients may remain asymptomatic for several years, by which time many of the vascular complications may already be present at the time of diagnosis. The classic triad of polyuria, polydipsia and polyphagia is less common in type 2 diabetes but can occur if the degree of hyperglycaemia is severe.

Case Study

An 11-year-old boy is brought to the emergency department experiencing worsening nausea, vomiting, abdominal pain and lethargy. Over the past week, he reported feeling increasingly thirsty and passing copious amounts of urine. Physical examination reveals a thin, dehydrated boy with deep rapid breathing and tachycardia, with confused verbal response. He has an acute abdomen, and an initial blood gas analysis reveals the following.

pH 7.24
HCO_3 14 (mmol/l)
PCO_3 (3.6 kPa)
Na 130 (mmol/l)
K 5.0 (mmol/l)
Lactate 1.9 (mmol/l)

After reading the section on diabetes, return to this case study and explain this presentation using your understanding of the pathophysiology.

Learning Event

Using the further reading at the end of this chapter, review your understanding of the role of insulin in metabolism. Consider the role of insulin in carbohydrate, lipid and protein metabolism.

Aetiology and Pathogenesis of Type 1 Diabetes

Type 1 diabetes is characterised by absolute insulin deficiency resulting from autoimmune destruction of the insulin-secreting beta cells of the pancreatic islets.

Autoimmunity occurs when the immune system targets the body's own tissues or organs (self-antigens). Autoimmunity represents the failure of 'self-tolerance'. Self-tolerance is a property of the adaptive immune system and ensures that the components of the adaptive immune response (namely, the T- and B-lymphocyte response, and the antibodies produced by B lymphocytes) do not target the body's own antigens. The immune system produces both T and B lymphocytes that may recognise and respond to the body's own antigens. Self-tolerance mechanisms ensure that these self-reactive T and B lymphocytes are 'deleted' or 'suppressed'. *Deletion* refers to the destruction of self-reactive T or B lymphocytes probably in childhood when the immune system is developing. *Suppression* is a means of inhibiting self-reactive B and T lymphocytes and is carried out by a subset of T lymphocytes called regulatory T cells (T_{REG}).

A breakdown in self-tolerance occurs in autoimmune diseases. Self-reactive T lymphocytes begin to attack the body's tissues, and self-reactive B cells produce autoantibodies which can bind to self-antigens and trigger immune damage. The damage usually arises through an inflammatory response within the tissues targeted by the auto-reactive T lymphocytes and autoantibodies. The mechanisms by which self-tolerance is first induced to fail require both genetic and environmental factors. An important genetic risk factor is associated with individual human leucocyte antigen (HLA) genes, especially those of class II (Jose et al. 2014). The most significant environmental association is infection. Many autoimmune diseases arise following infection, although it has been difficult to conclusively demonstrate the role of a specific pathogen in triggering autoimmune disease.

In type 1 diabetes, autoimmune destruction of the beta cells of the pancreas is driven by a breakdown in T cell self-tolerance, with involvement of both CD4+ T helper and CD8+ cytotoxic T cells in beta cell destruction. Autoantibodies against a variety of B-cell antigens are also produced and may contribute to islet damage. The most commonly found autoantibody is against glutamic acid decarboxylase. After around 80–90% of the beta cells have been destroyed, hyperglycaemia develops and diabetes becomes apparent (Eisenbarth and Jeffrey 2008).

The most important genetic association (risk factor) in type 1 diabetes is with specific variants of the class II major histocompatibility complex (MHC) HLA locus DR and DQ. Environmental factors associated with type 1 diabetes include diet, vitamin D exposure, obesity and viral infection. The strongest association with the onset of type 1 diabetes is the human enterovirsuses (Hyöty 2016). Although the clinical onset of type 1 diabetes is usually abrupt, the immunological abnormalities comprising the auto-immune attack of the beta cells can be detected many years before the onset of diabetes.

Latent autoimmune diabetes in adults (LADA) is becoming increasingly recognised in clinical practice. LADA is a form of autoimmune diabetes defined by adult onset and the presence of diabetes-associated autoantibodies. LADA patients are often misdiagnosed as having type 2 diabetes; 4–14% of those with type 2 diabetes have autoimmune antibodies such as glutamic acid decarboxylase 65 autoantibodies. LADA patients tend to have a lower mean age at diabetes onset, lower body mass index and more frequent need for insulin treatment than patients with type 2 diabetes. The uncertainty is whether the underlying pathophysiology is distinct from childhood-onset type 1 diabetes or is part of a clinical spectrum encompassing all forms of autoimmune diabetes (Davies 2021).

Aetiology and Pathogenesis of Type 2 Diabetes

Type 2 diabetes results from the combination of insulin resistance and beta cell failure. This causes a relative insulin deficiency and the onset of hyperglycaemia and diabetes. Most people (80%) with type 2 diabetes are obese and there is a close link between central obesity and insulin resistance. Insulin resistance results from alterations in insulin signalling pathways and leads to reduced uptake of glucose by the liver and muscle tissue, and a decreased response in adipose tissue to insulin (Banday et al. 2020). Excess peripheral adipose tissue promotes insulin resistance through various inflammatory mechanisms, including increased free fatty acid (FFA) release and adipokine dysregulation (Galicia-Garcia et al. 2020).

In response to insulin resistance, there is an initial compensatory increase in insulin secretion. Beta cell function begins to decline and as a result, normoglycaemia can no longer be maintained (Figure 5.4).

Fields of Practice – Paediatrics

The onset of type 2 diabetes is usually in adulthood but there is an increasing incidence in childhood and adolescence.

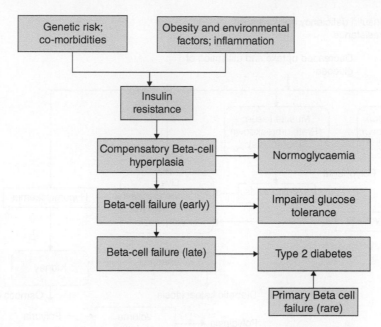

FIGURE 5.4 The pathogenesis of type 2 diabetes. *Source*: Adapted from Kumar et al. (2017).

Acute Complications of Diabetes

The acute complications of diabetes are diabetic ketoacidosis (DKA), hyperosmolar hyperglycaemic state (HHS) and hypoglycaemia (Kumar et al. 2017). The biochemical disturbances resulting from a deficiency of insulin are shown in Figure 5.5.

Insulin deficiency leads to decreased utilisation of glucose by the tissues and hyperglycaemia. Adipose tissue and skeletal muscle tissue are 'insulin dependent' which means they require insulin for glucose uptake and utilisation. In addition, glucose uptake by the liver is stimulated by insulin. In the absence of insulin, adipose tissue begins to break down (lipolysis) and free fatty acids are released into the bloodstream. Muscle tissue breaks down (proteolysis), releasing amino acids into the blood. In the absence of insulin, the liver utilises the amino acids and free fatty acids to make short-term fuels, namely glucose and ketone bodies (acetoacetate, beta-hydroxybutyric acid). Excess glucose in the blood spills over into the kidney tubules, leading to osmotic diuresis, which causes polyuria and volume depletion. Polyuria and volume depletion lead to dehydration and thirst. The cause of polyphagia in diabetes is less well understood but may result from the decreased use of carbohydrate by the cells and/or the presence of fat and protein breakdown. These are postulated to signal a 'negative energy balance' and hunger (Kumar et al. 2017).

The continued absence of insulin can progress rapidly to DKA which is a severe and life-threatening acute metabolic complication of type 1 diabetes. DKA is a form of metabolic acidosis caused by the build-up of acidic ketone bodies in the blood. Clinical manifestations include fatigue, nausea and vomiting, severe abdominal pain and laboured Kussmaul breathing. DKA is less frequent in type 2 diabetes due to the residual insulin secretion which inhibits ketone formation.

The long-term complications of diabetes are due to macrovascular and microvascular disease (Ohiagu et al. 2021). Microvascular diseases include diabetic retinopathy, nephropathy and neuropathy. Long-term hyperglycaemia is a major factor, although insulin resistance and dyslipidaemia contribute. Glycosylation of proteins in tissue and plasma, the production of sorbitol and free radical damage are also implicated. Macrovascular disease is an accelerated atherosclerosis and can lead to myocardial infarction, stroke and peripheral artery disease (see section above on cardiovascular disease and stroke).

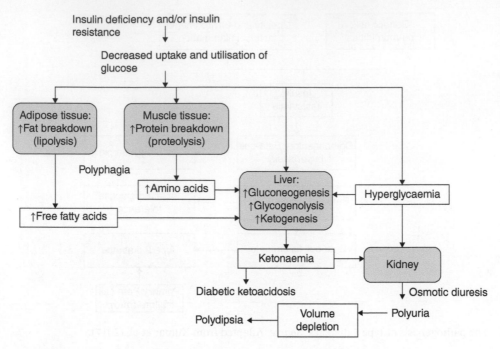

FIGURE 5.5   Summary of the metabolic disturbances resulting from a deficiency of insulin.

INVESTIGATIONS

Diabetes can be diagnosed using either venous plasma glucose or glycated haemoglobin (HbA1c). HbA1c reflects the average blood glucose levels over a 2–3-month period, reflecting the half-life of haemoglobin. HbA1c concentration is expressed in mmol/mol of glycated haemoglobin or as a percentage of glycated haemoglobin. An HbA1c of 48 mmol/mol (6.5%) or greater is diagnostic of diabetes according to the World Health Organization.

HbA1c is also used to monitor the level of glycaemic control in diabetes.

HbA1c test is not suitable for patients with inherited structurally variant haemoglobin as is present in haemoglobinopathies.

ORANGE FLAGS: PSYCHOLOGICAL CONSIDERATIONS AND FIELDS OF PRACTICE – MENTAL HEALTH

- Psychological problems are common in people with diabetes, but most can be overcome with support and education.
- Diabetes is more common in those with chronic mental illness.
- Problems range from those of adjustment to more serious depressive illness and maladaptive coping behaviours.
- Screening for depression using validated assessment tools should be part of routine surveillance.
- Psychological health is key to successful self-management.
- Family cohesion and agreement about management responsibilities improve metabolic control.

RESPIRATORY DISEASE

In this section, we focus on the pathophysiology of asthma and COPD which are two of the most common respiratory conditions in the UK. Both asthma and COPD arise through chronic inflammatory mechanisms (Table 5.1). We examine allergic (or atopic asthma) which is an example of a hypersensitivity reaction ('Immunopathology' in Table 5.1).

Asthma

Asthma is a chronic inflammatory condition affecting the airways. Typical symptoms include breathlessness, tightness in the chest, coughing and wheezing. Asthma is a heterogeneous collection of diseases with the common underlying characteristics detailed in Figure 5.6.

Aetiology and Pathogenesis of Asthma

Various classification systems have been proposed for asthma. These have been based on clinical presentation (asthma phenotypes) and underlying aetiological mechanism (so-called asthma endotypes) (Kuruvilla et al. 2019). In this section we focus on atopic asthma. Atopy is defined as a genetic predisposition to develop allergy. Allergies are a form of hypersensitivity reaction, where 'hypersensitivity' refers to an exaggerated or inappropriate immunological response occurring in response to an antigen or allergen (Table 5.1).

Atopy is caused by a type 1 hypersensitivity reaction (Justiz Vaillant et al. 2022). Type 1 hypersensitivity is also known as an immediate reaction and involves IgE-mediated release of antibodies against the soluble antigen. This results in mast cell degranulation and release of histamine and other inflammatory mediators. The same mechanism is responsible for a range of allergic reactions including asthma, allergic rhinitis (or hay fever), allergic conjunctivitis, atopic dermatitis (a type of eczema) and anaphylaxis. Type 1 hypersensitivity is driven by a subset of T helper lymphocytes known as TH2 cells. In response to allergen, TH2 cells secrete a specific subset of cytokines (IL-4, IL-5 and IL-13). These cytokines induce B lymphocytes to produce IgE antibody which coats the mast cells and 'primes' them for release of inflammatory mediators following subsequent exposure to allergen.

Atopic asthma usually begins in childhood, and there may be a family history of related allergic conditions including eczema, allergic rhinitis and urticaria. The disease is triggered by environmental allergens, such as house dust, pollen and cat hair. In the airways, there is a sensitisation to the inhaled allergen. This stimulates the TH2 cell response and leads to the production of IgE antibodies. IgE antibody binds to mast cells within the mucosa of the airways, priming them for an immediate response to subsequent allergen inhalation.

Subsequent exposure to the inhaled allergen elicits an immediate response and a late-phase reaction. In the *immediate response*, the allergen cross-links the IgE-coated mast cells and triggers them to release a cocktail of inflammatory mediators including histamine and leukotrienes. This causes airway swelling and oedema (inflammation) with increased mucus secretion. Bronchospasm is provoked through direct stimulation of the smooth muscle cells by the allergen, and by local stimulation of vagal (parasympathetic) receptors present on smooth muscle of the airways, causing bronchoconstriction. The resultant airway swelling from oedema, bronchoconstriction and increased mucus secretion leads to wheezing, cough, chest tightness and breathlessness characteristic of an asthma exacerbation. The *late-phase reaction*, which occurs 8–12 hours later, is characterised by infiltration of eosinophils into

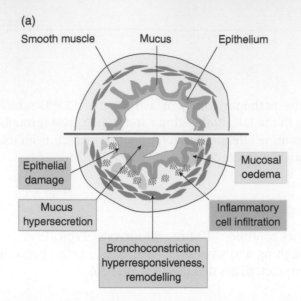

(a)

Smooth muscle   Mucus   Epithelium

Epithelial
damage

Mucosal
oedema

Mucus
hypersecretion

Inflammatory
cell infiltration

Bronchoconstriction
hyperresponsiveness,
remodelling

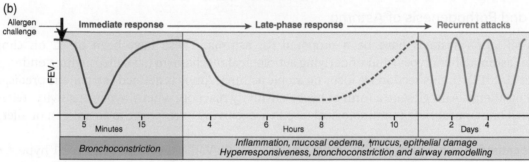

(b)

Allergen
challenge

Immediate response   Late-phase response   Recurrent attacks

FEV_1

5   15
Minutes

4   6   8   10
Hours

2   4
Days

Bronchoconstriction   *Inflammation, mucosal oedema, ↑mucus, epithelial damage*
Hyperresponsiveness, bronchoconstriction and airway remodelling

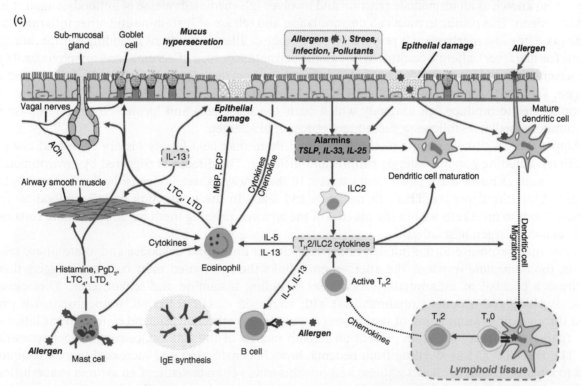

(c)

Sub-mucosal
gland   Goblet
cell   *Mucus*
hypersecretion   *Allergens ( ), Strees,*
Infection, Pollutants   *Epithelial damage*   *Allergen*

Vagal nerves   *Epithelial*
damage   Mature
dendritic cell

ACh   IL-13   **Alarmins**
TSLP, IL-33, IL-25   Dendritic cell maturation

Airway smooth muscle LTC_4, LTD_4 MBP, ECP   Cytokines Chemokine   ILC2

Cytokines   IL-5
IL-13 T_H2/ILC2 cytokines

Histamine, PgD_2,
LTC_4, LTD_4 Eosinophil   IL-4, IL-13   Active T_H2

Allergen   IgE synthesis   B cell   *Allergen*   Chemokines T_H2 T_H0

Mast cell   *Lymphoid tissue*

FIGURE 5.6 (a) Changes occurring in the airways during an asthma exacerbation. (b) Typical response of an atopic asthmatic to an inhaled antigen. (c) Cellular mechanisms of an atopic asthmatic in response to an inhaled antigen. *Source*: Ward J.P.T. et al. The Respiratory System at a Glance. John Wiley & Sons, 2015.

the airways. The eosinophils can amplify and sustain the inflammatory response through their release of mediators, especially leukotrienes. Over the long term, eosinophils have been implicated in tissue damage through oxidative stress. This is believed to play a role in harmful airway remodelling (Kumar et al. 2017).

The treatment and management of asthma include patient and family education. Various pharmacological treatments are used. One of the goals of the NHS Long Term Plan on asthma is to improve the use of medication and the correct use of inhalers (NHS 2019).

Pharmacological Principles

The following drugs are used in the management of asthma.

- Beta-2 agonists
- Corticosteroids
- Leukotriene receptor agonists
- Xanthines
- Corticosteroids

Learning event

Using the information from this chapter, the further reading and your own research into the literature, explain the action of the drugs used in asthma. What are the principles of asthma management? Link the action of the drugs to the pathophysiology of asthma to explain their mechanism of action.

Chronic Obstructive Pulmonary Disease

Chronic obstructive pulmonary disease (COPD) is a diffuse inflammatory disease of the lung tissue and airways. It is characterised by airflow obstruction that is not fully reversible. The term COPD includes two main conditions: chronic (long-term) bronchitis or inflammation of the bronchi, and emphysema in which there is destruction in the air sacs (or alveoli). Most patients have a mixture of the two conditions.

Aetiology and Pathogenesis of COPD

Smoking is the main risk factor for COPD, although other environmental pollutants can also cause it. COPD is often described as a combination of chronic bronchitis and emphysema (Figure 5.7). Chronic bronchitis is a clinical concept referring to inflammation of the airways and the presence of a productive cough over two or more years. Emphysema results from the breakdown of the walls of the alveoli. There is a rare genetic form of emphysema, in which patients inherit a deficiency in the antiprotease alpha-1-antitrypsin. The role of antitrypsin is described below.

Inflammation in the lungs, particularly the small airways, is part of the normal immune response to smoking. However, in COPD, the response to inhaled smoke or other toxins is magnified and causes damage to the lung tissue. Inflammation of the bronchial tubes can result and is characterised by a productive cough. The cough results from increased mucus secretion from goblet cells lining the airways and hypertrophy of the mucus glands within the wall of the airway. Airway inflammation results in swelling and oedema and contributes to airway obstruction.

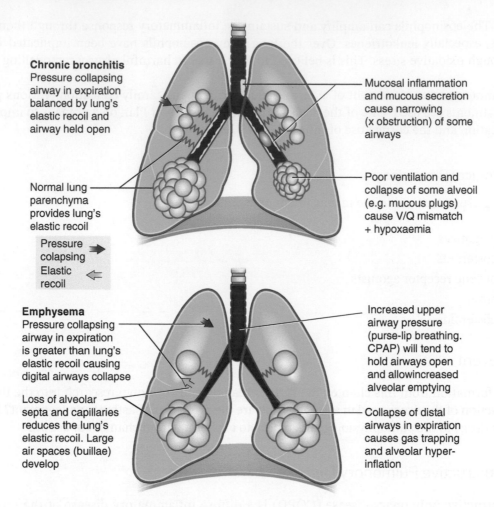

Chronic bronchitis
Pressure collapsing airway in expiration balanced by lung's elastic recoil and airway held open

Normal lung parenchyma provides lung's elastic recoil

Pressure colapsing →
Elastic recoil ⇐

Mucosal inflammation and mucous secretion cause narrowing (x obstruction) of some airways

Poor ventilation and collapse of some alveoil (e.g. mucous plugs) cause V/Q mismatch + hypoxaemia

Emphysema
Pressure collapsing airway in expiration is greater than lung's elastic recoil causing digital airways collapse

Loss of alveolar septa and capillaries reduces the lung's elastic recoil. Large air spaces (buillae) develop

Increased upper airway pressure (purse-lip breathing. CPAP) will tend to hold airways open and allowincreased alveolar emptying

Collapse of distal airways in expiration causes gas trapping and alveolar hyper-inflation

FIGURE 5.7   Pathophysiology of chronic bronchitis and emphysema. *Source*: Ward J.P.T. et al. The Respiratory System at a Glance. John Wiley & Sons, 2015.

Emphysema is characterised by enlargement of the airspaces beyond the terminal bronchioles due to destruction of the alveolar walls. This leads to the development of air spaces (or bullae) in the lungs. This reduces both ventilation and perfusion of the affected area which can cause poor oxygenation of the blood and retention of carbon dioxide. In addition, the loss of elastic tissue within the alveolar walls reduces the elastic recoil of the lungs during exhalation. This makes it more difficult to exhale and can lead to closure of the small airways.

Current theory proposes that harmful chemical imbalances develop in the lungs of those with COPD: a protease/antiprotease imbalance and an oxidant/antioxidant imbalance. These lead to the eventual tissue destruction characteristic of emphysema. Cigarette smoke and other environmental irritants activate the epithelial cells lining the airways and macrophages in the lungs to release chemotactic factors. These factors attract CD8+ lymphocytes and neutrophils from the circulation. Neutrophils and macrophages produce proteases, which are enzymes that break down proteins, particularly the elastic and collagen fibres of lung tissue. In normal lungs, there is a significant presence of antiprotease enzymes, especially alpha-1-antitrypsin. The antiproteases normally act to balance the proteases and limit their destructive effects. In emphysema, the balance is tipped in favour of the proteases, partly because of the infiltration of neutrophils.

Airway obstruction and collapse can lead to arterial hypoxaemia (low arterial blood oxygen levels) in advanced disease, largely through ventilation–perfusion mismatches. Hypoxaemia can present with or without hypercapnia (increased levels of carbon dioxide in the blood). Some patients maintain blood oxygen levels by increasing their respiratory effort. Other patients fail to maintain respiratory effort and develop hypercapnia. This raised carbon dioxide (and associated respiratory acidosis) normally stimulates breathing rate. However, over time, patients with hypercapnia develop insensitivity to raised carbon dioxide levels in the blood.

In advanced COPD, patients may develop pulmonary hypertension (Figure 5.8). Blood vessels supplying parts of the lung which remain unventilated automatically constrict. This causes increased resistance to blood flow and raises the pulmonary blood pressure. Pulmonary hypertension (PH) can eventually lead to enlargement of the right ventricle (*cor pulmonale*) due to the increased work needed to pump blood through the pulmonary system. This results in weakness of the right ventricle and right ventricular failure.

Patients may experience exacerbations in COPD in which symptoms worsen or flare up. Eventually, increased airway inflammation and reduced gas exchange can lead to severe respiratory failure and death.

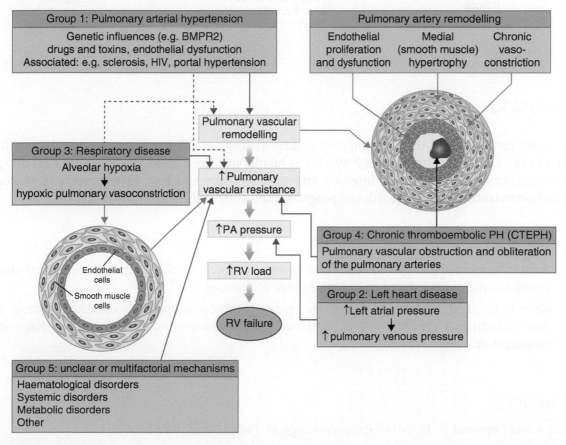

FIGURE 5.8 Pathophysiology of pulmonary hypertension. *Source*: Ward J.P.T. et al. The Respiratory System at a Glance. John Wiley & Sons, 2015.

GREEN FLAGS – SOCIAL CONSIDERATIONS

Treatment plans in both COPD and PH should encompass the multifactorial impact that the disease can have upon patients, including psychological and social considerations.

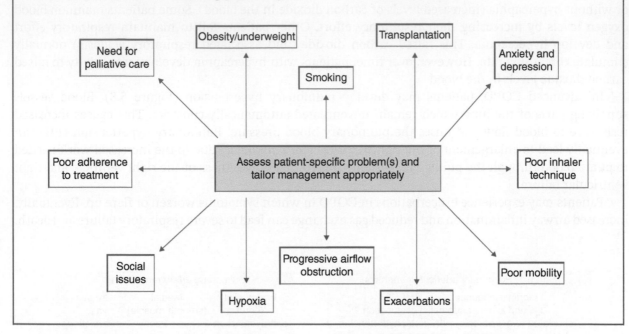

CONCLUSION

This chapter has examined the underpinning pathophysiology of the top five major health conditions outlined in the NHS Long Term Plan (2019). It has highlighted the disease mechanisms of carcinogenesis, atherosclerosis, inflammation, infection and autoimmunity and how developments in genomics enhance understanding of disease risk and prognosis, and personalised therapeutic options.

Take Home Points
- A small number of pathophysiological mechanisms (infection, inflammation, immunopathology, neoplasia and genetics) underpin a wide range of diseases.
- Knowledge and understanding of the basic pathophysiological mechanisms enable an understanding of the disease and its clinical manifestations, but also the related diagnostic investigations and treatment.

REFERENCES

Banasik, J. and Copstead, L.-E. (2018). *Pathophysiology*, 6e. Philadelphia: Elsevier.

Banday, M.Z., Sameer, A.S., and Nissar, S. (2020). Pathophysiology of diabetes: an overview. *Avicenna Journal of Medicine* 10 (4): 174–188.

CRUK (2022). Cancer statistics for the UK. www.cancerresearchuk.org/health-professional/cancer-statistics-for-the-uk#heading-Zero

Davies, S. (2021). Latent autoimmune diabetes in adults (LADA): what do primary care professionals need to know? Journal of diabetes. *Nursing* 25: JDN191.

Dobrek, L. (2021). An outline of renal artery stenosis pathophysiology – a narrative review. *Life* 11 (3): 208.

Eisenbarth, G.S. and Jeffrey, J. (2008). (2008) The natural history of type 1A diabetes. *Arquivos Brasileiros de Endocrinologia e Metabologia* 52 (2): 146–155.

Faculty of Intensive Care Medicine (2015). Critical Care Curriculum. www.ficm.ac.uk/careersworkforceaccps/accp-curriculum

Galicia-Garcia, U., Benito-Vicente, A., Jebari, S. et al. (2020). Pathophysiology of type 2 diabetes mellitus. *International Journal of Molecular Sciences* 21 (17): 6275.

Genome UK (2020). The future of healthcare. www.gov.uk/government/publications/genome-uk-the-future-of-healthcare

Hanahan, D. (2022). Hallmarks of cancer: new dimensions. *Cancer Discovery* 12 (1): 31–46.

Hanahan, D. and Weinberg, R.A. (2011). Hallmarks of cancer: the next generation. *Cell* 144 (5): 646–674.

Health Education England (2017). Multi-professional framework for advanced clinical practice in England. www.hee.nhs.uk/sites/default/files/docuemtns/HEE%20ACP%Framework.pdf

Health Education England (2020a). Advanced practice credential specification in autism. https://healtheducationengland.sharepoint.com/Comms/Digital/Shared%20Documents/Forms/AllItems.aspx?id=%2FComms%2FDigital%2FShared%20Documents%2Fhee%2Enhs%2Euk%20documents%2FWebsite%20files%2FAdvanced%20Practice%20website%2FCredentials%2FFinal%20Credentials%20Documents%2FAdvanced%20practice%20credential%20specification%20in%20autism%2Epdf&parent=%2FComms%2FDigital%2FShared%20Documents-%2Fhee%2Enhs%2Euk%20documents%2FWebsite%20files%2FAdvanced%20Practice%20website%2FCredentials%2FFinal%20Credentials%20Documents&p=true&ga=1

Health Education England (2020b). Core Capabilities Framework for Advanced Clinical Practice (Nurses) Working in General Practice/Primary Care in England. https://www.hee.nhs.uk/sites/default/files/documents/ACP%20Primary%20Care%20Nurse%20Fwk%202020.pdf

Health Education England (2020c). Surgical Advanced Practitioner Curriculum and Assessment Framework. https://advanced-practice.hee.nhs.uk/surgical-advanced-practitioner-curriculum-and-assessment-framework/

Health Education England (2022a). Advanced Clinical Practice in Acute Medicine Curriculum. https://healtheducationengland.sharepoint.com/sites/APWC/Shared%20Documents/Forms/AllItems.aspx?id=%2Fsites%2FAPWC%2FShared%20Documents%2FCredentials%2FCredentials%20Endorsement%20Documents%2FAdvanced%20clinical%20practice%20in%20acute%20medicine%20curriculum%20framework%2Epdf&parent=%2Fsites%2FAPWC%2FShared%20Documents%2FCredentials%2FCredentials%20Endorsement%20Documents&p=true&ga=1

Health Education England (2022b). Advanced Practice in Mental Health Curriculum and Capabilities Framework. https://healtheducationengland.sharepoint.com/sites/APWC/Shared%20Documents/Forms/AllItems.aspx?id=%2Fsites%2FAPWC%2FShared%20Documents%2FCredentials%2FCredentials%20Endorsement%20Documents%2FAdvanced%20practice%20in%20mental%20health%20curriculum%20and%20capabilities%20framework%2Epdf&parent=%2Fsites%2FAPWC%2FShared%20Documents%2FCredentials%2FCredentials%20Endorsement%20Documents&p=true&ga=1

Health Education England (2022c). Advanced Clinical Practice in Older People Curriculum Framework. `https://healtheducationengland.sharepoint.com/sites/APWC/Shared%20Documents/Forms/AllItems.aspx?id=%2Fsites%2FAPWC%2FShared%20Documents%2FCredentials%2FCredentials%20Endorsement%20Documents%2FAdvanced%20clinical%20practice%20older%20people%20curriculum%20framework%20%20%2Epdf&parent=%2Fsites%2FAPWC%2FShared%20Documents%2FCredentials%2FCredentials%20Endorsement%20Documents&p=true&ga=1`

Hippisley-Cox, J., Coupland, C., and Brindle, P. (2017). Development and validation of QRISK3 risk prediction algorithms to estimate future risk of cardiovascular disease: prospective cohort study. *BMJ* 357: j2099.

Hyöty, H. (2016). Viruses in type 1 diabetes. *Pediatric Diabetes* 17 (Suppl 22): 56–64.

Jose, J., Naidu, R.M., Sunil, P.M., and Varghese, S.S. (2014). Pathogenesis of autoimmune diseases: a short review. *Journal of Oral and Maxillofacial Pathology* 5 (1): 434–436.

Justiz Vaillant, A.A., Vashisht, R., and Zito, P.M. (2022). *Immediate Hypersensitivity Reactions*. Treasure Island, FL: StatPearls.

Kumar, V., Abbas, A., and Aster, J. (ed.) (2017). *Robbins Basic Pathology*, 10e. Philadelphia, PA: Saunders Elsevier.

Kuruvilla, M.E., Lee, F.E., and Lee, G.B. (2019). Understanding asthma phenotypes, endotypes, and mechanisms of disease. *Clinical Reviews in Allergy and Immunology* 56 (2): 219–233.

Liberti, M.V. and Locasale, J.W. (2016). The Warburg effect: how does it benefit cancer cells? *Trends in Biochemical Sciences* 41 (3): 211–218.

Lilly, L. (ed.) (2021). *Pathophysiology of Heart Disease: An Introduction to Cardiovascular Medicine*, 7e. Philadelphia, PA: Wolters Kluwer.

McDonaugh, B. and Whyte, M. (2020). The evolution and future direction of the cardiac biomarker. *EMJ Cardiology* 8 (1): 97–106.

Morley, R.L., Sharma, A., Horsch, A.D., and Hinchliffe, R.J. (2018). Peripheral artery disease. *BMJ* 360: j5842.

Murphy, M., Srivastava, R., and Deans, K. (2019). *Clinical Biochemistry: An Illustrated Colour Text*, 6e. Edinburgh: Elsevier.

NHS (2019). The NHS Long Term Plan. `www.longtermplan.nhs.uk`

NICE (2010). Metastatic malignant disease of unknown primary origin in adults: diagnosis and management. CG104. `www.nice.org.uk/guidance/cg104`

NICE (2011). Ovarian cancer: recognition and initial management. CG122. `www.nice.org.uk/guidance/cg122`

NICE (2023). Cardiovascular disease: risk assessment and reduction, including lipid modification. CG181. `www.nice.org.uk/guidance/cg181`

NICE (2019). Prostate cancer: diagnosis and management. NG131. `www.nice.org.uk/guidance/ng131`

Ohiagu, F., Chikezie, P., and Chikezie, C. (2021). Pathophysiology of diabetes mellitus complications: metabolic events and control. *Biomedical Research and Therapy* 8 (3): 4243–4257.

Royal College of Emergency Medicine (2022a). Emergency Care – Adult. `https://rcem.ac.uk/wp-content/uploads/2022/09/ACP_Curriculum_Adult_Final_060922.pdf`

Royal College of Emergency Medicine (2022b). Emergency Care – Child. `https://rcem.ac.uk/wp-content/uploads/2022/09/ACP_Curriculum_Children_Final_060922.pdf`

FURTHER READING

Kumar, V., Abbas, A., and Aster, J. (ed.) (2017). *Robbins Basic Pathology*, 10e. PA: Saunders Elsevier. Philadelphia.

SELF-ASSESSMENT QUESTIONS

1. List the main hallmarks of cancer. How does the genetic basis of cancer help understanding of diagnosis and treatment?
2. Describe the development of an advanced atheromatous plaque and how atherosclerosis can result in clinical complications.
3. Compare and contrast the pathophysiology of type 1 and type 2 diabetes.
4. Compare and contrast the pathophysiology of asthma and COPD.

GLOSSARY

Aetiology   The cause, set of causes or manner of causation of a disease or condition.

Allergen   A substance that causes an allergic reaction.

Antigen   A substance, usually a protein, that stimulates the production of antibodies.

Arterial stenosis   Abnormal narrowing of an artery leading to reduced blood flow.

Autoantibody   An antibody produced by the immune system and targeted against one of the body's own antigens.

CD4+ T helper cell   A type of T lymphocyte expressing a surface protein called CD4. CD4+ T helper cells help activate B cells to secrete antibodies and macrophages to destroy ingested microbes, but they also help activate cytotoxic T cells to kill infected target cells.

CD8+ cytotoxic T cell   A type of T lymphocyte expressing a surface protein called CD8. CD8+ cytotoxic T cells kill cells infected with a virus, and can kill foreign cells and cancer cells.

Endothelial cells   Endothelial cells form a single cell layer that lines all blood vessels and regulates exchanges between the bloodstream and the surrounding tissues.

Leucocyte   A type of blood cell made in the bone marrow and found in the blood and lymph tissue. Leucocytes are part of the body's immune system.

Low-density lipoprotein (LDL)   Lipoproteins are complex particles that have a central hydrophobic core of non-polar lipids, primarily cholesterol esters and triglycerides. LDL particles are the main carriers of cholesterol in the human bloodstream. Clinically, an abnormally elevated level of LDL in human blood has been confirmed to be a main independent risk factor for the process of atherosclerosis.

Major histocompatibility complex (MHC)   The MHC is a group of genes that code for proteins found on the surfaces of cells that help the immune system recognise foreign substances. MHC proteins are found in all higher vertebrates. In humans, the complex is also called the human leucocyte antigen (HLA) system.

Necrosis   Necrosis is death of a cell or tissue. It is a pathological process arising following irreversible injury.

Pathogenesis   The processes and mechanisms of disease development.

Thrombus   An abnormal blood clot within a blood vessel.

CHAPTER 6

Principles of Pharmacology

Ihab Ali and Phil Broadhurst

Aim

The aim of this chapter is to help the learner understand the pharmacokinetics and pharmacodynamics of drugs.

LEARNING OUTCOMES

After reading this chapter the reader will:

1. understand the basics of pharmacokinetics and pharmacodynamics
2. have an awareness of the importance of protein binding and volume of distribution
3. be able to consider pharmacological interventions across different fields of practice
4. understand about monitoring requirements for drugs, including being aware of adverse drug reactions, interactions and trough levels.

INTRODUCTION

Pharmacology is the study of the complex processes that occur between living organisms and chemical substances that alter the way that they function through enhancing or inhibiting pathophysiological processes (Atkinson 2022; Brenner and Stevens 2017). Within healthcare, this is used to achieve positive outcomes to optimise patients' health, although an understanding of how and why the processes occur is critical to help the AP to improve clinical outcomes whilst reducing the chances of increased risks including adverse drug reactions, interactions and other unwanted side-effects.

The Advanced Practitioner: A Framework for Practice, First Edition. Edited by Ian Peate,
Sadie Diamond-Fox, and Barry Hill.
© 2024 John Wiley & Sons Ltd. Published 2024 by John Wiley & Sons Ltd.

Multi-Professional Framework for Advanced Clinical Practice (MPFfACP)

This chapter relates to the following areas of the MPFfACP:
1.7, 2.9, 2.11

(HEE 2017)

Accreditation Considerations

This chapter is applicable to the following specialist curricula:

- Acute Medicine (HEE 2022a)
- Critical Care (ACCP) (FICM 2015)
- Emergency Care – Adult and Child (RCEM 2022)
- Learning Disability and/or Autism (HEE 2020a)
- Mental Health (HEE 2022b)
- Older People (HEE 2022c)
- Primary Care (HEE 2020c)
- Surgical Care (HEE 2020b)

This is an ever evolving field and work continues to agree various competence and capability frameworks for advanced clinical practice in other clinical specialties, therefore the readers is encouraged to refer to https://advanced-practice.hee.nhs.uk/credentials

PHARMACOTHERAPY

Pharmacotherapy is described as treatments or interventions that utilise pharmaceutical drugs. It is classically split into four main processes: pharmacokinetics, pharmacodynamics, therapeutic and pharmaceutical (Figure 6.1).

PHARMACOKINETICS (PK)

Pharmacokinetics is the study of the movement of drugs through the body. This includes absorption, distribution, metabolism and excretion (Eusuf and Thomas 2021).

Absorption is largely affected by route of administration, for example via the oral route, intramuscular (IM) or intravenous (IV). Different routes of administration will have different rates of absorption, with IM and IV being the most rapid (Barber and Robertson 2012). In some cases, the amount of drug that reaches the site of action can be significantly lower than the amount originally administered. This is known as reduced bioavailability. Bioavailability is particularly decreased with some drugs when they are administered orally due to first-pass metabolism. This is because once the drug is absorbed by the

Process	Question for consideration	Factors that may affect the process
Pharmaceutical	Is the drug getting into the patient?	• Patient concordance with therapy • The physicochemical properties of the drug formulation: — Amount of active drug — Drug molecule size — Bulking agents used — Rate of disintegration of an orally given tablet — Rate of dissolution of drug particles in the intestinal fluid after oral administration • Bioavailability – fraction of an administered drug that reaches the systemic circulation and therefore is able to reach the site of action
Pharmacokinetic	Is the drug getting to its site of action?	A – Drug absorption and systemic availability (bioavailability): • Drug-related factors • Patient-related factors • Environmental-related factors D – Drug distribution: • Drug–protein binding complexes • Tissue distribution, dependent on: — Vascular permeability — Regional blood flow — Cardiac output — Perfusion rate of the tissue in question M – Drug metabolism: • Patient age, alcohol consumption and smoking • Cytochrome P450 enzymes • Phase 1 reactions • Phase 2 reactions • Liver, gut, kidney and/or lung function E – Drug excretion: • Renal function (blood flow, glomerular filtration rate [GFR], urine flow rate and urinary pH) • Gastrointestinal tract (GIT) and liver function
Pharmacodynamic	Is the drug producing the required pharmaceutical effect?	• Drug-receptor effects (most commonly via protein molecules located within the cell membrane) • Inhibition of transport processes and/or enzymes • Drug potency and receptor affinity • Drug efficacy • Drug interactions
Therapeutic	Is the pharmacological effect being translated into a therapeutic effect?	• Positive or adverse effects • Pharmacological effects and rate of onset and duration • Drug-disease interactions • Tolerance, tachyphylaxis and desensitisation • Withdrawal

FIGURE 6.1   An overview of the four main processes of pharmacotherapy. *Source*: Peate I, Hill B. 2022/ John Wiley & Sons.

stomach, it enters the hepatic portal system and is partially metabolised by the liver before entering the systemic circulation (McKay and Walters 2013). One example of where first-pass metabolism is particularly problematic is with GTN as it is completely metabolised by the liver, therefore giving it no bioavailability when taken orally. This is why it is usually administered sublingually or intravenously (Barber and Robertson 2012). Drugs administered intravenously will always have 100% bioavailability as they bypass the first-pass metabolism (Batchelder et al. 2011).

Stomach acidity can also play a role in the rate of absorption of orally administered drugs, and some drugs can be enterically coated to protect them from early breakdown whilst others, such as metronidazole, require stomach acid for activation (Alqahtani et al. 2021) (Figure 6.1).

Fields of Practice – Paediatrics

Drug metabolism often involves the cytochrome P450 system, most importantly CYP3A4 and CYP1A2 enzymes (Kearns et al. 2003). The most important liver enzyme responsible for drug metabolism is CYP3A4; however, activity of this enzyme is very low in neonates, increasing in the first year of life (de Wildt et al. 1999). There are many enzymes that affect drug metabolism, and activity is often decreased in neonates but increases in infancy. Other processes of drug metabolism include glucuronidation and sulfation, metabolising drugs such as paracetamol and morphine (de Wildt et al. 2003). Glucuronidation is reduced in neonates and increases during infancy while sulfation is increased in neonates due to the immaturity of the enzyme system (Choonara and Sammons 2014). Table 6.3 highlights the different rates at which the metabolic pathways develop with age (Choonara and Sammons 2014).

Distribution is associated with how drugs pass across cell membranes and is affected by solubility, molecular size and ability to bind to proteins (Eusuf and Thomas 2021). Drugs mainly rely on protein binding for distribution via plasma proteins, which then carry the drug systemically around the body (Mukherjee 2022). Different drugs have different levels of protein binding; for example, phenytoin is highly protein bound. When a drug is bound to protein, it is not active, and the protein-bound quantity creates a reservoir of the drug that can become active once it is freed (Barber and Robertson 2012).

Another consideration in drug distribution is volume of distribution. Although some drugs, such as heparin, have large molecules that leave them unable to leave the capillaries, other drugs are soluble in fat or water. The volume of distribution (Vd) helps prescribers to consider a drug's ability to leave the plasma and enter other body tissues by considering how much of a drug is in a bodily fluid at any time. In other words, Vd is the amount of plasma that would be needed to store the entire quantity of a drug if it was all being stored in the plasma (Monsoor and Mahabadi 2021; Rang et al. 2019).

Elimination happens by removing a drug from the body through the mechanisms of renal excretion and hepatic metabolism (McKay and Walters 2013). Within the liver, drugs undergo a process of biotransformation, whereby their composition is altered. This can increase or decrease the efficacy of the drug, or even be responsible for activating the drug and causing it to be therapeutic (Barber and Robertson 2012). With some drugs, the liver causes biliary excretion into the intestine. Although this does ultimately lead to excretion of the drug, it can also increase the therapeutic ability of drugs due to the reabsorption rate (Neal 2012).

The main mode of elimination of drugs from the body is by renal excretion. Smaller molecule drugs will be filtered out by the glomeruli, with the exception of those which are protein bound. Tubular secretion, on the other hand, is effective at clearing protein-bound drugs and is responsible for the majority of drug clearance. Finally, a small number of non-lipid-bound drugs become concentrated and excreted through the process of water reabsorption at the renal tubule (Rang et al. 2019).

PHARMACODYNAMICS (PD)

Pharmacodynamics is the study of the biochemical and physiological effects of drugs on the body. PD includes factors such as a drug's mechanism of action, its binding sites, drug efficacy, potency and toxicity.

Drugs alter biochemical processes of cells by interacting with target structures in the body, such as receptors (Rang et al. 2019). Pharmacodynamics is the relationship between the drug concentration at the site of action and its effect, which is notably determined by the drug's ability to bind to receptors. Receptors can be present in many tissues around the body, each exhibiting different effects, e.g. opioid receptors in the central nervous system affect pain. Factors that affect this ability to cause an effect include the concentration of the drug at the site of action, the density of the receptors, how a signal is transmitted or regulatory factors that control gene translation and protein production (ASHP 2017).

Pharmacodynamics: Drug–Receptor Interactions

Drug–receptor interactions either enhance or inhibit downstream biochemical processes. A drug that activates a receptor is characterised as an 'agonist' while drugs that inhibit a receptor are characterised as 'antagonists'. Agonists mimic the natural endogenous molecules found in the body (sometimes referred as 'ligands') whereas antagonists are inhibitors of receptors (Figure 6.2). The extracellular binding of the drug on the cell's surface receptor will activate an intracellular process, causing different effects based on its location in the body. Agonists work in two ways: binding to the receptor to produce a similar effect to the natural endogenous ligand (termed 'direct agonists') or increasing the signalling effects of endogenous ligands (termed 'indirect agonists'). On the other hand, antagonists are used to impair these processes and are called either 'competitive' or 'non-competitive'.

A competitive antagonist competes with the endogenous ligand for binding at the receptor site, reducing the amount of signalling molecules that bind onto the receptor which will reduce the cell's ability to elicit an effect. Non-competitive antagonists bind to a site other than the usual receptor binding site, which causes structural changes of the receptor binding site which in turn will reduce or eliminate the ability of the endogenous ligand to bind to the receptor. Furthermore, there are some drugs that are termed 'partial agonists' as they bind directly to the receptor site that generates a weaker signal compared to the endogenous ligand.

To summarise, there are seven main effects that drugs can have on the body (PsychDB, 2021).

- **Stimulating action** – direct receptor agonisms, e.g. levo-dopa in Parkinson's disease.
- **Depressing action** – direct receptor agonism and downstream effects.
- **Blocking action** – binds to receptor but does not activate an effect.
- **Stabilising action** – acts as neither a stimulant nor depressant.
- **Exchanging substances** – accumulating substances to form a reserve.
- **Direct beneficial chemical reaction** – e.g. free radical scavenging.
- **Direct harmful chemical reaction** – damage to cells through induced lethal damage, e.g. chemotherapy.

Pharmacodynamics: Drug Concentration

For a drug to elicit a response, its concentration at the site of action needs to be adequately high. Therefore a drug's efficacy and potency are calculated using drug concentrations in plasma. The correlation between a drug and the response can be estimated using a dose–response curve (Figure 6.3). The efficacy is the maximum effect a drug is capable of eliciting based on its medicinal purpose (Amboss 2019). The ED_{50} value is the dose required to produce half of the maximum possible response, indicating a drug's potency (Amboss 2019). The potency of a drug is based on its efficacy as well as its binding affinity at the receptor target site. Therefore, a drug with high potency will require a lower dose while a drug with low potency will require a higher dose.

However, a highly potent drug does not always cause more adverse effects, as can be seen from the toxicity curve in Figure 6.3. The toxicity curve indicates that any drug can cause a toxic effect if given in large enough amounts. The lethal dose (LD) is the amount of drug that is lethal in 100% of the exposed

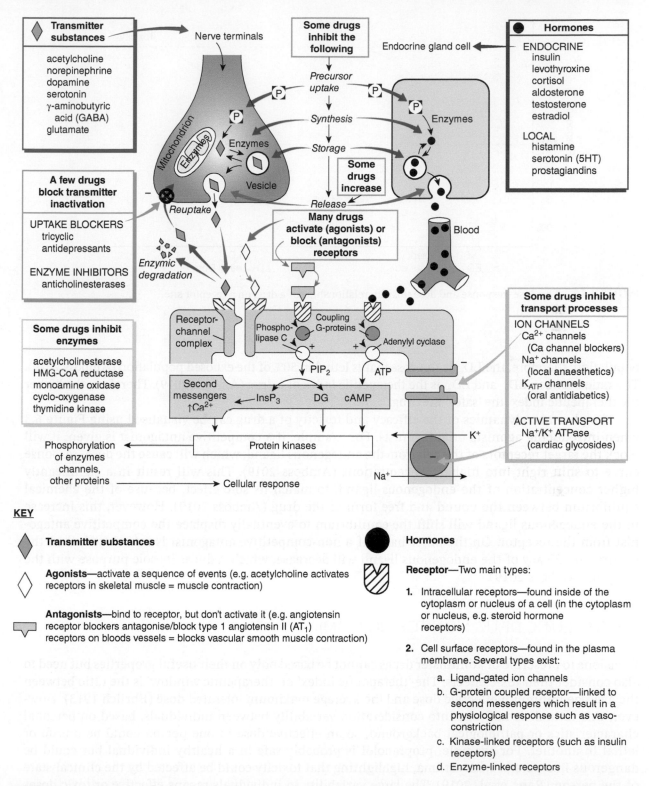

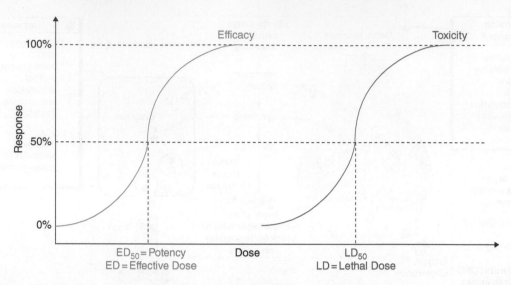

FIGURE 6.3   The dose–response and dose–toxicity relationships of a drug on a receptor site.

population; therefore, the LD_{50} is the dose that is lethal in 50% of the exposed population (Amboss 2019). The ratio between ED_{50} and LD_{50} is the therapeutic index of a drug (Amboss 2019). Therefore, the higher the therapeutic index, the 'safer' the drug.

The pharmacodynamics of the efficacy and toxicity of a drug can be visualised using Figure 6.3 when introducing agonists or antagonists. For example, if a competitive antagonist is given, it will block the target receptors of the cell from the endogenous ligand, which will cause the dose–response curve to shift right into higher concentrations (Amboss 2019). This will result in a significantly higher concentration of the endogenous ligand, to match its sole effect, because of the chemical equilibrium between the bound and free form of the drug (Amboss 2019). However, this increase in the endogenous ligand will shift the equilibrium to eventually displace the competitive antagonist from the receptor. On the other hand, if a non-competitive antagonist is introduced, then the maximum efficacy of the endogenous ligand will decrease, which reduces its sole purpose with the receptor (Amboss 2019).

THERAPEUTIC DRUG MONITORING (TDM)

Decisions to prescribe or administer drugs cannot be based only on their useful properties but need to also consider their toxic effects. The 'therapeutic index' or 'therapeutic window' is the ratio between the average minimum effective dose and the average maximum tolerated dose (Ehrlich 1913). However, this ratio does not take into consideration variability between individuals, based on personal characteristics or pathological background, so an effective dose in one person could be unsafe or lethal in another. For example, propranolol is probably safe in a healthy individual but could be dangerous in a person with asthma, highlighting that toxicity could be affected by the clinical state of the person (Rang et al. 2019). The large variability in individuals means effective or toxic doses are less predictable, especially in an acute clinical situation (Rang et al. 2019). To ensure doses are effective and safe, drug plasma concentration must be above the subtherapeutic level but below the toxic level (Figure 6.4).

CLINICAL INVESTIGATIONS – THERAPEUTIC DRUG MONITORING (TDM)

TDM is a concept used to measure the plasma concentrations of drugs in the blood to identify if a dose is deemed effective or toxic. TDM is primarily used in drugs with a narrow therapeutic index as the ratio between effective and toxic dose is small. Most drug dosages are altered based on patient responses (e.g. amlodipine dose is reduced if blood pressure is too low). However, there are few drugs that require specific plasma concentration levels to identify their efficacy vs toxicity; these drugs are commonly known as 'narrow therapeutic window drugs'.

The properties of individual drugs, and when best to take the plasma concentration level, are based on the drug's pharmacological properties. For example, gentamicin is heavily dose dependent to ensure plasma concentrations are above the subtherapeutic level and within the peak concentration to carry out its bactericidal activities, very similar to Figure 6.4. The plasma level of gentamicin is heavily dose dependent so larger doses will push the drug to the toxic level, exhibiting adverse effects such as ototoxicity and nephrotoxicity.

Ototoxicity occurs due to the progressive destruction of sensory cells in the cochlea and vestibular organ of the ear, resulting in possibly irreversible ataxia, vertigo, loss of balance and deafness (Rang et al. 2019). On the other hand, low plasma concentrations of gentamicin are ineffective, often requiring a further dose to be administered. Similarly, this is why the plasma concentration of gentamicin is taken immediately before the next dose is given, a 'trough' level, to ensure it is not within the toxic range. Gentamicin is eliminated almost entirely by the kidneys, so in patients with renal impairment, peak plasma concentration is raised with prolonged elimination time (EMC 2021a). This is why many guidelines only allow for a 'one-off' dose of gentamicin in patients with renal impairment because essentially it is 'still in the system'. Furthermore, this highlights the importance of taking plasma concentrations at the right time, based on the individual drug, because incorrect timing could result in false positives, i.e. plasma level suggesting toxicity but the level was taken post-dose rather than pre-dose. Table 6.1 highlights some common drugs that require therapeutic drug monitoring (Joint Formulary Committee 2021; Wiffen et al. 2017).

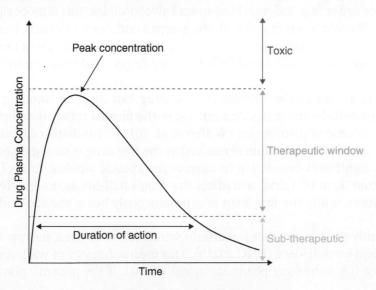

FIGURE 6.4 The therapeutic window of a drug administered with time.

TABLE 6.1   Common drugs that require therapeutic drug monitoring.

Drug	Therapeutic Plasma Concentration Range	Level Sampling Timing
Carbamazepine	4–10 mg/l	Trough level before dose
Digoxin	0.8–2 mcg/l	6 h post dose
Gentamicin (once daily)	Trough: <2 mg/l	Trough: immediately before dose
Lithium	0.4–1 mmol/l	12 h post dose
Phenytoin	10–20 mg/l	Trough level before dose
Theophylline	10–20 mg/l	Trough level before dose

Plasma Protein Binding

It has been determined that drugs require, in general, a non-uniform distribution in the body or tissue to exhibit their pharmacological effects (Ehrlich 1913). In modern pharmacology, it is believed that drugs are bound to plasma proteins and the efficacy of the drug is dependent on the degree to which they are bound – termed 'plasma protein binding' (Rang et al. 2019). A chemical equilibrium exists between the bound and free forms of the drug:

$$Protein + Drug \leftrightarrow Protein\text{-}Drug\ Complex$$

There are two forms of a drug in the blood – 'bound' and 'free'. A fraction of the drug is bound to plasma proteins while the rest is free or 'unbound'. Some drugs have a higher protein-binding affinity than others, therefore exhibiting various pharmacological effects. It is said that the free or unbound drug is the form that exhibits the pharmacological effect and is the fraction of the drug that will be metabolised or cleared (Sun and Zhao 2016). The protein–drug complex will then transfer to the tissue where it will dissociate back to the drug and protein. Common blood proteins to which drugs bind include albumin, lipoprotein, glycoprotein and some globulins (Sun and Zhao 2016). Acidic drugs (e.g. aspirin) bind to albumin while alkaline drugs (e.g. codeine) bind to acid glycoproteins; this is more significant in medical conditions that affect albumin levels (e.g. dehydration, sepsis and shock). Equally, it is significant in older underweight people in whom albumin levels decrease, leading to higher levels of the free form of highly protein-bound drugs, e.g. non-steroidal anti-inflammatory drugs (NSAIDs), warfarin and sulfonylureas (Wiffen et al. 2017).

Protein binding is a competitive process so one drug can displace another; this interaction is significant in highly protein-bound drugs that remain in the plasma rather than being transferred into tissue, causing a low volume of distribution (Wiffen et al. 2017). This displacement causes a small rise in drug levels before chemical equilibrium is reached as the free drug is now metabolised and excreted, potentially causing a significant interaction in narrow therapeutic window drugs (Wiffen et al. 2017). Furthermore, the bound form of a drug will affect the drug's half-life as it will release a proportion of the drug to the free form, while the free form is simultaneously being metabolised and excreted (Sun and Zhao 2016).

One drug commonly used in practice is warfarin which not only has a narrow therapeutic window but is also highly protein bound, ~99% (EMC 2021b). This means that 99% of warfarin is bound to plasma proteins and 1% is free (i.e. exhibiting pharmacological effects). If the patient's plasma protein reduces, warfarin binding will be saturated, resulting in higher free form warfarin transported into the tissue. As warfarin is a narrow therapeutic window drug, any small increase in warfarin levels could push the plasma concentration to the toxic range, resulting in higher risk of adverse effects, the most significant being haemorrhage.

Pharmacodynamic drug interactions between protein-bound drugs can also increase the concentration of free form drugs, potentially leading to a higher risk of adverse effects. This is because another drug can competitively displace the first drug from the drug–protein complex, leading to higher free form concentrations of the first drug.

Table 6.2 highlights the protein-binding displacement interactions between two drugs. Drug A is 99% protein bound (e.g. warfarin) which means 99% is bound to plasma proteins. If drug B is then administered, this will displace a fraction of drug A from plasma proteins, leading to a higher free form drug A level. In this example, if only 1% of bound drug A is displaced, this leads to a 100% increase in the free form whereas drug B only exhibits a 10% increase in free form. In the case of warfarin, and all narrow therapeutic window drugs, this 1% increase can significantly increase the pharmacological effects of warfarin, and similarly adverse effects, as it has been established that free form versions of a drug exhibit the effects. In the case of warfarin, measuring a patient's INR level gives an indication of how the drug is working, making it slightly more appreciable in clinical practice. However, this interaction is not straightforward, as a higher percentage of free form drug A leads to increased metabolism and excretion, which in turn reduces the concentration of drug A. Nevertheless, care must be taken with some drugs depending on their pharmacology, e.g. phenytoin has zero order kinetics so any small increase in its plasma concentration of phenytoin can cause substantial toxic effects (Table 6.3).

TABLE 6.2   An example of how free form drug plasma concentrations can rise between an interaction with two protein-bound drugs.

	Before Displacement	After Displacement	% Increase in Free Form Drug
		Drug A	
% Bound	99	98	
% Free	1	2	**100**
		Drug B	
% Bound	90	89	
% Free	10	11	**10**

TABLE 6.3   How drug metabolic pathways develop with age.

Age	CYP3A4	CYP1A2	Glucuronidation	Sulfation
Preterm neonates	+	+	+	+++
Term neonates	+	+	+	+++
Infants	+++	++	++	++
Children	+++	+++	+++	+
Adolescents	++	+++	+++	+

Drug-induced Adverse Effects

Dopamine is an important neurotransmitter involved in several central nervous system disorders, including schizophrenia and Parkinson's disease. Many of the drugs that treat these conditions have an impact on dopamine transmission. Dopaminergic neurons recapture dopamine that is released from the nerve terminals using specific dopamine transporters (Rang et al. 2019). Dopamine works within all these pathways by interacting with receptors that mediate the functional effects of dopamine. There are five types of receptors found in these pathways, D1–D5. Psychotic disorders have a high abundance of D1 and D2 receptors.

Antipsychotic drugs mainly act by blocking the D2 receptors on dopaminergic neurons in all four pathways of the brain – termed 'dopamine antagonists'. 'Typical' or 'first-generation' antipsychotics are not selective and therefore will block D2 receptors in all four pathways, causing a range of symptoms. Examples of 'typical' antipsychotics include chlorpromazine, haloperidol and zuclopenthixol. These typical dopamine antagonists will cause positive and negative symptoms depending on which pathway is affected (mesolimbic, mesocortical, nigrostriatial or tuberofundibular) (Speed Pharmacology 2018).

'Atypical' or 'second-generation' antipsychotics act on a range of receptors, not just D2, and therefore are associated with a lower risk of acute extrapyramidal symptoms and tardive dyskinesia. However, they have a higher incidence of metabolic effects such as weight gain and glucose intolerance (Joint Formulary Committee 2022). Examples of 'atypical' antipsychotics include amisulpride, clozapine, olanzapine, quetiapine and risperidone.

Examination Scenarios

When examining patients on antipsychotic drugs, or any dopamine antagonist (e.g. metoclopramide), it is important to be vigilant for the following physical signs of antipsychotics-induced adverse effects, caused by the reasons mentioned above (Wiffen et al. 2017; Wyatt et al. 2020).

- Acute dystonia
- Akathisia
- Parkinsonism
- Tardive dyskinesia

Salbutamol is a drug that is often used to manage acute exacerbations of asthma or bronchospasm (Joint Formulary Committee 2022). It is a beta-2-adrenergic receptor agonist, meaning that it stimulates these receptors within smooth muscle, causing bronchodilation due to an increase in cAMP that leads to relaxation of smooth muscle (Lackie and Nation 2019; Batchelder et al. 2011). Salbutamol is a relatively short-acting drug as it can only bind briefly to its receptor before diffusing back into the microcirculation (Sears and Lötvall 2005). Due to its close relationship to adrenaline (although it is more selective), at high doses salbutamol can also agonise beta-1-adrenergic receptors and cause tachycardia (Neal 2012; Rang et al. 2019), although this is usually seen in more acute situations where salbutamol is administered at higher doses or intravenously (McKay and Walters 2013; Reactions Weekly 2018).

One of the adverse effects most widely associated with the use of beta-2-adrenergic receptor agonists is a fine muscle tremor. Although the reason is still not fully understood, it is believed to be caused by the increase in adrenaline (or adrenergic receptor agonists) leading to an increase in discharge from muscle spindles (Rang et al. 2019). Tremors are believed to affect between 2% and 4% of patients who are taking beta-2-adrenergic receptor agonists but increase to 2–14% in acute bronchitis (Cazzola and Matera 2012).

Salbutamol can also cause activation of cholinergic terminals in the nerves. It is believed that beta-2-adrenergic receptors in skeletal muscle control the permeability of cells to potassium, and that by giving the associated agonist, sodium-potassium-ATPase can hyperpolarise the cells, causing potassium to enter the cell but then being unable to complete its discharge, hence causing hypokalaemia (Brown et al. 1983; Rang et al. 2019). Some of the signs and symptoms of hypokalaemia include cardiac arrhythmias, ECG changes, leg cramps, metabolic acidosis and respiratory failure (Kardalas et al. 2018).

Fields of Practice – Mental Health

Selective serotonin reuptake inhibitors (SSRIs) are commonly used in the management of depression; they include citalopram, fluoxetine, sertraline and paroxetine (Joint Formulary Committee 2022). They work by increasing the level of serotonin (5-HT) at the synaptic space by inhibiting its reuptake through the neurons, thus improving neurotransmission by downregulating 5-HT$_{1A}$ receptors (Draper and Berman 2008; McKay and Walters 2013). SSRIs are predominantly administered via the oral route, where they undergo substantial first-pass metabolism. They are extensively protein bound, therefore reducing their distribution volume, and this should be borne in mind when prescribing other drugs which are highly protein bound or if protein levels drop as this could cause a higher risk of serotonin syndrome (EMC 2021c).

SSRIs are generally deemed to be safe and have fewer side-effects than other drugs that could be used to treat depression (Barber and Robertson 2012). However, prescribers should consider interactions with other drugs; for example, the Joint Formulary Committee (2022) recommends caution when prescribing ondansetron to a patient receiving SSRIs. Ondansetron is commonly used postoperatively to prevent nausea and vomiting. It works by antagonising serotonin (5-HT$_3$) receptors in the GI tract and central nervous system (EMC 2022b). For this reason, there is an increased risk of serotonin syndrome when used concomitantly with SSRIs and helps to explain why nausea can often be an unwanted side-effect of SSRI usage.

Fields of Practice – Learning Disabilities

People with learning difficulties often live with multiple co-morbidities, which means receiving significant amounts of drugs and being at higher risk of drug interactions and side-effects (Hannah and Brodie 1998; Lee et al. 2021). Alongside multiple drugs that affect the cholinergic systems, people with learning difficulties can often be prescribed antiepileptic drugs due to a higher incidence of seizures amongst this population (Hannah and Brodie 1998), leading to a risk of interaction with other medications the patient may be using.

One example of this is carbamazepine, which works by inhibiting the sodium channels in the neurons (McKay and Walters 2013). Although this can help to control seizures, it can also lead to behavioural changes. Furthermore, it can cause hyponatraemia when given alongside some other drugs (for example, antidepressants) and reduce the efficacy of some medications, including risperidone due to increased enzyme induction and metabolism (Mula and Monaco 2002; Ono et al. 2002), Therefore, in this situation one should consider prescribing an alternative such as levetiracetam, which is renally excreted and only produces minimal enzymatic activation (EMC 2021d).

Learning Events

There are many situations where skills and knowledge are required to resolve pharmaceutical issues. Two examples are given below.

- A Muslim teenager with severe infected eczema required oral flucloxacillin four times a day. The patient refused the medication for two reasons: the capsules contain gelatine and he could not have it four times a day due to fasting. Changing the formulation to a suspension will not resolve the issues as the frequency will remain the same. An alternative, azithromycin tablets once daily, was prescribed – an example of the social and cultural considerations that arise when treating patients.

- A patient presented with symptoms of acute confusion, reduced oral intake, vomiting and tremor. She was diagnosed with dehydration and UTI as the most likely causes. However, she was recently started on bumetanide for ankle oedema as well as continuing her usual lithium for bipolar disease. The interaction between the two drugs pushed the patient into lithium toxicity which was potentiated by a dehydrated state and underlying infection. This highlights the importance of monitoring drugs with a narrow therapeutic window, especially if they interact with other drugs, as well as looking out for physical signs of toxicity (e.g. tremor in lithium).

RED FLAGS – PATHOLOGICAL CONSIDERATIONS

Adverse Drug Reactions (ADRs)

There are different classifications of ADRs. The two most common types of ADRs are as follows (MHRA 2015; Wiffen et al. 2017).

1. Type A Reactions (Augmented)

    These reactions are caused by an accelerated pharmacological effect of two drugs by potentiating similar effects. The reactions are common manifestations of the drug's toxicological properties that are often dose related and predictable, with low mortality. Examples of type A reactions include hypotension in patients taking ramipril, bleeding with naproxen or hypoglycaemia with insulin. For example, apixaban is a highly selective inhibitor of factor Xa causing inhibition of free and clot-bound factor Xa, resulting in prevention of thrombin generation and thrombus development (EMC 2021e). This mechanism of action is the reason why apixaban is used to prevent formation of venous thromboembolism but this same mechanism causes inhibition of clotting factor Xa, resulting in higher incidence of haemorrhagic adverse effects.

2. Type B Reactions (Bizarre/Idiosyncratic)

    Type B reactions are unrelated to the drug's pharmacological and toxicological properties and cannot be predicted from the drug's pharmacological characteristics. These reactions are often immunological and dose independent and are quite rare. Examples of type B reactions include anaphylaxis with penicillin, hepatotoxicity with isoflurane and toxic epidermal necrolysis with lamotrigine. For example, serious hypersensitivity reactions can occur in people taking amoxicillin; however, they are often likely to occur in people with a history of penicillin sensitivity or in atopic individuals, highlighting that the ADR is related to an immune response rather than a pharmacological effect.

Drug Interactions

With many different drug variables and factors, pharmacodynamic interactions between drugs do occur. Classifications include the following (Wiffen et al. 2017).

- **Additive** – e.g. increased sedation with alcohol and hypnotics such as benzodiazepines.
- **Synergism** – e.g. ethambutol increases the effectiveness of other tuberculosis drugs.
- **Antagonism** – e.g. propranolol diminishes effectiveness of salbutamol.

Although drug–receptor interactions are the most common pharmacodynamic drug actions, other factors must be taken into consideration when prescribing or administering drugs. One factor is age, as older people are at higher risk of adverse effects due to polypharmacy interactions and a natural loss of cellular activity which can increase or decrease drug sensitivity (Wiffen et al. 2017). Likewise, pharmacodynamics of drugs vary for each drug as some can interact with cell DNA, some interfere with osmotic cell balance and some act on ions or G proteins. For example, carbamazepine has been shown to be strongly associated with an increased risk of developing Stevens–Johnson syndrome in people of Han Chinese and Thai origin due to the HLA-B*1502 allele, often requiring prescreening investigations to be done before initiating the drug (EMC 2021f).

Contraindications

Contraindications do not only occur between drugs but can occur when a drug interacts with the body – these are termed 'drug–disease interactions'. Table 6.4 demonstrates examples of these interactions (Richards and Aronson 2008; Rang et al. 2019; Joint Formulary Committee 2022).

TABLE 6.4   Common drug–disease interactions with a rationale for contraindications.

Drug–Disease Interaction Example	Rationale
Metformin in acute kidney injury (AKI)	Can cause lactic acidosis due to increased glycolysis and inhibition of gluconeogenesis from lactate in the liver. This effect is potentiated in renal impairment due to reduced drug elimination from the kidneys and reduced tissue oxygenation. Metformin is contraindicated in patients with GFR <30 ml/min
Paracetamol in liver impairment	Paracetamol produces a highly reactive metabolite, N-acetyl-p-benzoquinoneimine (NAPQI) by CYP enzymes in liver and kidneys – completely detoxified by conjugation with glutathione. NAPQI is toxic to the liver so in liver impairment, there are decreased amount of proteins (glutathione) to conjugate with NAPQI, to clear it from the body. This increased NAPQI concentration in the blood will lead to increased risk of toxicity including jaundice and hepatitis, which can be potentially fatal
Sodium valproate in pregnancy	Sodium valproate crosses the placenta into the fetus. Many studies have reported that sodium valproate serum concentration in the umbilical cord is the same or higher than that of the mother. Sodium valproate is highly teratogenic and evidence supports that use in pregnancy leads to neurodevelopmental disorders (approx. 30–40% risk) and congenital malformations (approx. 10% risk)

(Continued)

TABLE 6.4   (Continued)

Drug–Disease Interaction Example	Rationale
Amiodarone during breastfeeding	Amiodarone is an iodine-containing drug that is present in milk which passes through the breast tissue to the infant. Metabolism of amiodarone releases free iodine which can be transferred to the infant, potentially causing neonatal hypothyroidism. Amiodarone has a significantly long half-life because it is extensively stored in body fat
Quinolones (e.g. ciprofloxacin) in epilepsy	Quinolones can lower the seizure threshold by inhibiting the GABA receptor complex. This is more significant in people with epilepsy as quinolones are more likely to cause central nervous system adverse effects
Aminoglycosides (e.g. gentamicin) in neuromuscular disorders	Aminoglycosides can impair neuromuscular transmission by inhibiting the calcium uptake necessary for the exocytotic release of acetylcholine. This effect is potentiated if aminoglycosides are given with non-depolarising muscle relaxants (e.g. rocuronium). Likewise, these neuromuscular blocking properties can also exacerbate other neuromuscular diseases such as myasthenia gravis and Parkinson's disease

ORANGE FLAGS – PSYCHOLOGICAL CONSIDERATIONS

Overdose

The mode of action of SSRIs has already been briefly explored within this chapter, but this is a long way from being the sole medication used to support people's mental health. Although SSRIs are generally deemed to be safe in the event of overdose (Barber and Robertson 2012), other drugs can be less so. Amitriptyline, for example, is a tricyclic antidepressant used to inhibit serotonin and noradrenaline uptake, but is less specific than SSRIs, meaning it can also cause unwanted side-effects including drowsiness, arrhythmias, constipation, increased weight and seizures (EMC 2022a). These happen due to tricyclics' role in blocking cardiac sodium channels and alpha-1-adrenergic receptors (Toxbase 2022). Tricyclics are not alone in causing serious side-effects in the case of overdose and practitioners should consider which drugs would be most appropriate.

Excipients

Formulations of drugs do not just contain the active drug itself but also the excipients used to make it up. For example, tablets contain the active drug but can also include excipients used to stabilise the drug, bulk it up or facilitate absorption of a drug (Bhattacharyya et al. 2006; Borbas et al. 2016). Table 6.5 highlights some of the common excipients seen in practice and the real-life implications they can have on patients (Joint Formulary Committee 2022; Sweetman 2014).

Adherence

Drug prescribing is the most common intervention carried out by healthcare professionals. However, although effective consultations are key to ensuring effective medication optimisation, there are many factors affecting the adherence of drugs. One of the most influential is the patient's individual social

TABLE 6.5 Common excipients present in some drugs and potential effects on patients.

Excipients	Examples of Drug	Potential Effects
Alcohol	Contained in some liquid or injection preparations, e.g. chlorphenamine syrup	Avoided in certain religious or social groups so choice of formulation needs to be reviewed
Arachis (peanut)/soya	Arachis oil enema, some brands of desogestrel, isotretinoin, benzylpenicillin injections, propofol	Higher risk of allergic reactions in hypersensitive patients
Aspartame (E951)	Montelukast chewable tablets, ondansetron orodispersible tablets	Patients with autosomal recessive phenylketonuria need to avoid aspartame
Gelatine	Most hard-shell capsules, e.g. amoxicillin	Usually derived from animals – should be avoided by some religious/social/vegan individuals
Lactose	Most tablet formulations	Might cause problems in lactose-intolerant patients
Porcine	Low molecular weight heparins (e.g. enoxaparin)	Derived from porcine intestinal mucosa – should be avoided by some religious/social/vegan individuals
Sucrose	Methadone (333 mg sucrose per 1 ml), antibiotic suspensions, some cough medicines	Can increase risk of developing diabetes mellitus or hyperglycaemia in patients who might not have the best physical health

and cultural beliefs regarding drugs and treatments. For example, one study showed that students with Asian backgrounds were significantly more likely to perceive medicines as being harmful, addictive and to be avoided compared to students with a European background (Horne et al. 2004). However, there have been studies that highlight a higher adherence to traditional Chinese medication compared to self-management therapies (Eh et al. 2016). This is similar to another study showing that some patients believe traditional herbal medications are safer than inhalers in treating asthma (Chiu et al. 2014).

Route of administration is another social and cultural issue that can affect drug adherence. Some European patients prefer to take medications rectally, via suppositories, rather than orally due to the faster mechanism of action. Some patients in developing countries also prefer rectal suppositories over oral medications due to the lack of clean water. However, most Western cultures prefer oral medications, especially if it is for paediatric patients. Similarly, as mentioned above, some patients prefer parenteral or transdermal routes of administration over oral due to their religious background, e.g. fasting during Ramadan.

GREEN FLAGS – SOCIAL AND CULTURAL CONSIDERATIONS

Addiction

Some drugs, through their modes of action, can cause desensitisation, tolerance or addiction to the product. One example of this is morphine. Morphine is an agonist that binds to opioid receptors, creating analgesic effects by blocking calcium channels within the neurons and therefore inhibiting pain conduction across the synapse (Barber and Robertson 2012; Khan et al. 2022). It is thought that when morphine is prescribed regularly, there can be a reduction in the density or affinity of opioid receptors, therefore causing tolerance to morphine (Peck and Harris 2021). Due to this, upregulation of opioid receptors occurs, meaning that the number of receptors increases and therefore a higher quantity of drug is required to achieve the same level of analgesia. This in turn causes dependency and, if the drug is abruptly stopped, withdrawal symptoms can occur (Rang et al. 2019). It is no surprise, therefore, that continuous use of morphine can lead to addiction, especially when the associated euphoria is considered that is associated with morphine use in the absence of chronic pain (Barber and Robertson 2012; Peck and Harris 2021; Rang et al. 2019). When used appropriately, however, dependency on and addiction to morphine are less likely to occur (Barber and Robertson, 2012). Indeed, in palliative care increased dosages have not been observed routinely and where required are usually attributed to a natural increase in pain rather than an increased tolerance (Neal 2012).

Case Study

Drug Interaction

Patient X, a 42-year-old male, is being treated for osteomyelitis with oral rifampicin tablets 600 mg twice a day. Patient X has started rifampicin in hospital and is being discharged to continue the antibiotic course for another six months. He has no known drug allergies. He only takes methadone oral solution 80 mg once daily and paracetamol oral tablets 1 g four times a day. He has been on methadone for more than 10 years.

A few days after patient X completed his rifampicin, he was admitted to hospital with respiratory depression.

- What are the pharmacokinetic and pharmacodynamic properties of methadone and rifampicin?
- What are the potential issues with this management plan?
- What monitoring should be carried out?

Overdose

A patient has been admitted to the emergency department with a reduced GCS and tachycardia. Prior to his admission, the paramedic noted several empty medication boxes in his home, including amitriptyline, propranolol and gabapentin.

- What are the pharmacokinetic and pharmacodynamic properties of these drugs?
- What side-effects could be caused by these drugs?
- How could these drugs interact with each other and how would this affect your management plan?
- What clinical examinations should be considered?

Side-effects

A patient presents to her GP with a new wheeze. She is usually fit and well and has no history of respiratory disease. Over the last few months, she has started purchasing aspirin for migraines, which she has continued to take on a daily basis.

- What is the mode of action of aspirin?
- What side-effects can occur with aspirin, and why do these happen?
- Look up and explain the oxygenase/leukotriene pathways – where does aspirin fit into this and what could an increase in its substrate cause?
- Consider the management plan for this patient – what would you propose?

CONCLUSION

Pharmacology is the study of how drugs move through and are processed by the body. These can be affected by multiple factors and it is important for clinicians to consider drugs' modes of action and evaluate any risk of interactions, adverse reactions and the affinity and efficacy of any drug prescribed. The pharmacological properties of drugs patients can often have not just physiological effects but also psychological and social consequences, and steps should be taken to recognise and mitigate these where appropriate.

Take Home Points
- Pharmacology is the study of how drugs interact with the body. It is divided into two subcategories: pharmacokinetics and pharmacodynamics.
- Drugs can interact with each other and fight for binding sites on plasma proteins. This can cause adverse drug reactions and changes to volumes of distribution.
- The mode of action of a drug is determined by its ability to bind to receptors, activate enzymes, block or activate ion channels, or enhance or inhibit transduction of a ligand-originated signal across a membrane.

REFERENCES

Alqatani, M.S., Kazi, M., Alsenaidy, M.A., and Ahmed, M.Z. (2021). Advances in Oral drug delivery. *Frontiers in Pharmacology* 12: 618411.

Amboss: Medical Knowledge Distilled (2019). Pharmacodynamics – Part 2: Dose–response Relationship. www.youtube.com/watch?v=Vzrvk1X5Wmw

American Society of Health-System Pharmacists (2017). Introduction to Pharmacokinetics and Pharmacodynamics. www.ashp.org/-/media/store%20files/p2418-sample-chapter-1.pdf

Atkinson, A.J. (2022). Chapter 1 – Introduction to clinical pharmacology. In: *Atkinson's Principles of Clinical Pharmacology*, 4e (ed. S.M. Huang, J.J.L. Lertora, P. Vincini, and A.J. Atkinson). San Diego: Elsevier.

Barber, P. and Robertson, D. (2012). *Essentials of Pharmacology for Nurses*, 2e. Berkshire: Open University Press.

Batchelder, A., Rodrigues, C., and Alrifai, Z. (2011). *Rapid Clinical Pharmacology a Student Formulary*. Chichester: Wiley Blackwell.

Bhattacharyya, L., Schuber, S., Sheehan, C., and William, R. (2006). Excipients: Background/introduction. In: *Excipient Development for Pharmaceutical, Biotechnology and Drug Delivery Systems* (ed. A. Katdare and M. Chaubal). Boca Raton: CRC Press.

Borbas, E., Sinko, B., Tsinman, O. et al. (2016). Investigation and mathematical description of the real driving force of passive transport molecules from supersated solutions. *Molecular Pharmaceutics* 13 (11): 3816–3826.

Brenner, G.M. and Stevens, C. (2017). *Pharmacology*, 5e. Philadelphia: Elsevier.

Brown, M.J., Brown, D.C., and Murphy, M.B. (1983). Hypokalemia from Beta2-receptor stimulation by circulating epinephrine. *New England Journal of Medicine* 309 (23): 1414–1419.

Cazzola, M. and Matera, M.G. (2012). Tremor and ß$_2$-adrenergic agents: is it a real clinical problem? *Pulmonary Pharmacology and Therapeutics* 24 (1): 4–10.

Chiu, K.C., Boonsawat, W., Cho, S.H. et al. (2014). Patients' beliefs and behaviors related to treatment adherence in patients with asthma requiring maintenance treatment in Asia. *Journal of Asthma* 51 (6): 652–659.

Choonara, I. and Sammons, H. (2014). Paediatric clinical pharmacology in the UK. *Archives of Disease in Childhood* 99: 1143–1146.

Draper, B. and Berman, K. (2008). Tolerability of selective serotonin reuptake inhibitors. Issues relevant to the elderly. *Drugs and Ageing* 25 (6): 501–519.

Eh, K., McGill, M., Wong, J., and Krass, I. (2016). Cultural issues and other factors that affect self-management of type 2 diabetes mellitus (T2D) by Chinese immigrants in Australia. *Diabetes Research and Clinical Practice* 119: 97–105.

Ehrlich, P. (1913). Address in pathology on chemotherapeutics: scientific principles, methods and results. *Lancet* 181 (4668): 445–451.

Electronic Medicines Compendium (2021a). Eliquis 5 mg film-coated tablets. www.medicines.org.uk/emc/product/2878/smpc

Electronic Medicines Compendium (2021b). Gentamicin 40mg/ml Solution for Injection/Infusion. www.medicines.org.uk/emc/product/12877/smpc

Electronic Medicines Compendium (2021c). Sertraline 100mg Film Coated Tablets. www.medicines.org.uk/emc/product/13524/smpc#DOCREVISION

Electronic Medicines Compendium (2021d). Desitrend 100mg/ml concentrate for solution for infusion. www.medicines.org.uk/emc/product/7345/smpc#DOCREVISION

Electronic Medicines Compendium (2021e). Tegretol 100mg Tablets. www.medicines.org.uk/emc/product/1040

Electronic Medicines Compendium (2021f). Warfarin 0.5mg Tablets. www.medicines.org.uk/emc/product/3064

Electronic Medicines Compendium (2022a). Amitriptyline 25mg tablets BP. www.medicines.org.uk/emc/product/5699/smpc#UNDESIRABLE_EFFECTS

Electronic Medicines Compendium (2022b). Ondansetron 2mg/ml Solution for Injection. www.medicines.org.uk/emc/product/6469/smpc#DOCREVISION

Eusuf, D.V. and Thomas, E. (2021). Pharmacokinetic variation. *Anaesthesia and Intensive Care Medicine*. 23 (1): 50–53.

Faculty of Intensive Care Medicine (2015). Curriculum for Training for Advanced Critical Care Practitioners. www.ficm.ac.uk/sites/ficm/files/documents/2021-10/ACCP%20Curriculum%20Part%20I%20-%20Handbook%20v1.1%202019%20Revision.pdf

Hannah, J.A. and Brodie, M.J. (1998). Treatment of seizures in patients with learning difficulties. *Pharmacology and Therapeutics* 78 (1): 1–8.

Health Education England (2017). Multi-professional framework for advanced clinical practice in England. www.hee.nhs.uk/sites/default/files/docuemtns/HEE%20ACP%2Framework.pdf

Health Education England (2020a). Advanced Clinical Practice: Capabilities framework when working with people who have a learning disability and/or autism. www.skillsforhealth.org.uk/wp-content/uploads/2020/11/ACP-in-LDA-Framework.pdf

Health Education England (2020b). Surgical Advanced Clinical Practitioner (SACP) Curriculum and Assessment Framework. www.iscp.ac.uk/media/1141/sacp_curriculum_dec20_accessible-1.pdf

Health Education England (2022a). Advanced Clinical Practice in Acute Medicine Curriculum Framework. https://healtheducationengland.sharepoint.com/sites/APWC/Shared%20Documents/Forms/AllItems.aspx?id=%2Fsites%2FAPWC%2FShared%20Documents%2FCredentials%2FCredentials%20Endorsement%20Documents%2FAdvanced%20clinical%20practice%20in%20acute%20medicine%20curriculum%20framework%2Epdf&parent=%2Fsites%2FAPWC%2FShared%20Documents%2FCredentials%2FCredentials%20Endorsement%20Documents&p=true&ga=1

Health Education England (2022b). Advanced Practice Mental Health Curriculum and Capabilities Framework. https://healtheducationengland.sharepoint.com/sites/APWC/Shared%20Documents/Forms/AllItems.aspx?id=%2Fsites%2FAPWC%2FShared%20Documents%2FCredentials%2FCredentials%20Endorsement%20Documents%2FAdvanced%20practice%20in%20mental%20health%20curriculum%20and%20capabilities%20framework%2Epdf&parent=%2Fsites%2FAPWC%2FShared%20Documents%2FCredentials%2FCredentials%20Endorsement%20Documents&p=true&ga=1

Health Education England (2022c). Advanced Clinical Practice in Older People Curriculum Framework. https://healtheducationengland.sharepoint.com/sites/APWC/Shared%20Documents/Forms/AllItems.aspx?id=%2Fsites%2FAPWC%2FShared%20Documents%2FCredentials%2FCredentials%20Endorsement%20Documents%2FAdvanced%20clinical%20practice%20older%20people%20curriculum%20framework%20%20%2Epdf&parent=%2Fsites%2FAPWC%2FShared%20Documents%2FCredentials%2FCredentials%20Endorsement%20Documents&p=true&ga=1

Health Education England, NHS England and Skills for Health (2020c). Core Capabilities Framework for Advanced Clinical Practice (Nurses) Working in General Practice/Primary Care. www.hee.nhs.uk/sites/default/files/documents/ACP%20Primary%20Care%20Nurse%20Fwk%202020.pdf

Horne, R., Graupner, L., Frost, S. et al. (2004). Medicine in a multi-cultural society: the effect of cultural background on beliefs about medications. *Social Science and Medicine* 59 (6): 1307–1313.

Joint Formulary Committee (2021). *British National Formulary*. London: BMJ Group and Pharmaceutical Press.

Joint Formulary Committee (2022). *Children British National Formulary*, 83e. London: BMJ Group and Pharmaceutical Press.

Kardalas, E., Paschou, S.A., Anagnostis, P. et al. (2018). Hypokalemia: a clinical update. *Endocrine Connections* 7 (4): R135–R146.

Kearns, G.L., Abdel-Rahman, S.M., Alander, S.W. et al. (2003). Developmental pharmacology – drug disposition, action, and therapy in infants in children. *New England Journal of Medicine* 349: 1157–1167.

Khan, D., Asher, Y.G., and Benzon, H.T. (2022). Management of acute and chronic pain. In: *Cliincal Anaesthesia Fundamentals*, 2e (ed. B.F. Cullen, M.C. Stock, R. Ortega, et al.). London: Wolters Kluwer.

Lackie, J. and Nation, B. (2019). *Oxford Dictionary of Biomedicine*, 2e. Oxford: Oxford University Press.

Lee, C., Ivo, J., Carter, C. et al. (2021). Pharmacist interventions for persons with intellectual disabilities: a scoping review. *Research in Social and Administrative Pharmacy* 17 (2): 257–272.

McKay, G.A. and Walters, M.R. (2013). *Clinical Pharmacology and Therapeutics. Lecture Notes*, 9e. Chichester: Wiley.

Medicines and Healthcare products Regulatory Agency (2015). Guidance on adverse drug reactions. www.mhra.gov.uk

Monsoor, A. and Mahabadi, N. (2021). Volume of distribution. www.ncbi.nlm.nih.gov/books/NBK545280/

Mukherjee, B. (2022). *Pharmacokinetics Basics to Applications*. Singapore: Springer.

Mula, M. and Monaco, F. (2002). Carbamazepine-risperidone interactions in patients with epilepsy. *Clinical Neuropharmacology* 25 (2): 97–100.

Neal, M.J. (2012). *Medical Pharmacology at a Glance*. Chichester: Wiley.

Ono, S., Mihara, K., Suzuki, A. et al. (2002). Significant pharmacokinetic interaction between risperidone and carbamazepine: its relationship with CYP2D6 genotypes. *Psychopharmacology* 162 (1): 50–54.

Peate, I. and Hill, B. (2022). *Fundamentals of Critical Care*. Oxford: Wiley-Blackwell.

Peck, T. and Harris, B. (2021). *Pharmacology for Anaesthesia and Intensive Care*, 5e. Cambridge: Cambridge University Press.

Psychiatry Database (2021). Introduction to pharmacology. www.psychdb.com/meds/pharmacology/home#introduction-to-pharmacology

Rang, H.P., Dale, M.M., Ritter, J.M., and Flower, R.J. (2019). *Rang and Dale's Pharmacology*, 9e. Edinburgh.: Elsevier.

Richard, D. and Aronson, J. (2008). *Oxford Handbook of Practical Drug Therapy*. Oxford: Oxford University Press.

Royal College of Emergency Medicine (2022). Emergency Care Advanced Clinical Practitioner Curriculum - Adult. https://rcem.ac.uk/wp-content/uploads/2022/09/ACP_Curriculum_Adult_Final_060922.pdf

Sears, M.R. and Lötvall, J. (2005). Past, present and future – ß$_2$-adrenoceptor agonists in asthma management. *Respiratory Medicine* 99 (2): 152–170.

Speed Pharmacology (2018). Pharmacology - ANTIPSYCHOTICS (MADE EASY). www.youtube.com/watch?v=nKkIh1B2Js8

Sun, H. and Zhao, H. (2016). Physiologic drug distribution and protein binding. In: *Applied Biopharmaceutics & Pharmacokinetics*, 7e (ed. L. Shargel and A.B.C. Yu). New York: McGraw Hill.

Sweetman, S.C. (2014). *Martindale: The Complete Drug Reference*. London: Pharmaceutical Press.

Toxbase (2022). Amitriptyline. www.toxbase.org/poisons-index-a-z/a-products/amitriptyline----------------/ (paywall)

Weekly, R. (2018). Salbutamol: palpitations: case report. *Reactions Weekly* 1719 (1): 211.

Wiffen, P., Mitchell, M., Snelling, M., and Stoner, N. (2017). *Oxford Handbook of Clinical Pharmacy*. Oxford: Oxford University Press.

de Wildt, S.N., Kearns, G.L., Leeder, J.S. et al. (1999). Glucuronidation in humans. Pharmacogenetic and developmental aspects. *Clinical Pharmacokinetics* 36: 439–452.

de Wildt, S.N., Johnson, T.N., and Choonara, I. (2003). The effect of age on drug metabolism. *Paediatric and Perinatal Drug Therapy* 5: 101–106.

Wyatt, J.P., Taylor, R.G., Wit, K., and Hotton, E.J. (2020). *Oxford Handbook of Emergency Medicine*. Oxford: Oxford University Press.

FURTHER READING

Barber, P. and Robertson, D. (2012). *Essentials of Pharmacology for Nurses*, 2e. Berkshire: Open University Press.

Brenner, G.M. and Stevens, C. (2017). *Pharmacology*, 5e. Philadelphia: Elsevier.

Eusuf, D.V. and Thomas, E. (2021). Pharmacokinetic variation. *Anaesthesia and Intensive Care Medicine*. 23 (1): 50–53.

Horne, R., Graupner, L., Frost, S. et al. (2004). Medicine in a multi-cultural society: the effect of cultural background on beliefs about medications. *Social Science and Medicine* 59 (6): 1307–1313.

Neal, M.J. (2012). *Medical Pharmacology at a Glance*. Chichester: Wiley.

Peck, T. and Harris, B. (2021). *Pharmacology for Anaesthesia and Intensive Care*, 5e. Cambridge: Cambridge University Press.

Rang, H.P., Dale, M.M., Ritter, J.M., and Flower, R.J. (2007). *Rang and Dale's Pharmacology*. Edinburgh.: Elsevier.

Wiffen, P., Mitchell, M., Snelling, M., and Stoner, N. (2017). *Oxford Handbook of Clinical Pharmacy*. Oxford: Oxford University Press.

SELF-ASSESSMENT QUESTIONS

1. Describe the four principles of the pharmacological process.
2. Describe the mechanisms by which drugs exert their actions.
3. Describe the formula commonly used to calculate estimated glomerular filtration rate and why this is an important factor when considering renal clearance of certain drug groups.
4. Name a national resource that may be used if drug toxicity is suspected.

GLOSSARY

Absolute drug contraindication   A drug interaction that can cause a life-threatening state.

Absorption   The uptake of a drug by the body.

Addiction   Drug-seeking behaviour despite negative consequences.

Additive effect   The overall consequence which is the result of two chemicals acting together and which is the simple sum of the effects of the chemicals acting independently.

Adverse drug reaction (ADR)   An unwanted or harmful reaction to a drug.

Affinity   The willingness of a drug to bind to its receptor.

Agonist   Drug action that causes a receptor to produce its intended response.

Antagonism   Opposing effects.

Antagonist   Drug action that inhibits a receptor from producing its intended response.

Bioavailability   The availability of a drug for distribution following first-pass metabolism when taken via the oral route.

Contraindication   Opposite to 'indication' where it is harmful to give a drug or carry out a procedure in certain specific circumstances.

Dependence   The presence of withdrawal symptoms when a drug is stopped.

Distribution   The mechanism of transport of a drug in the body.

Efficacy   The maximum effect that a drug can produce regardless of dose.

Elimination   The excretion of a drug from the body.

Half-life   The time taken for half of the administered drug to be eliminated from the body.

Metabolism   The breakdown of a drug by the body.

Overdose   The process of receiving more than the intended dose of a drug. Can be intentional or accidental.

Potency   Measure of the quantity of drug needed to produce a maximal effect (e.g. 2 mg vs 200 mg).

Pharmacodynamics   The study of biochemical and physiological effects of a drug on the body.

Pharmacokinetics   The study of how the body absorbs, distributes, metabolises and eliminates a drug.

Pharmacology   The study of the processes that occur between drugs and biological organisms.

Relative drug contraindication   When two or more drugs interact with each other that can potentially cause harm if the benefit outweighs the risk.

Serotonin   A neurotransmitter.

Synergism   Similar to additive effect but the combination of drugs has a significantly greater effect.

Tolerance   Decreased effect of a drug over time when the same dose is administered.

CHAPTER 7

Supplementary and Independent Prescribing

Brigitta Fazzini, Esther Clift, and Jill Bentley

Aim

The aim of this chapter is to introduce the reader to the core principles of prescribing for the advanced practitioner.

LEARNING OUTCOMES

After reading this chapter the reader will understand:

1. supplementary and independent prescribing with relevant legislation
2. prescribing in different fields of practice
3. special considerations including antibiotic stewardship and authorisation of blood components
4. principles of de-prescribing.

INTRODUCTION

Prescribing medications was traditionally limited to medical practitioners. However, this has since changed and Table 7.1 details the legislation timeline allowing other healthcare practitioners to become prescribers.

The Medicines Act 1968 introduced the authority to prescribe in statute and it was followed by the Misuse of Drugs Act 1971 acknowledging that medications have differing severity, with the possibility of harm and/or addiction. These legislative Acts laid the legal foundations for modern0day prescribing. In 1986, the Cumberlege Report reviewed delivery of community healthcare, highlighting streamlined

TABLE 7.1   Professionals' eligibility to become independent and supplementary prescribers (correct at time of publishing).

Independent Prescribers	Supplementary Prescribers
• Pharmacists • Physiotherapists • Podiatrists • Nurses • Midwives • Paramedics • Therapeutic radiographers	• Nurses • Midwives • Optometrists • Pharmacists • Physiotherapists • Podiatrists • Radiographers • Paramedics • Dietitians

services by removing needless steps in a patient's journey, freeing resources and improving patient experience. Multiple exchanges of information between community nurses and general practitioners were not necessary if community nurses could prescribe. A key recommendation was for nurses to prescribe certain medications, dressings and appliances. It took three years for these to become part of legislation in the Crown Report.

In 1994, the Pharmaceutical Services Regulation allowed community pharmacists to dispense prescriptions by authorised nurse prescribers The first non-medical prescribing courses arose from this training need. Pilot sites were set up in 1994 with national implementation in 1998. A further Crown Report that year, Parts 1 and 2, made significant changes. Part 1 reviewed the progress of implementation and safety, making recommendations for Patient Group Directions (PGDs), enabling limited use of medication in specific situations by specified staff and highlighting that much more could be done. Part 2 articulated the need for other professional groups with expertise in specialist areas to prescribe. It recommended training both independent and dependent prescribers, later becoming supplementary. This significant change gave prescribers responsibility for the assessment and treatment planning for patients. By 2001, the Health and Social Care Act set out the required legislation for some other allied health professionals (AHPs) and pharmacists to train as prescribers.

Supplementary prescribing is defined as a 'voluntary partnership between an independent prescriber (must be doctor/dentist) and a supplementary prescriber (nurse, pharmacist or AHP) to implement an agreed patient specific clinical management plan' (RCN 2022). Independent prescribers 'take responsibility for the clinical assessment of the patient, establishing a diagnosis and the clinical management required, as well as for prescribing where necessary and the appropriateness of any prescription' (RCN 2022) (Figure 7.1).

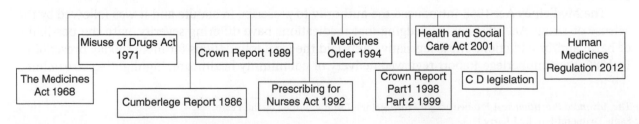

FIGURE 7.1   Key moments in prescribing – a timeline.

EDUCATION

Healthcare professionals who are legally eligible to undertake independent and/or supplementary prescribing need to undertake a specialist course at an accredited higher education institution (HEI). Entry requirements for these courses are governed by professional, statutory and regulatory bodies (PSRBs) requirements. These are organisations (for example, the Nursing and Midwifery Council) that work with HEIs on the approval, monitoring and review of programmes that lead to the professional qualification of independent and/or supplementary prescribing. Approved courses are aligned to the Royal Pharmaceutical Society's Competency Framework for all prescribers (RPS 2021).

Eligibility to become a registered independent or supplementary prescriber differs between professions (Table 7.1). Each regulatory body has its own entry requirements. On completion of the academic course, practitioners require a dedicated scope of practice to be able to prescribe in clinical areas.

Physiotherapists and paramedics are able to prescribe oral or injectable morphine, transdermal fentanyl and oral diazepam, dihydrocodeine tartrate, lorazepam, oxycodone hydrochloride or temazepam, with a key caveat of prescribing within their area of practice and their own competence. Discussions are well under way for extending the scope of practice to include other AHPs, but as this is a legal change, it is likely to be slow. However, this does not exclude other AHPs from undertaking full advanced practice accreditation. Some universities offer the same pharmacology training for AHPs which gives them the knowledge required to recommend and advise on medicines management, both prescribing and de-prescribing, but they are legally unable to register to write the script.

GENERAL PHARMACOLOGICAL PRINCIPLES

Pharmacology is the study of drugs, concentrating on the interactions with the human body, and is explored in detail in Chapter 6. As prescribers, it is essential that we do not just demonstrate a clear understanding of these principles but also can apply them to our prescribing practice. We need to be able to translate the actions of medicines into benefits for patients. Without understanding these key principles, we will not be able to determine how altered physiology affects our choice or dose of drug. Pharmacological principles are therefore taught as part of prescribing programmes and are integrated into the RPS Competency Framework for Prescribers (RPS 2021).

There are key special considerations within pharmacological principles that are discussed separately within the relevant sections of this chapter. For example, those relating to changes due to critical illness are discussed in the 'Prescribing in Critical Care' section of this chapter.

Prescribing in Paediatrics

It is important to emphasise that independent prescribers must work within their own level of professional competence and expertise regardless of professional background. Children present multiple challenges for prescribers and extra care should be taken when prescribing for neonates. Complex physiological and anatomical differences prove that they are not just small adults (Nuttall and Rutt-Howard 2020). They have altered pharmacokinetics and pharmacodynamics that affect absorption, metabolism, distribution and excretion of certain medications. Drugs are not extensively tested in children due to the ethics of clinical trials. As a result, many drugs used in this area remain unlicensed. The MHRA has clear guidance on the importance of reporting adverse reactions in children as well as adults utilising the Yellow Card system.

Dosages are often based on body weight but sometimes on age, depending on the drug. A good tool to know is the use of body surface area and also ideal body weight in obesity. It is recommended to check weight and height of children wherever possible. Doses should be calculated on an individual basis. Check the children's British National Formulary (BNFC) for the latest information if prescribing in the UK. Ages are classified as follows.

- Neonate – up to 28 days of life.
- Infant – up to 1 year of age.
- Child – up to 12 years of age However, children should be grouped by 1–5 years of age then 6–12 years of age.

Fields of Practice – Paediatrics

- Be extra vigilant for developmental differences in children of the same age.
- Principles of absorption in children under two are different from those of older children.
- When prescribing for children, it is important that prescribers be aware of excipients in the formulation they are prescribing. These can be associated with additional problems such as the presence of lactose for those who are intolerant (Nuttall and Rutt-Howard 2020).
- How does it taste? With children, there are additional considerations of appearance, taste and ease of administration.
- Regimes need to be simple and easy to follow with clear written instructions.

Prescribing in Mental Health

Fields of Practice – Mental Health and Examination Scenario

Deepak is an advanced practitioner in mental health who works in a dementia diagnosis clinic for older people. He assesses people with cognitive impairment to diagnose whether they are likely to have Alzheimer or mixed dementia and may benefit from a choline esterase inhibitor or a glutamate receptor antagonist. He undertakes a full physical assessment, including an ECG, to ensure the person is well enough to commence a new drug, and a full history and medication history to highlight any problematic interactions, before commencing them on a new drug. He will then monitor for any adverse effects, and to ensure efficacy of the pharmacological intervention. He will ensure concordance and understanding for the person, and manage family expectations.

Fields of Practice – Learning Disability, Mental Health and Paediatrics

STOMP (Stopping Overmedication of People with a learning disability, autism or both with psychotropic medicines) and STAMP (Supporting Treatment and Appropriate Medication in Paediatrics) are NHS England (2022a, 2022b) initiatives that should be considered when prescribing psychotropic medications in patients with a learning disability, autism or both.

Prescribing in Critical Care

Critical illness induces pathophysiological changes that cause significant alterations to drug pharmacokinetics and pharmacodynamics (PK-PD). Therapies designed to replace or support failing organs, including extracorporeal membrane oxygenation (ECMO) or renal replacement therapies (RRTs), affect drug PK-PD. The overall picture in critical illness is one of considerable PK-PD heterogeneity, which is highly dynamic with significant inter- and intraindividual variation.

Figure 7.2 describes the complex, dynamic interaction of critical illness-induced PK-PD changes. Numerous drugs used to support patients during critical illness can be titrated to a PD target (e.g. sedative and analgesic agents titrated to sedation and pain scores, or cardiovascular medicines titrated to haemodynamic goals).

Absorption

Absorption is dependent on drug bioavailability (F). Table 7.2 describes pathological changes observed in critical illness that affect absorption and bioavailability.

Distribution

Drug distribution occurs immediately after absorption into the systemic circulation and is dependent on patient, disease, drug and treatment/extracorporeal-related factors.

Table 7.3 summarises the changes of distribution during critical illness.

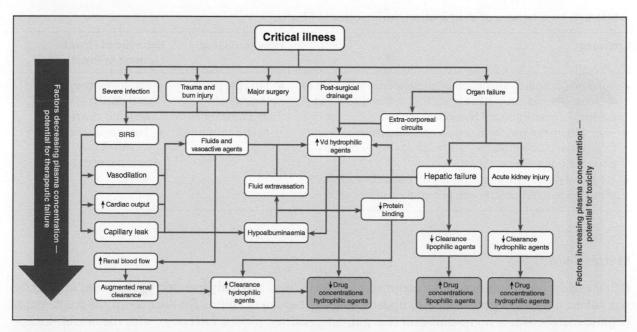

FIGURE 7.2   Critical illness-induced pharmacokinetic changes. SIRS, systemic inflammatory response syndrome. *Source*: Adapted from Blot et al. (2014).

TABLE 7.2   Pathological changes affecting absorption in critical illness.

Changes	How to Assess	Example of How to Manage These Changes
• Causes of decreased gastrointestinal blood flow can lead to ileus/enteral feed intolerance (i.e. from shock, sympathetic activation, lack of bolus feeding, vasopressin analogues and vasopressor administration, surgery, thromboembolic events or trauma) • Increased gastric pH can significantly reduce bioavailability of some medications • Nasojejunal feeding reduces bioavailability of medicine absorbed via duodenum • Increased GI transit time and delayed gastric emptying owing to high-dose opioids or alpha-2 agonist • Drug–enteral feed interaction resulting in reduced bioavailability (i.e. phenytoin, rifampicin). Calcium-containing medicines affect ciprofloxacin absorption	• Check nasogastric aspirate volume. If the gastric aspirate volume is less than gastric residual volume, this means that the content is passing the pylorus and facilitating absorption • Check for drug–drug interactions • Check site of absorption • Monitor for therapeutic effect • Review drug summary of product characteristics	• Consider interim parenteral administration of critical medicines (i.e. antimicrobials and antiepileptics) • Note differences in bioavailability (including first-pass elimination) between formulations and routes of administration (i.e. opioids, tacrolimus, antiepileptics, theophylline) • Transdermal administration may not be ideal as peripheral ischaemia can decrease bioavailability; in contrast, pyrexia may increase bioavailability and toxicity • Ensure appropriate use of drugs with narrow therapeutic index • Consider intravenous administration of medicines that require a break in enteral feeding

TABLE 7.3   Changes of distribution during critical illness.

Changes	How to Assess	Example of How to Manage in Practice
• Fluid resuscitation, vasodilation and capillary leak lead to increased apparent volume of distribution and reduced plasma concentration of hydrophilic drugs • Hypoalbuminaemia from sepsis and inflammation leads to increased free drug concentration for highly protein-bound drugs (i.e. phenytoin) • Reduced peripheral tissue perfusion secondary to shock state leads to reduced tissue penetration of free drug	• Vasopressor requirement and monitor for tissue oedema	• Higher loading dose and dosing in the first 48 h may be required • Therapeutic drug monitoring or calculated plasma levels

Metabolism

Renal and/or liver dysfunction are common in critical illness and daily monitoring is advised to mitigate risks of accumulation and toxicity, or underdosing and treatment failure. For the majority of drugs, extra-hepatic metabolism is non-significant (e.g. gut, lung, kidney, plasma esterases), with the notable exceptions of remifentanil (plasma esterase) and atracurium/cisatracurium. Table 7.4 summarises the changes of metabolism during critical illness.

TABLE 7.4   Changes of metabolism during critical illness.

Changes	How to Assess	Example of How to Manage in Practice
• Induction of hepatic enzymes by critical illness or drugs leading to increasing hepatic clearance of drugs with low hepatic extraction ratio • Inhibition of hepatic enzymes by critical illness or drugs leading to reduced hepatic clearance of drugs with low hepatic extraction ratio • Acute reduction in hepatic blood flow leading to reduced hepatic clearance of drugs with high hepatic extraction ratio	• Medication chart review, titration to effect and therapeutic drug monitoring	• Caution with narrow therapeutic index drugs • Titrate to effect or use therapeutic drug monitoring • Drugs such as propofol which have high hepatic extraction ratio are at high risk to cause adverse effects in shock

Excretion

Most drugs and metabolites are excreted or eliminated via the kidney. Acute kidney injury (AKI) is common in critical illness, and renal blood flow is a major contributing factor. Table 7.5 summarises the changes of excretion during critical illness.

CLINICAL INVESTIGATIONS

The NHS campaign 'Think Kidneys' provides useful resources regarding which investigations to utilise in the event of AKI: www.thinkkidneys.nhs.uk/aki/resources

---

Assessing Drug Therapy in Critical Illness

A conceptual framework can be used to assess the effects of critical illness on drug PK-PD and whether a change to pharmacotherapy is recommended, as summarised in Figure 7.3.

TABLE 7.5   Changes of excretion during critical illness.

Changes	How to Assess	Example of How to Manage in Practice
• Augmented renal clearance leading to increased clearance of renally eliminated drugs • AKI leading to reduced clearance of renally eliminated drugs • Renal replacement therapy leading to varied effects of clearance depending on the medication • Acute on chronic kidney injury –likely to have prolonged elimination	• Consider augmented renal clearance if eGFR>130 ml/min/1.73 m² • Consider urine creatinine collection if not on renal replacement therapy • Apply AKI classification	• Consider need for increasing • Consider therapeutic drug monitoring or decreased dosing (i.e. antibiotics) • Be aware of caveats regarding use of Cockcroft–Gault creatinine clearance formula in critical illness

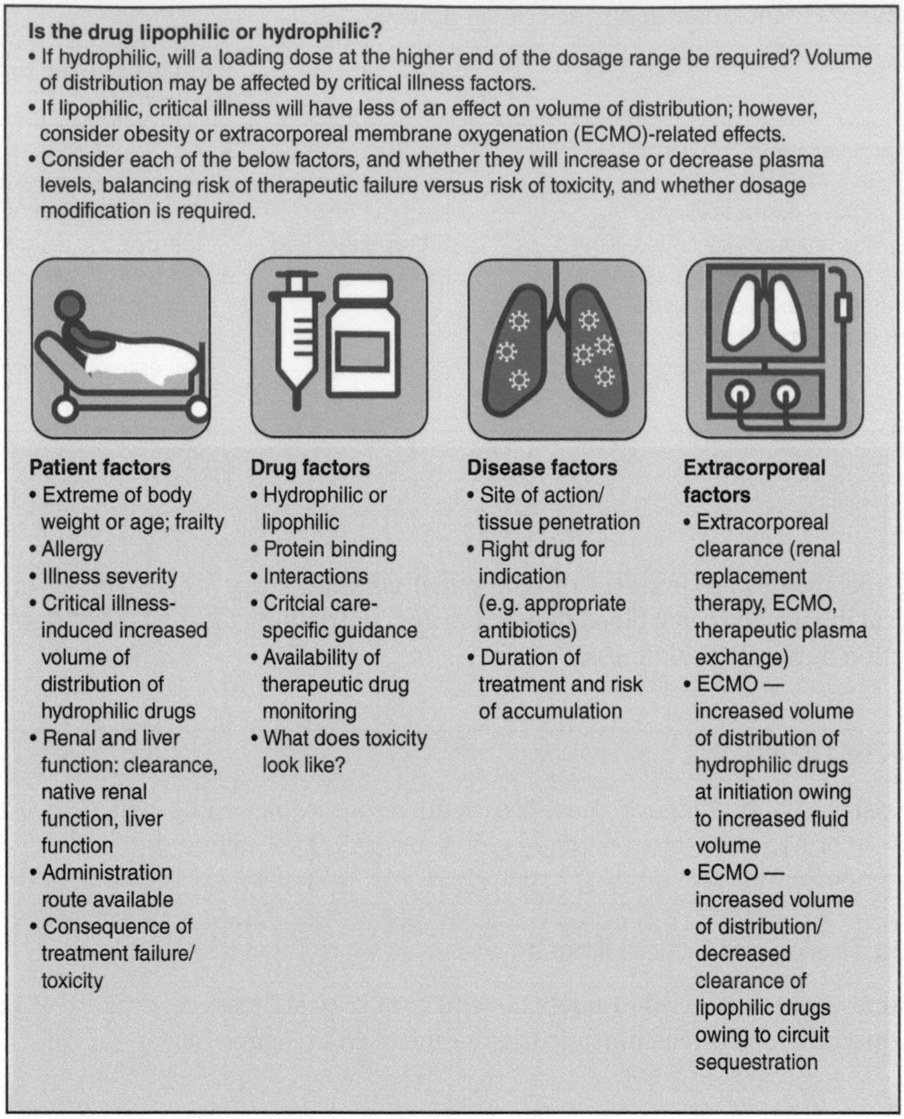

Is the drug lipophilic or hydrophilic?
- If hydrophilic, will a loading dose at the higher end of the dosage range be required? Volume of distribution may be affected by critical illness factors.
- If lipophilic, critical illness will have less of an effect on volume of distribution; however, consider obesity or extracorporeal membrane oxygenation (ECMO)-related effects.
- Consider each of the below factors, and whether they will increase or decrease plasma levels, balancing risk of therapeutic failure versus risk of toxicity, and whether dosage modification is required.

Patient factors	Drug factors	Disease factors	Extracorporeal factors
• Extreme of body weight or age; frailty • Allergy • Illness severity • Critical illness-induced increased volume of distribution of hydrophilic drugs • Renal and liver function: clearance, native renal function, liver function • Administration route available • Consequence of treatment failure/toxicity	• Hydrophilic or lipophilic • Protein binding • Interactions • Critical care-specific guidance • Availability of therapeutic drug monitoring • What does toxicity look like?	• Site of action/tissue penetration • Right drug for indication (e.g. appropriate antibiotics) • Duration of treatment and risk of accumulation	• Extracorporeal clearance (renal replacement therapy, ECMO, therapeutic plasma exchange) • ECMO — increased volume of distribution of hydrophilic drugs at initiation owing to increased fluid volume • ECMO — increased volume of distribution/decreased clearance of lipophilic drugs owing to circuit sequestration

FIGURE 7.3   Conceptual framework for assessing the influence of patient factors, drug factors, disease factors and extracorporeal factors. ECMO, extracorporeal membrane oxygenation.

Prescribing in Older People

Prescribing for older people, especially those living with frailty, requires specific consideration. Older people often receive multiple drugs for a number of long-term conditions, which greatly increases the risk of drug interactions and iatrogenic reactions. They may have multiple factors which make drug concordance problematic, such as practical administration or cognitive constraints.

Medication Reviews

Regular medications reviews for older people are encouraged in primary care to assess concordance and review medication regimes to ensure they are still beneficial.

Prophylactic medications may be deemed inappropriate as an underlying poor prognosis may outweigh any possible benefit. Older people should be offered and not denied medications which may be of benefit, such as anticoagulation, antiplatelets, antihypertensives, statins and osteoporosis interventions, but they should be fully consulted as to the purpose of the medication, and enabled to participate fully in the decision as to whether to take the medication or not, clearly sharing the decision around benefit and harm, and number needed to treat data. However, many of the drug trials undertaken to develop the evidence base for prescribing exclude older people, and specific trials for older people are scant.

Pharmacokinetics

It is important to consider the medicine form when prescribing in this area. Older people may struggle to swallow, so a clear understanding of the physical ability to swallow the prescribed medication should be established, or a liquid formulation offered instead. The principles of pharmacokinetics are also an important consideration as older people may experience significant changes in tissue concentration, especially those with severe frailty and renal impairment. A reduction in renal clearance leads to slower excretion and higher susceptibility to nephrotoxic drugs. This is often exacerbated by acute illness and dehydration which may radically transform a normally stable medication regime, for example digoxin, and result in a toxic dose. Older people also experience a reduction in liver volume which results in reduced hepatic metabolism of lipid-soluble drugs, which needs careful review for drugs with a narrow therapeutic window.

Examination Scenario

Prescribing and De-prescribing for Older People

Doris presents to you, an independent prescriber, having had two falls in the last week. She has not lost consciousness but she is fearful of falling again, so is no longer leaving the house.

    Past medical history: ischaemic heart disease, atrial fibrillation, gout and hypertension

Drug history:

    Aspirin 75 mg
    Bendroflumethiazide 5 mg mane
    Simvastatin 10 mg
    Codeine phosphate 30 mg QDS
    Amitriptyline 25 mg nocte

    What additional information might you want to know before de-prescribing?
    What drug would you reduce or discontinue first?

Answer:

    Check indication for codeine and amitriptyline but if no clear indication, reduce codeine; substitute paracetamol if renal function good, stop amitriptyline.
    Check eGFR and electrolytes and review fluid balance, lying and standing blood pressure, and heart function – oedema, JVP, before changing bendroflumethiazide but could reduce in discussion with heart failure team.

Guidelines on Drug Prescription for Older People

The following principles may be used as a guide when prescribing for this patient population.

1. Always consider first whether a drug is indicated at all, or if a non-pharmacological measure may be more appropriate for common symptoms such as headache, insomnia and dizziness. Try relaxation techniques, apps and sleep hygiene as well as Cawthorne Cooksey or Brandt-Darroff exercises for benign positional paroxysmal vertigo. Anxiety and depression may be better addressed with talking therapies, exercise and social prescribing.

2. 'Start low, go slow' – always commence any new medication on the lowest therapeutic dose, and titrate up incrementally.

3. Be thoroughly familiar with the evidence base for any medication which you are commencing for older people.

4. Review medications regularly, to ensure they are still indicated and any repeat prescriptions are being taken. Wasted medication is a significant burden to the NHS, and disposal has a significant environmental impact.

5. Simplify regimes where possible, if there are formal carers involved to support the older person or concordance may be problematic. A regime for twice-daily medication that is actually taken is better than prescribing four times daily and seeing many doses missed. If cognition is significantly impaired, consider requesting medication in a NOMAD or pod tray in conjunction with the pharmacy. There may be a cost to this. Alternative dispensing technology devices are available which can prompt medication to be taken within a specified window, but these often need to be loaded by a family member or carer (but can run for 28 days).

6. Always give very clear instructions for prescribed medication with the reason, as well as the directions, for taking the medication, so family and carers can support. This should be indicated clearly on every prescription, even repeats, to ensure that everyone is fully appraised of the purpose and intended reason for the prescription.

7. Ensure older people are very clear about requesting only required medications, and how to dispose of any untaken medication.

RED FLAGS – PATHOLOGICAL CONSIDERATIONS

Prescribing in Older People

The prescriber should proceed with caution when considering prescribing the following drug groups.

1. **Hypnotics**: benzodiazepines (such as diazepam, lorazepmam, etc.) but including non-benzo hypnotics, such as zopiclone, and antihistamines such as promethazine hydrochloride. These should be avoided because they have a long half-life, and often serious hangover effects such as drowsiness, unsteady gait and slurred speech with confusion. These may lead to increased falls risk and catastrophic functional change

2. **Non-steroidal anti-inflammatory drugs (NSAIDs)**: bleeding associated with aspirin and NSAIDs is more common in older people, with potentially fatal outcomes. A short course of low-dose NSAID should only be offered after considering non-pharma analgesia, such as

heat pads, mobility aids for short-term support and appropriately prescribed exercise such as stretching. Counselling for weight loss may also be appropriate.

3. **Diuretics** are often overprescribed for older people, and should not be prescribed for dependent oedema without ensuring an exercise regime and positional pumping or support stockings are used appropriately first.

4. **Warfarin** should be actively de-prescribed in older people and alternative oral anticoagulation sought, as often the intensity of monitoring and titrating warfarin is an unnecessary burden for older people.

Other drugs which cause adverse reactions include **antihypertensives** and **parkinsonian drugs**.

Antibiotics Stewardship

Antimicrobial resistance is a global heath emergency. Antimicrobial drug development is challenging and costly; improving antibiotic prescribing is critical to effectively treat infections, protect patients from harms caused by unnecessary antibiotic use, prevent and combat antibiotic resistance, and improve patient outcomes. Antibiotic stewardship is the effort to measure and improve how antibiotics are prescribed by clinicians and used by patients. This has been defined as 'the optimal selection, dosage, and duration of antimicrobial treatment that results in the best clinical outcome for the treatment or prevention of infection, with minimal toxicity to the patient and minimal impact on subsequent resistance' (Gerding 2001).

There are three goals of antimicrobial stewardship.

1. *Prescribe the most appropriate antimicrobial agent with the correct dose and duration.* This can be done following the 4 Ds approach for optimal antimicrobial therapy: right **D**rug, right **D**ose, **D**e-escalation to pathogen-directed therapy, and right **D**uration of therapy.

2. *Prevent antimicrobial overuse, misuse and abuse.* Both in the hospital setting and the outpatient community; antibiotics are often prescribed when not entirely necessary. Abuse of antibiotics is more difficult to define, but the term might be used to describe the use of one particular antibiotic preferentially over others by a practitioner as a result of aggressive detailing by the pharmaceutical representative or, worse, because of financial interest.

3. *Minimise the development of resistance.* Patients exposed to antibiotics are at higher risk of becoming colonised or infected by resistant organisms. A primary focus is prevention of the indiscriminate use of broad-spectrum antibiotics. The rationale for this strategy is twofold. First, broad-spectrum antibiotics, as well as being effective against a wide range of bacteria, are also frequently active against multidrug-resistant (MDR) bacteria and must be held in reserve for when they are genuinely needed. Antimicrobial resistance is associated with increased morbidity and mortality, excess duration of hospital stay, and significant hospital and societal costs. Second, broad-spectrum agents cause extensive destruction of normal commensal flora, thereby compromising host immune function and rendering patients vulnerable to opportunist pathogens such as MRSA and *Clostridium difficile*. The importance of this is increasingly recognised, as the presence of the human microbiota interferes with colonisation by potential pathogens by depletion of nutrients, production of enzymes and toxic metabolites, and modulation of the innate immune response. These resistant organisms can become transmitted to other individuals within the hospital or in the patient's community.

All practitioners who prescribe antibiotics have a responsibility to their patients and for public health to prescribe optimally. Guidance for effective antibiotic prescribing includes the following 10 steps.

1. Consider each case individually and institute antibiotic treatment immediately in patients with life-threatening infection.
2. Prescribe in accordance with local policies and guidelines, avoiding broad-spectrum agents when possible.
3. Clearly document the indication for prescribing antibiotics in the clinical notes.
4. Send appropriate specimens to the microbiology laboratory (i.e. the common septic panel would include blood, urine and sputum cultures) and consider additional sources of infection which are not visible. Consider source control and if indicated, drain pus and remove foreign bodies.
5. Use antimicrobial susceptibility data to de-escalate, substitute and add agents, and to switch from intravenous to oral therapy.
6. Prescribe the shortest antibiotic course likely to be effective.
7. Always select agents to minimise collateral damage (i.e. selection of multiresistant bacteria).
8. Monitor antibiotic drug levels when relevant (i.e. vancomycin, amikacin, gentamicin).
9. Use single-dose antibiotic prophylaxis wherever possible.
10. Consult the local microbiology team or infection experts for early advice on treatment and management.

At the organisational level, stewardship refers to evidence-based programmes and interventions to monitor and direct antimicrobial use. Table 7.6 summarises examples of antibiotic stewardship interventions commonly deployed in hospitals.

TABLE 7.6   Examples of antibiotic stewardship interventions commonly deployed in hospitals.

Intervention	Example

Governance structures	• Organisational strategy for antibiotic stewardship
	 • Antibiotic prescribing policy which may include:
	   – 48 h review
	   – Intravenous to oral switch
	   – Automatic stop order
	   – Compulsory order forms
	   – Expert approval
	   – Dedicated antibiotic prescription chart
	   – Removal by restriction
	   – Therapeutic substitution
	   – Antibiotic cycling and rotation policy
	 • Antibiotic stewardship committee

Operational delivery	• Antibiotic formulary • Guidelines for initial treatment of common infections • Guidelines for perioperative prophylaxis for common surgical procedures • Reminder systems • Computerised order entry • Mobile device software application for point-of-care information and guidance

TABLE 7.6 (Continued)

Intervention	Example
Risk management	• Guidelines for management of infection in patients with allergy to antibiotics • Information on safe administration • Guidelines for dosing and monitoring serum levels of toxic antibiotics
Clinical microbiology/infectious disease specialist and laboratory support	• Validation and interpretation of microscopy, culture and susceptibility results for laboratory reporting • Surveillance and reporting of trends in antibiotic resistance • Telephone consultation for advice on infection management • Bacteraemia follow-up service • Antibiotic stewardship ward rounds • Point-of-care rapid test for bacterial infection • Advanced sepsis biomarkers (i.e. procalcitonin)
Controls and quality assurance	• Surveillance of antibiotic prescribing trends • Public reporting and benchmarking of antibiotics consumption data (i.e. who doses) • Audit and feedback of adherence to prescribing policies/guidelines
Education and training	• Induction training on antibiotics stewardship • Revalidation training • Distribution of printed educational materials • Educational meeting and electronic learning • Nominated clinical champions for antimicrobial stewardship • Provision of patient information and counselling

Authorisation of Blood Components and Products

The Blood Safety and Quality Regulations (2005) define blood components as 'a therapeutic constituent of blood', i.e. whole blood, red blood cells, platelets, fresh frozen plasma (FFP) (excluding Octaplas™), cryoprecipitate and granulocytes. Blood components are excluded from the legal definition of medicinal products and therefore must be 'authorised' rather than 'prescribed'. Blood products are produced by pharmaceutical processes, are classed as medicines, must be prescribed, and are covered by the Medicines Act (1968). Examples of blood products include prothrombin complex concentrate (PCC) (Octaplex®, Beriplex®), solvent detergent FFP (SDFFP) (Octaplas) and albumin.

LEGAL ASPECTS AND GOVERNANCE

There are no legal barriers to any appropriately trained, competent, locally designated and approved registered regulated healthcare professional being able to authorise blood component administration. Specific recommendations are in place and advanced clinical practitioners should follow the British Society for Haematology guidelines, key points of which are summarised below.

1. The practitioner's decision to transfuse must be based on a thorough clinical assessment of the patient and his or her individual needs, including an evaluation of the patient's age, body weight, symptoms and concomitant medical conditions, and documented in the patient's clinical record.

2. All public or private healthcare organisations involved in the transfusion of blood components should implement the recommendations on patient consent from the General Medical Council and the Advisory Committee on the Safety of Blood Tissues and Organs.

3. Blood components should only be authorised by an appropriately trained, competent and locally designated healthcare practitioner.

4. Advanced clinical practitioners wishing to prescribe transfusion of blood, platelets, fresh frozen plasma, cryoprecipitate or anti-D immunoglobulins should include this as part of their prescribing scope of practice. Practitioners must have up-to-date mandatory trust blood transfusion training and are required to renew their training accreditation before it expires (at least every two years). Local trusts may also require completion of the non-medical authorisation course from NHS Blood and Transfusion; therefore, practitioners should refer to their local supplementary and independent prescribing policy within the trust or healthcare institution.

5. Practitioners should not prescribe transfusion of blood, platelets, fresh frozen plasma, cryoprecipitate or anti-D immunoglobulins if this is not specified within their scope of practice. Specifically, this should be also in liaison with the parent team.

6. There are no special training requirements for non-medical prescribers wishing to include normal immunoglobulins, albumin or recombinant blood products (e.g. erythropoietin, factor VIII) in their scope of practice.

Patient Consent

An informed and valid consent should be obtained for all patients (adults or children) prior to authorisation/prescription and administration. Consent should be documented in the clinical record and when it is not possible to gain consent (i.e. unconscious patients or in emergency scenarios), the clinical documentation should highlight best interest as per the Mental Capacity Act (2005).

Clinical practitioners not familiar with consent can find guidance on obtaining consent for blood and blood components transfusion from the Advisory Committee on the Safety of Blood Tissues and Organs. These principles apply for adults and children. Additional standardised information resources indicating the key issues to be discussed when obtaining valid consent from a patient for a blood transfusion are also available online and leaflets can be printed for patients. This guideline does not intend to provide specific guidance related to the intricacies of consent or treatment refusal and this should be assessed as a specific individual case with a holistic approach. Local policies detailing specific actions should be followed and alternative treatment options such as erythropoietin, intravenous and oral iron supplementation, cell salvage and tranexamic acid can be offered if appropriate.

Clinical Decision Making

Clinical decision-making algorithms should be implemented locally to decide whether a patient needs transfusion of blood products. The key six steps are as follows.

1. Consider if the patient needs a blood transfusion.
2. Consider if alternatives to blood transfusion could be an option.

3. Identify the appropriate component/product to be transfused. Specific guidelines/local protocol must be in place regarding:
   - major haemorrhage
   - acute coronary syndrome
   - sickle cell disease
   - regular bloods transfusion in chronic anaemia
   - autoimmune/immunological compromise and thrombocytopenia.
     In these cases, careful advice and support from senior specialists should be followed as well as use of thromboelastogram and its adequate interpretation.
4. Obtain appropriate verbal or written consent from the patient and/or carer or family.
5. Follow the recommendation for each component/product based on the specific clinical situation.
6. Monitor the patient for any adverse reaction.

DE-PRESCRIBING

De-prescribing is the planned process of reducing or stopping medications that may no longer be of benefit or may be causing harm. The goal is to reduce medication burden or harm while improving quality of life. Best practice is for all prescribers to undertake a medicine review during consultations. De-prescribing is often well received by patients with changes being made between 72% and 91% cases (Ibrahim et al. 2021).

Polypharmacy is often defined as taking five or more medications (Masnoon et al. 2017), but these medications may all be indicated and efficacious, so a more nuanced approach is needed. De-prescribing becomes urgent when symptoms change or when the goal of treatment changes, for example when approaching end of life.

Approximately 30% of admissions to hospital for older people are due to adverse medicine responses. This causes a significant burden to the health system, but also can cause serious harm to older people.

There are numerous validated tools for de-prescribing and every advanced practitioner should use the most appropriate validated tool in their area of specialism. Commonly used tools include the Beers criteria or STOPP (Screening Tool of Older Peoples Prescriptions), an explicit tool to facilitate medication review in multi-morbid older people (www.bgs.org.uk/resources/6-cga-in-primary-care-settings-medication-review), or the shorter NO TEARS mnemonic which was designed to review medication in primary care.

- **N**eed and indication
- **O**pen questions
- **T**ests and monitoring
- **E**vidence and guidelines
- **A**dverse events
- **R**isk reduction or prevention
- **S**implification and switches

HEALTH PROMOTION

As healthcare providers, we are in a unique position to support public health agendas, ideally placed to educate in relation to health promotion and to introduce and support the concept of well-being. We can also highlight health inequalities and tackle these head on. Health is about our social well-being, our physical and mental health so we should be trying to support all of these, not just treating physical disease when it occurs.

ORANGE FLAGS – PSYCHOLOGICAL CONSIDERATIONS

Health promotion is the process of enabling people to increase control over and to improve their health, using behaviour change models and techniques based in psychology to ensure change is delivered effectively and sustained. Health promotion considers the population as whole, enhancing health beliefs and taking action to change. There is a real emphasis on behaviour change to empower individuals to take responsibility, focusing on self-care and lifestyle, not just taking medicines. A large portion of our role involves review and de-prescribing as much as prescribing. The management of complex health conditions involves more of a holistic approach to health needs.

Why is This Important to Us as Prescribers?

Health inequalities continue to be apparent, highlighted in recent times by the pandemic that hit in 2020. Although life expectancy has risen, so has the number of people living with long-term diseases. Mortality remains higher in men and regional variations continue in terms of morbidity and mortality.

Health promotion by care providers relies on them having sufficient knowledge of health inequality, government targets for health and what local policies/agendas are in place. Moving beyond clinical assessment and understanding the wider context of healthcare factors will directly affect health. The challenge remains not to lose the individual in all this, to carefully balance the benefit for the patient versus society as a whole. This is evident when prescribing antimicrobials, for example.

GREEN FLAGS – SOCIAL CONSIDERATIONS

Wider social factors include access to medicines and supportive care. The escalating cost implications of prescriptions are also key factors that affect public health on a large scale.

As health professionals, we should always strive to improve practice and the care we deliver. Empowering those around us to be more autonomous with their health will ensure a valuable commodity remains available to those who need it, when they need it.

So What Can We Do?

All health professionals have multiple interactions daily with members of the public and as prescribers we are able to monitor the health state of others. Our consultations provide a holistic picture of the individuals we see. Therefore, we consider health much more broadly and utilise risk screening tools in our daily practice. As prescribers, we build a rapport with the patient, families and carers to ensure they feel comfortable to disclose and engage. This requires strong communication skills and expertise at handling sensitive conversations.

This is linked to the knowledge of the prescribers. You will need knowledge of the activities that help individuals but also understanding of the wider factors that affect individuals to engage with these activities. Making Every Contact Count (MECC) is a Health Education England initiative using local providers to support people with making positive changes to their mental and physical health. It partners with multiple agencies at all levels to support providers in this, focusing on the links between behaviour factors and long-term disease processes and through clinicians' trusted relationships often built up over multiple interactions.

MECC focuses on the lifestyle issues that, when addressed, can make the greatest improvement to an individual's health.

- Stopping smoking
- Drinking alcohol only within the recommended limits
- Healthy eating
- Being physically active
- Keeping to a healthy weight
- Improving mental health and well-being

It follows a simple 4 As approach to consultations to tackle these areas.

- ASK – about mental health, smoking, alcohol intake, activity levels and diet.
- ASSESS – the impact of these on the individual's health and risk factors.
- ADVISE – offer support, educate why these changes will bring benefits, encourage a willingness to change.
- ASSIST – consider referral to other services and information in a format suitable to the individual.

SOCIAL PRESCRIBING

Social prescribing is defined as a community referral, which recognises that people's health and well-being are determined by a range of social, economic and environmental factors. Social prescribing is designed to support people with a wide range of social, emotional or practical needs. Some schemes focus more on health and well-being and others on loneliness and social isolation. Most schemes involve a local link worker, often in primary care (care navigator, community connector or health advisor) who may be able to link in with a wide variety of local, formal or third sector groups or activities. There is a growing evidence base for improved outcomes for anxiety and social isolation from these interventions. The rise of isolation and loneliness has only been exacerbated with the COVID-19 pandemic, and there is strong evidence for worse health outcomes for those who are lonely and isolated, with significantly higher morbidity and mortality rates.

The NHS Long Term Plan (2019) incorporated social prescribing as part of the comprehensive model of personalised care, and for advanced practitioners in any sphere of practice, there is a need to understand and integrate appropriately with colleagues and support systems for patients in our care. Care navigators will have a good understanding of local provision for lunch clubs, exercise groups and accessible spiritual resources, which is invaluable and often rapidly changing.

CONCLUSION

Advanced clinical practitioners have a solid legislative ground which allows them to prescribe safely for patients. Practitioners must undertake a dedicated academic course and be registered with their regulatory body in order to prescribe effectively. Practitioners must prescribe within their scope of practice, be able to undertake patient assessment and test interpretation, be updated with evidence and have governance in place. Safe and effective prescribing allows timely treatment initiation for patients as well as discontinuation of unnecessary medications.

Take Home Points

- AP prescribers need to be aware of the special considerations when prescribing in certain groups such as the critically ill and elderly due to altered physiology.
- Variations due to professional backgrounds mean AP prescribers must have extensive knowledge of legislation around what and how they can prescribe and ensure they are up to date with changes to legislation.
- Early identification of scope of practice and supervision to extend this is key to new prescribers.

REFERENCES

Blood Safety and Quality Regulations (BSQR) (2005). Statutory Instrument 2005/50. www.opsi.gov.uk/si/si2005/20050050.htm

Blot, S.I., Pea, F., and Lipman, J. (2014). The effect of pathophysiology on pharmacokinetics in the critically ill patient – concepts appraised by the example of antimicrobial agents. *Advanced Drug Delivery Reviews* 77: 3–11.

Gerding, D.N. (2001). The search for good antimicrobial stewardship. *Joint Commission Journal on Quality Improvement* 27 (8): 403–404.

Ibrahim, K., Cox, N., Stevenson, J. et al. (2021). A systematic review of the evidence for deprescribing interventions among older people living with frailty. *BMC Geriatrics* 21: 258.

Masnoon, N., Shakib, S., Kalisch-Ellett, L. et al. (2017). What is polypharmacy? A systematic review of definitions. *BMC Geriatrics* 17: 230.

NHS (2019). The NHS Long Term Plan. www.longtermplan.nhs.uk/wp-content/uploads/2019/08/nhs-long-term-plan-version-1.2.pdf

NHS England (2022a). Stopping over medication of people with a learning disability, autism or both (STOMP). www.england.nhs.uk/learning-disabilities/improving-health/stomp/

NHS England (2022b). Supporting Treatment and Appropriate Medication in Paediatrics (STAMP). www.england.nhs.uk/learning-disabilities/improving-health/stamp/

Nuttall, D. and Rutt-Howard, J. (2020). *The Textbook of Non-Medical Prescribing*. Chichester: Wiley Blackwell.

Royal College of Nursing (2022). Types of nurse prescriber. www.rcn.org.uk/get-help/rcn-advice/non-medical-prescribers

Royal Pharmaceutical Society (2021). Prescribing Competency Framework. www.rpharms.com/resources/frameworks/prescribers-competency-framework

FURTHER READING

Gangannagaripalli, J., Porter, I., and Davey, A. (2021). STOPP/START interventions to improve medicines management. *Health Services and Delivery Research* 9 (23).

Masnoon, N., Shakib, S., Kalisch-Ellett, L. et al. (2017). What is polypharmacy? A systematic review of definitions. *BMC Geriatrics* 17: 230.

www.bgs.org.uk/resources/6-cga-in-primary-care-settings-medication-review

www.longtermplan.nhs.uk/

SELF-ASSESSMENT QUESTIONS

1. How will I evidence that I continue to maintain competency in prescribing?
2. Do you know the difference between independent and supplementary prescribers?
3. Can non-medical prescribers authorise blood and blood products?

GLOSSARY

Extracorporeal membrane oxygenation (ECMO)   The use of a modified heart–lung machine to provide respiratory, circulatory, or both support within critical care or a perioperative environment.

Hydrophilic drug   A drug which has the ability to dissolve in water.

Independent prescribing   Independent prescribers 'take responsibility for the clinical assessment of the patient, establishing a diagnosis and the clinical management required, as well as for prescribing where necessary and the appropriateness of any prescription'.

Lipophilic drug   A drug which has the ability to dissolve in a lipid-containing medium.

Lipophilicity   An important physicochemical property of a drug that contributes to absorption, distribution, metabolism, excretion and toxicity.

Patient Group Directions   Allow healthcare professionals to supply and administer specified medicines to predefined groups of patients, without a prescription. Further information can be accessed here: www.nice.org.uk/guidance/mpg2/chapter/recommendations#using-patient-group-directions

Plasma esterases   Enzymes of drug metabolism.

Social prescribing   A community referral, which recognises that people's health and well-being are determined by a range of social, economic and environmental factors.

Supplementary prescribing   Supplementary prescribing is defined as a 'voluntary partnership between an independent prescriber (must be doctor/dentist) and a supplementary prescriber (nurse, pharmacist or AHP) to implement an agreed patient specific clinical management plan'.

Vasopressor   A drug which causes the constriction of blood vessels.

CHAPTER 8

Core Procedural Skills

Mark Cannan, Kirstin Geer, and Stuart Cox

Aim

The aim of this chapter is to identify the core, more advanced procedural skills in the context of advanced clinical practice. It is not to replace local agreed practice or guide infection prevention.

LEARNING OUTCOMES

After reading this chapter the reader will be able to:

1. identify consideration for obtaining consent for procedures in advanced clinical practice
2. identify core procedural skills for advanced practice using an ABCDE approach
3. identify that procedural success requires application of assessment, clinical skills and clear communication as well as technical skills.

INTRODUCTION

Clinical procedures play a vital role in a patient's healthcare journey. They aid in diagnosis, provide access, enable monitoring and allow therapeutic (sometimes life-saving) interventions, thereby attempting to improve the clinical situation. What was typically a 'doctor's role' is now being undertaken by the advanced practitioner throughout the United Kingdom in primary, secondary and tertiary care. The approach, application and follow-up of clinical procedures are multifaceted and not just limited to knowledge, technical skills and dexterity. It should encompass ethics, consent, physiological and

The Advanced Practitioner: A Framework for Practice, First Edition. Edited by Ian Peate, Sadie Diamond-Fox, and Barry Hill.
© 2024 John Wiley & Sons Ltd. Published 2024 by John Wiley & Sons Ltd.

psychological considerations. This clinical procedures chapter will give the advanced practitioner the knowledge and understanding of common clinical procedures to provide a foundation which can be built upon in clinical practice in a supervised and independent manner.

CONSENT/ASSENT

Consent is a key responsibility for advanced practitioners, and links most closely to the pillar of clinical practice. Advanced practitioners are a resource for information and ideally placed to provide meaningful discussion with patients to facilitate informed consent and should take a proactive approach in engaging patients with effective consent processes (Farmer 2017). The practitioner administering treatment is the person responsible for seeking consent and should have the knowledge and skills to explain the procedure, including any risks (Dennhey and White 2012). If adequate information is not provided, consequences could potentially include litigation (Farmer 2017). The information patients require to make an informed decision are the risks and benefits of the procedure/investigation, hazards, potential outcomes positive and negative as well as alternative options (Farmer 2017).

The Mental Capacity Act (2005) is designed to protect and empower patients who lack capacity and provides clear instructions for practitioners to follow to uphold this. Capacity assessment must be based on the patient's ability to make a specific decision at a specific time.

To be deemed to have capacity, the patient needs to be able to:

- understand information given to them relevant to the decision
- retain information long enough to make the decision
- use or weigh up the information as part of the decision-making process
- communicate their decision (DoH 2009).

If a patient lacks capacity, the treating clinician can make best interest treatment decisions. However, consideration must not just be based on medical issues but be non-discriminatory and consider the patient's known wishes previously expressed to relatives or other third parties (Dennhey and White 2012).

Advanced practitioners should have an awareness of legal aspects of consent, including advanced decision making, living wills, power of attorney and the role of the independent mental capacity advocate (IMCA). IMCAs should be involved in decisions regarding serious medical treatment where no one other than paid healthcare professionals is available (DoH 2009). NICE (2018) provides guidance for managing these situations.

Fields of Practice – Mental Health

The Royal College of Psychiatrists provides useful resources regarding assessing capacity in individuals with mental illnesses: www.rcpsych.ac.uk/mental-health/treatments-and-wellbeing/mental-capacity-and-the-law

Fields of Practice – Learning Disabilities and Autism

The University of Hertfordshire provides an list of resources surrounding obtaining consent from those with a learning disability and autism: www.herts.ac.uk/intellectualdisability/how-to-guides/articles/consent-and-people-with-an-intellectual-disability-the-basics-2021

Fields of Practice – Paediatrics

The Care Quality Commission published a useful guide for assessing capacity and competence in patients under the age of 18years: www.cqc.org.uk/sites/default/files/Brief_guide_Capacity_and_consent_in_under_18s%20v3.pdf

---

GREEN FLAGS – SOCIAL CONSIDERATIONS

Critical to informed consent is ensuring that sufficient information has been given to the patient to ensure they understand the procedure. Practitioners should be mindful of the Equality Act 2010 (UK Government 2010) and make reasonable adjustments, particularly when sharing written information to patients, to ensure patients are not being discriminated against because of a protected characteristic.

CLINICAL COMPETENCE FOR PROCEDURES

Clinical competence refers to the practitioner's ability to undertake the procedure in a safe manner, having undergone sufficient education and training pertinent to the procedure. Gone are the days of 'see one, do one, teach one'. Education for acquisition of clinical skills should include theory, practice and simulation. Procedure-specific physiology and pathophysiology, equipment, technique and postprocedure safety checks should be included as well as the consenting processes. Certain skills will be utilised in multiple procedures, such as asepsis and safe administration of local anaesthetic.

Healthcare practitioners are bound by the ethics of non-maleficence (to do no harm), but many procedures that are part of the advanced practitioner role can have serious consequences, including patient death, if not conducted appropriately and proficiently. According to Nutbeam and Daniels (2010), each new practical procedure competency, such as intravenous cannulation, requires a minimum of 30 episodes before the psychomotor process is learned, and the greater the difficulty of the process (e.g. central venous catheterisation), the greater the number of performances required (50–80) before an adequate level of failure/complication rate (5%) is reached, thus allowing the practitioner to navigate procedure-relevant complications safely. A logbook is a good way of keeping track and identifying gaps in practice so that either simulation practice or more supervision in practice by your education/practice supervisor can be sought, which can also allow opportunities for individual assessment.

PREPARATION: POSITIONING

Preparation prior to any procedure is just as important as carrying out the procedure itself, and if done incorrectly, can lead to increased stress levels and frustration for both the patient and the staff involved and may lead to procedural complications/errors. Ensuring all the necessary equipment is available (including back-up equipment in case the procedure does not go as planned) and that the user is competent and familiar in its use are paramount. If the procedure requires specimen analysis or postprocedure checks, consideration must be taken for external teams such as laboratory staff and radiology. However, a caveat to preparation is the urgency with which the procedure is required such as emergency life-saving interventions. Kit boxes for specific procedures such as central venous catheters and chest drains can save time but robust restocking and checking systems must be in place.

Correct patient positioning and practitioner ergonomics are directly related to procedural success (Hughes and Mardell 2009). The purpose of positioning the patient is to maximise first-time success whilst not distorting the patient's anatomy. Each procedure will have its own recommended patient position. Likewise, the ergonomics of the practitioner undertaking the procedure needs to be comfortable and natural; if they are straining, this will detract the practitioner's attention from the job at hand. Consideration must be given to additional technical equipment such as ultrasound machines or video screens, which ideally should be placed within the practitioner's line of sight and be an extension of the operative field.

In 2015, NHS England produced a National Safety Standard for Invasive Procedures (NatSSIP) to improve patient safety. These NatSSIPs were intended to be the foundation on which local hospital trusts could then develop Local Safety Standards for Invasive Procedures (LocSSIP), specific to the individual trust, taking into account human factors, communication and team working and thus harmonising practice across the organisation such that patients undergoing invasive procedures receive a consistent approach (NHS England 2015). This was initiated on the background of the World Health Organization's (WHO) Safer Surgical Checklist (Figure 8.1) initiative which provided multiple checkpoints in which numerous questions were asked specific to patient safety, and as a result, reduced intraoperative errors. These LocSSIPs/NatSSIPs were intended to improve multidisciplinary team working and communication, both of which are paramount in safe practice.

World Health Organization

SURGICAL SAFETY CHECKLIST (FIRST EDITION)

Before induction of anaesthesia ▶▶▶▶▶▶▶▶▶	Before skin incision ▶▶▶▶▶▶▶▶▶▶▶▶	Before patient leaves operating room
SIGN IN	**TIME OUT**	**SIGN OUT**
☐ **PATIENT HAS CONFIRMED** • IDENTITY • SITE • PROCEDURE • CONSENT ☐ **SITE MARKED/NOT APPLICABLE** ☐ **ANAESTHESIA SAFETY CHECK COMPLETED** ☐ **PULSE OXIMETER ON PATIENT AND FUNCTIONING** **DOES PATIENT HAVE A:** **KNOWN ALLERGY?** ☐ NO ☐ YES **DIFFICULT AIRWAY/ASPIRATION RISK?** ☐ NO ☐ YES, AND EQUIPMENT/ASSISTANCE AVAILABLE **RISK OF >500 ML BLOOD LOSS (7 ML/KG IN CHILDREN)?** ☐ NO ☐ YES, AND ADEQUATE INTRAVENOUS ACCESS AND FLUIDS PLANNED	☐ **CONFIRM ALL TEAM MEMBERS HAVE INTRODUCED THEMSELVES BY NAME AND ROLE** ☐ **SURGEON, ANAESTHESIA PROFESSIONAL AND NURSE VERBALLY CONFIRM** • PATIENT • SITE • PROCEDURE **ANTICIPATED CRITICAL EVENTS** ☐ **SURGEON REVIEWS:** WHAT ARE THE CRITICAL OR UNEXPECTED STEPS, OPERATIVE DURATION, ANTICIPATED BLOOD LOSS? ☐ **ANAESTHESIA TEAM REVIEWS:** ARE THERE ANY PATIENT-SPECIFIC CONCERNS? ☐ **NURSING TEAM REVIEWS:** HAS STERILITY (INCLUDING INDICATOR RESULTS) BEEN CONFIRMED? ARE THERE EQUIPMENT ISSUES OR ANY CONCERNS? **HAS ANTIBIOTIC PROPHYLAXIS BEEN GIVEN WITHIN THE LAST 60 MINUTES?** ☐ YES ☐ NOT APPLICABLE **IS ESSENTIAL IMAGING DISPLAYED?** ☐ YES ☐ NOT APPLICABLE	**NURSE VERBALLY CONFIRMS WITH THE TEAM:** ☐ **THE NAME OF THE PROCEDURE RECORDED** ☐ **THAT INSTRUMENT, SPONGE AND NEEDLE COUNTS ARE CORRECT** (OR NOT APPLICABLE) ☐ **HOW THE SPECIMEN IS LABELLED** (INCLUDING PATIENT NAME) ☐ **WHETHER THERE ARE ANY EQUIPMENT PROBLEMS TO BE ADDRESSED** ☐ **SURGEON, ANAESTHESIA PROFESSIONAL AND NURSE REVIEW THE KEY CONCERNS FOR RECOVERY AND MANAGEMENT OF THIS PATIENT**

THIS CHECKLIST IS NOT INTENDED TO BE COMPREHENSIVE. ADDITIONS AND MODIFICATIONS TO FIT LOCAL PRACTICE ARE ENCOURAGED.

FIGURE 8.1 Surgical safety checklist (1st edition). *Source*: Lister et al. (2021) The Royal Marsden Manual of Clinical Nursing Procedures. Wiley-Blackwell.

ORANGE FLAGS – PSYCHOLOGICAL CONSIDERATIONS: PREPARATION FOR PROCEDURES

The psychological preparation of patients via the supplying of information, cognitive coping strategies, relaxation and hypnosis, reassurance and support, and rehearsal has been shown to have postoperative benefits (Powell et al. 2016). These benefits extended to a reduction of postoperative pain, enhanced behavioural recovery, reduced negative effects of an operation and reduced length of stay. It is recommended that all aspects of procedures are fully explained to patients to allow them to prepare psychologically.

Practitioners should have an awareness of how human factors may affect clinical performance; this can include equipment, workspace, organisational culture and fatigue (Catchpole 2010). The use of NatSSIPs and LocSSIPs can help to facilitate this.

CORE PROCEDURAL SKILLS

Prior to all procedures, the practitioner should introduce themselves to the patient (if able to), gain consent and prepare equipment. Postprocedure sharps must be disposed of safely and equipment decontaminated. All procedures must be documented in medical notes and should include consent, assistant if applicable, summary of procedure, untoward events and postprocedure checks. Infection prevention guidelines must be adhered to according to local policy.

Airway: Basic Manoeuvres and Adjuncts

Multiple manoeuvres and adjuncts may be utilised when trying to relieve an obstructed airway (Figure 8.2). Head tilt and chin lift manoeuvres should not be utilised where there is concern about cervical spine injury. Nasopharyngeal adjuncts should not be used where there is concern about basilar skull/base-of-skull fracture.

Airway: Supraglottic Airway Devices

Supraglottic airway devices (SADs) (Figure 8.3), such as an iGel, are ideal airway adjuncts in a cardiac arrest situation owing to their quick and easy insertion, causing minimal disruption to chest compressions and almost guaranteeing effective ventilation. Placement is confirmed using the end-tidal carbon dioxide ($EtCO_2$) trace. SADs are also recommended in the Difficult Airway Society guidelines following a failed intubation attempt (Difficult Airway Society 2015). Sizes are based on weight: size 3 for <50 kg, size 4 for 50–90 kg and size 5 for >90 kg, or if there is excessive leak with a size 4.

The patient should be positioned with the head extended and neck flexed, 'sniffing the morning air' position. Lubricate the back of the device, hold the airway at the bite block so the coloured part with the opening is facing the patient's chin. Press the chin down to open the mouth and insert the airway without using excessive force. Glide the airway along the back of the soft palate with gentle continuous pressure until you feel resistance and a 'bounce' (sometimes requiring a slight rotation to navigate the tongue). Attach the $EtCO_2$ and a bag valve mask. An $EtCO_2$ trace should be obtained, with chest rise and bilateral air entry on auscultation.

Any patient requiring airway support needs to be referred to and assessed by the critical care team.

Breathing: Intercostal Drain Insertion

An intercostal drain (ICD) is a flexible plastic tube that is inserted through the chest wall into the pleural space. Indications for ICD insertion generally include removal of fluid (e.g. haemothorax) or air (e.g. pneumothorax), or to facilitate pleurodesis. Contraindications to insertion include coagulopathy and local infection to the entry site. Prior to insertion, practitioners should consider whether the drain is truly indicated (Table 8.1), review clinical signs and radiology and consider the most appropriate location for the procedure to take place (e.g. interventional radiology).

Preprocedure Set-up and Equipment for ICD Insertion

- Set up sterile trolley.
- Prepare drain appropriate for the indication. Chest drain sizes range from 8 to 40F in adults. Large-bore drains (>24F) are recommended for draining blood and require blunt dissection. Small-bore chest drains may be inserted by Seldinger technique.

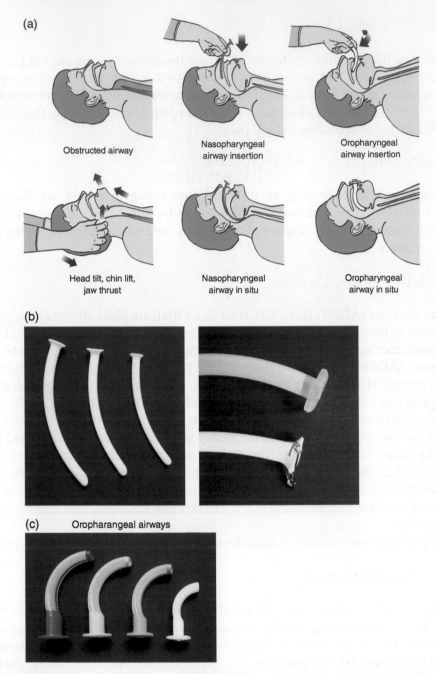

FIGURE 8.2   (a–c) Simple airway manoeuvres and adjuncts. *Source*: Thomas et al. (2015)/John Wiley & Sons.

- Pour sterile water/saline into the chest drain bottle up to the prime line.
- Attach the chest drain tubing, ensuring the end stays within the package and remains sterile.
- Review imaging and examine the patient to confirm side of insertion using a local agreed protocol.
- Position the patient leaning forward with arms outstretched or sitting at 90° with arm lifted and hand resting behind their head.

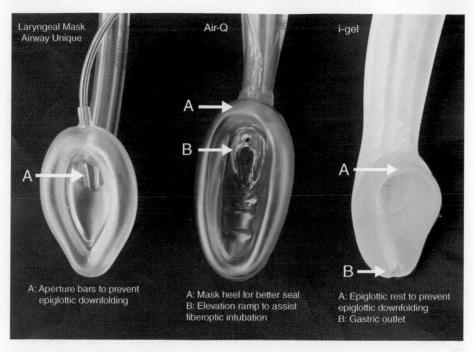

FIGURE 8.3   Supraglottic airway devices (SADs). *Source*: Huang et al. (2020)/John Wiley & Sons.

TABLE 8.1   Indications and contraindications for ICD insertion (Yousuf and Rahman 2018).

Indications	Contraindications
• Tension pneumothorax • Primary and secondary spontaneous pneumothoraces (>2 cm in size) • Haemothorax • Empyema • To facilitate pleurodesis	• Coagulopathy (not an absolute) • Lack of experienced staff • Patient refusal to consent

- If drain is for a pleural effusion, then ultrasound the area to identify insertion site.
- Check that your marked site of insertion is correct (Oxford Medical Education 2021).

Procedure for ICD Insertion (Seldinger) – Small Bore

This is a strictly aseptic technique so ensure eye protection, sterile gown and gloves.

1. Wash hands and don sterile gown and gloves.
2. Clean insertion site: either the site identified by ultrasound or, for pneumothorax, insert drain in the 'safe triangle' (Figure 8.4): lower border of axilla to the fifth intercostal space; the lateral edge of pectoralis major; and the lateral edge of latissimus dorsi.
3. Apply sterile field.

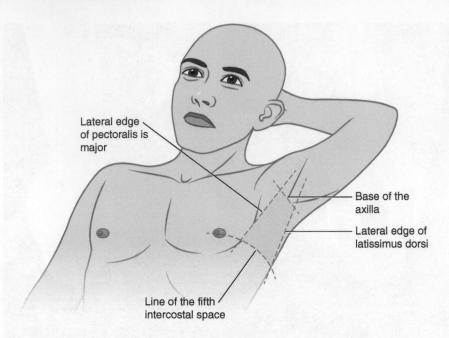

Lateral edge
of pectoralis is
major

Base of the
axilla

Lateral edge of
latissimus dorsi

Line of the fifth
intercostal space

FIGURE 8.4   The 'triangle of safety' for inserting an intercoastal drain. *Source*: Rahman et al. (2018).

4. Insert local anaesthetic (1% lidocaine) cutaneously, subcutaneously and then into the pleural space. Sedation can be considered if the patient requires it.
5. Fluid or air should be able to be aspirated with the green needle.
6. Take the Seldinger needle and attach this to the 10 ml syringe provided.
7. Insert needle in the same plane as the lidocaine, aspirating as you advance. Insert needle to the same distance as air was aspirated with the green needle. Once air is aspirated, inset 0.5 cm further and confirm ongoing air aspiration.
8. Remove the 10 ml syringe, ensuring you place your thumb over the open needle.
9. Take the Seldinger wire and insert through the needle. Ensure you always hold the wire and needle.
10. Remove Seldinger needle over the wire.
11. Take a scalpel and make a 0.5 cm incision in the skin. The sharp edge of the scalpel should always be facing away from the wire.
12. Take the Seldinger dilator and pass it over the wire; gently but firmly insert the dilator over the wire through the skin and intercostal muscles.
13. Once dilated, remove the dilator and pass the chest drain over the wire.
14. Ensure that you hold the wire out the end of the drain before advancing.
15. Insert the drain over the wire and remove the wire.
16. Attach a three-way tap to the drain and ensure it is closed.
17. Then confirm air or fluid aspiration with a syringe via the three-way tap.
18. Close the three-way tap once position is confirmed and suture drain in place. This needs to be firm but not pinch the skin or occlude the drain.
19. Dress the drain so the insertion site is visible.
20. Attach drain to chest drain tubing.

Pharmacological Principles – Lidocaine Toxicity

Proximal infiltration of lidocaine to neural tissue results in a transient loss of sensory, motor and autonomic function (Torp and Simon 2022). Practitioners should be cognisant of the toxicokinetics of lidocaine which can result in dramatic neuro- and cardiovascular effects. The usual maximum dose of plain lidocaine is 4.5 mg/kg.

Procedure for ICD Insertion – Large Bore (Lloyd 2019)

1. This is a strictly aseptic technique so ensure eye protection, sterile gown and gloves.
2. Wash hands and don sterile gown and gloves.
3. Clean insertion site: either the site identified by ultrasound or, for pneumothorax, insert drain in the 'safe triangle' (Figure 8.1): lower border of axilla to the fifth intercostal space; the lateral edge of pectoralis major, and the lateral edge of latissimus dorsi.
4. Apply sterile field.
5. Insert lidocaine cutaneously, subcutaneously and then into the pleural space. Sedation can be considered if the patient requires it.
6. When the anaesthesia has taken effect, make the incision. Use blunt dissection with curved clamp.
7. Pierce the pleura and widen the pleural breach.
8. Undertake a 360° finger sweep with caution.
9. Insert the drain by mounting the tip of the chest drain on a clamp and guiding it into the pleural cavity.
10. Ensure the proximal drain hole lies within the chest cavity.
11. Attach the connecting tube to the underwater seal.
12. Confirm that the drain lies within the chest wall cavity by noting fogging of the tube.
13. Secure the drain, which needs to be firm but not pinch the skin or occlude the drain and ideally with a horizontal mattress suture.

Postprocedure Checks

1. Place drain on free drainage but monitor closely with guidance on how much is drained to reduce the risk of re-expansion pulmonary oedema.
2. Apply analgesia which may be topical or systemic.
3. Postprocedure CXR is essential.
4. Document procedure clearly and document length of drain inserted and if the drain is oscillating (swinging), draining or leaking air (bubbling), or a combination.
5. Document if the drain needs to be on suction and the kilopascal of suction required.

Pearls and Pitfalls

- Preparation – use a maximum of 3 mg/kg 1% lidocaine.
- Seldinger approach: warn the patient they will feel some pushing; do not be too forceful as you will kink the wire. If the dilator is not advancing, this may indicate you are pushing in the wrong plane or against bone.

- Stop if you cannot aspirate air, fluid or blood and reconsider your clinical diagnosis.
- Large-bore tube: caution with a 360° finger sweep with fractured ribs.
- Appropriate sterile gloves should be used as there is a risk of sharps injury.
- Chest drain position: if the drain points upwards for the haemothorax or conversely downwards it does not matter. It is likely to be effective and should not be repositioned solely because of the X-ray position.
- Underwater drainage bottle: the underwater seal needs to always remain below the insertion site otherwise the contents start to empty into the chest.
- Accidental disconnection: keep chest drain clamps at the bedspace. Clamp the drain tubing at the patient end, clean end of drain (in accordance with local policy) and connect new drainage system. Ensure clamp is removed when the problem is resolved.
- Transport: if the patient needs to be transferred to another department or is ambulant, the suction should be disconnected and left open to air. Do not clamp the drain.

Circulation: Venepuncture

Venepuncture is the procedure of entering a vein with a needle for various indications (Table 8.2). It is a skill that is mastered early in many advanced practice roles. Figure 8.5 details the various types of equipment that may be used to perform this procedure and Figure 8.6 shows some of the commonly used veins in the arm and hand. Unlike peripheral intravenous cannulation, it is suggested to start proximal (i.e. antecubital fossa) as this will increase first-pass success, then work distal if unsuccessful. Insertion in the patient's non-dominant hand is preferable and care should be taken to avoid important structures that run parallel to the vein such as arteries and nerves.

Practitioner Safety

In 2013, the Health and Safety Executive produced a legal directive which stipulated that healthcare providers in the UK should move to safer sharps which have mechanisms to prevent and minimise the risk of accidental injury. Mengistu et al. (2021) report that up to 1 million percutaneous needle stick injuries occur per year in Europe, which exposes the healthcare worker to increased risk of blood-borne viruses.

TABLE 8.2   Indications and contraindications for venepuncture.

Indications	Contraindications
<ul><li>To obtain venous blood for laboratory testing to aid diagnosis and testing (biochemistry, haematology, microbiology, virology or toxicology)</li><li>Venesection for the management of polycythaemia rubra vera</li></ul>	<ul><li>Cellulitis around proposed insertion site</li><li>Acute burns or acute trauma</li><li>Previous surgery to affected limb with axillary lymph node clearance</li><li>LymphoedemaThrombophlebitis</li><li>Patient refusal (if they have capacity)</li><li>Avoid blood sampling from same limb with IV infusion running</li></ul>

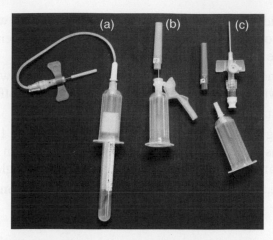

FIGURE 8.5 Examples of different equipment used for conducting venepuncture. (a) Butterfly needle with Vacutainer® adapter. (b) Vacutainer needle. (c) Cannula. *Source*: Thomas et al. (2015)/John Wiley & Sons.

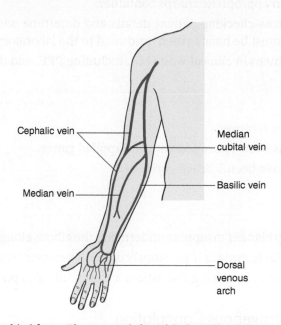

FIGURE 8.6 Veins of the antecubital fossa. Thomas et al. (2015)/John Wiley & Sons.

Technique

1. Wash hands with soap and water or bacterial handrub.
2. Apply apron and non-sterile, well-fitting gloves.
3. Apply tourniquet above the site of venepuncture and give sufficient time for the vein to engorge (this can be aided by asking the patient to make repetitive fist clenches).
4. Observe and palpate the area, feeling for a bouncy vessel, moving distally if no suitable vein can be identified,

5. Once a vein has been identified, wipe the skin with an antiseptic wipe, working in a circular motion from the insertion site outwards. Remember to allow sufficient time for the antiseptic to dry and do not repalpate – this is a non-touch technique.

6. With the practitioner's non-dominant thumb, stabilise the vein/skin with gentle pressure distal to the insertion site (this will prevent the vein from kinking or rolling off the needle).

7. Prewarn the patient that you are about to insert the needle.

8. With the bevel pointing upwards, insert the needle at an angle of 15–30° for superficial veins (steeper for deeper veins), passing through the skin and into the vein (some devices give a flash-back). It may be necessary to adjust the needle's direction and/or angle.

9. Stabilising the needle, attach the blood-collecting bottles (considering specimen bottle specific order).

10. Release tourniquet.

11. Remove needle and apply gauze with pressure (if the patient can, ask them to assist by applying pressure).

12. Apply tape.

13. Dispose of sharp into an appropriate sharps container.

14. Label all specimens, cross-checking patient details and date/time with request form (note that group and save bottles must be handwritten) and send to the laboratory.

15. Dispose of other equipment in clinical waste bin, including PPE, and disinfect hands.

Postprocedure Checks

1. Ensure the tourniquet is removed.
2. Check that bleeding has been controlled with the applied gauze.
3. Ensure all specimens have been labelled correctly.

Pearls and Pitfalls

- Use a pillow or rolled-up blanket to support underneath the elbow, elongating the antecubital fossa.
- Consider a reverse needle technique if previously difficult venepuncture/poor blood flows.
- Bedside manner is essential in gaining the patient's trust while also putting them at ease.

Circulation: Peripheral Intravenous Cannulation

In contrast to venepuncture, intravenous (IV) cannulation is best carried out working from distal to proximal. Patient comfort and convenience should be taken into consideration as it is likely that this device will remain in place for several days. Dorsal veins of the hand, median forearm vein, medial cubital vein, and cephalic and basilic veins of the upper arms are the most common sites. Lower limb veins such as the dorsal venous arch, lesser and greater saphenous veins have increased risk of phlebitis and thromboembolism. In an emergency, femoral veins and the external jugular vein can be used but care must be taken, and patients positioned in the Trendelenburg position when inserting an external jugular vein cannula. Areas to avoid include bony prominences such as wrists; likewise, cannulating the underside of the forearm is often painful. Indications and contraindications for this procedure can be found in Table 8.3.

TABLE 8.3   Indications and contraindications for peripheral venous cannulation.

Indications	Contraindications
• Intravenous fluid therapy • Continuous or intermittent intravenous drug therapy (including antibiotics and chemotherapy) • Blood transfusion (or blood products) • Radiological contrast administration for CT or MRI scans	• Cellulitis around proposed insertion site • Acute burns or acute trauma to affected limb • Previous surgery to affected limb • Previous axillary node clearance • Formation of arteriovenous (AV) fistula • Lymphoedema • Thrombophlebitis • Patient refusal (if they have capacity)

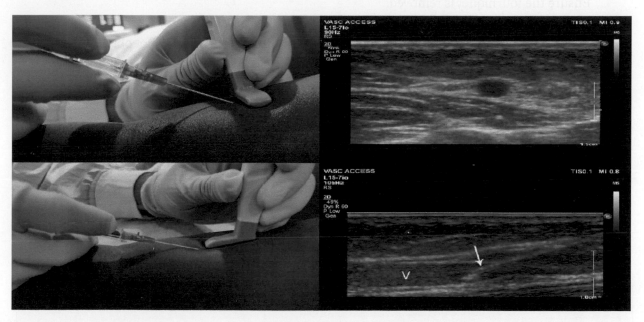

FIGURE 8.7   Ultrasound-guided peripheral venous cannular insertion. *Source*: Munshey et al. (2020)/John Wiley & Sons.

For practitioner and patient safety, all peripheral IV cannulation devices should have a sharp safe device attached. Extra equipment, for example ultrasonography (Figure 8.7) or a vein finder device, can facilitate successful cannulation. Practitioners must be trained in their use.

Technique

1. As per steps 1–7 in venepuncture.
2. With the bevel pointing upwards, insert the needle at an angle of 10–30° for superficial veins (steeper for deeper veins), passing through the skin and into the vein, looking for the flashback. It may be necessary to adjust the needle's direction and/or angle.
3. Once flashback has been seen, lower the cannula slightly and ensure the tip of the cannula is within the lumen of the vein (advancing a few millimetres further).

4. Withdraw the needle slightly (looking for secondary flashback) while at the same time advancing the cannula completely into the vein.
5. Release tourniquet.
6. Remove needle while applying gentle pressure to the end of the cannula to prevent blood from leaking; apply either the cannula cap or the flushed cannula extension line.
7. Flush the cannula and secure it in place with the dressing, ensuring asepsis is maintained (also date and time the dressing for monitoring purposes).
8. Ensure completion of a visual infusion phlebitis (VIP) chart according to local policy.

Postprocedure Checks

1. Ensure the tourniquet is removed.
2. Ensure the cannula has been flushed and there is no extravasation seen.
3. Ensure the cannula dressing is transparent and that the date sticker does not obscure the view of the insertion site.

Pearls and Pitfalls

- If the cannula won't advance, it is likely that it has hit a valve. This sometimes can be remedied by either advancing the needle past the valve and then looking for secondary flashback, or by removing the needle completely and attaching the 10 ml sodium chloride 0.9% flush and trying to gently flush the valves open while trying to advance (these methods are only recommended for advanced users and not for beginners).
- Ultrasound can be helpful but can also be a hindrance if it is used by a novice.

Examination Scenario – Obtaining Consent from Patient for Cannulation

A 64-year-old patient is admitted with acute kidney injury (AKI) secondary to dehydration due to diarrhoea and vomiting and continued used of ramipril.

Indication
- To administer fluid replacement to treat AKI and prevent further complications.

Consideration of alternatives
- Oral and/or nasogastric tube fluid replacement is not possible due to continued vomiting.

Patient consent
- Inform patient why IV access is required, risks of IV cannulation and risks of not receiving IV fluid replacement.
- Explain the procedure.
- Ascertain whether patient has any questions about the procedure and/or therapy.
- Confirm they have given consent.

Procedure
See above detailed description.

Actions and outcomes

- AKI evidence-based bundle of care initiated.
- IV fluids administered.
- Nephrotoxic medication (ramipril) suspended.
- Monitor urea and electrolytes and urine output to assess resolution of AKI and guide further therapy.

Circulation: Arterial Puncture and Cannulation

Indications and contraindications for these procedures can be found in Table 8.4. Unlike venepuncture and peripheral intravenous cannulas, arterial cannula needles do not yet encompass a safe sharp system. Blood gas syringe/needles, however, do. To that end, care when using these devices is imperative so as not to sustain a needle stick injury. Arterial puncture should be conducted using an arterial blood gas syringe which has been premanufactured with heparin already loaded within the syringe barrel. In difficult circumstances such as the hypotensive or oedematous patient, ultrasound can be beneficial in identifying the precise location of the artery and guiding the needle into the artery.

There are three main landmarks (with a fourth as a last resort) for arterial puncture and/or cannulation.

1. Radial artery – most frequently used. A modified Allen test should be performed prior to puncture (Figure 8.8) to assess patency of the ulnar artery.
2. Brachial artery.
3. Femoral artery.
4. Dorsalis pedis (least favoured option).

TABLE 8.4 Indications and contraindications for arterial puncture and cannulation.

Indications	Contraindications
• Assessment of oxygenation and acid–base status in the respiratory distresses or critically unwell/deteriorating patient • Quick assessment of electrolytes, haemoglobin and lactate • Patients requiring frequent blood sampling such as in diabetic ketoacidosis (DKA) • Patients on vasoactive drugs such as inotropic infusions or beta-blocker infusions where beat-by-beat arterial blood pressure monitoring is essential • To guide therapeutic interventions such as mechanical ventilation, supplementary oxygen delivery or intravenous fluid administration • Situations where pulse oximetry monitoring may be unreliable such as carbon monoxide poisoning	• Cellulitis • Previous arterial graft • Arteriovenous fistula • A positive Allen test • Acute burns or acute trauma • Caution in patients with coagulation defects • Patient refusal (if they have capacity)

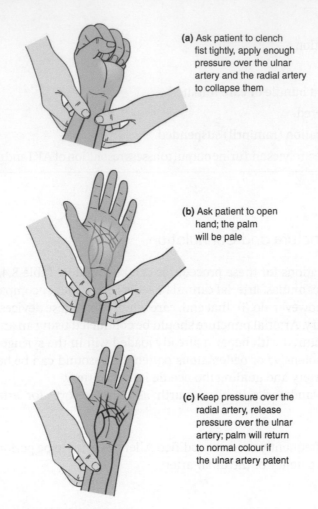

(a) Ask patient to clench fist tightly, apply enough pressure over the ulnar artery and the radial artery to collapse them

(b) Ask patient to open hand; the palm will be pale

(c) Keep pressure over the radial artery, release pressure over the ulnar artery; palm will return to normal colour if the ulnar artery patent

FIGURE 8.8   Performing the modified Allen test. *Source*: Thomas et al. (2015) Practical Medical Procedures at a Glance. John Wiley & Sons.

Technique

1. Prepare and stabilise the access site.
2. Palpate the artery (and conduct Allen test if opting for the radial artery).
3. After chlorhexidine wipe, inject 1–2 ml of local anaesthetic (LA) lateral to the pulsatile artery (taking care not to inject LA into the artery). Doing this early will allow the LA to take effect.
4. Open sterile field and put all equipment into the sterile field.
5. Conduct asepsis.
6. Palpate the artery using the first and second fingers of the non-dominant hand.
7. Once satisfied with the location of the artery, insert the needle in a proximal direction at a 45° angle until you enter the artery. It may be necessary to adjust the needle's direction and/or angle (if conducting an arterial puncture, the syringe should fill with blood).
8. a. If using a flow switch device, transfix the artery by advancing the needle through the posterior wall of the artery before pulling the needle back 2–3 mm then withdrawing the catheter until a

second flashback is seen. Lower the angle of the catheter and advance into the artery. Remove the needle and close the switch mechanism.

b. If using the Seldinger device, once flashback is evident, stabilise the needle with the non-dominant hand and insert the guidewire. Taking care not to lose the guidewire, remove the needle while keeping the guidewire in the vessel. Take the arterial catheter and place it over the guidewire, feed the guidewire back until it can be grasped and while holding the guidewire, insert the catheter into the artery. Remove the guidewire (confirming with your assistant that it has been removed).

9. Attach the flushed transducer set and flush the catheter.

10. Secure the catheter in place as per local policy.

11. Complete an arterial VIP chart according to local policy, which should clearly have a scoring system with necessary actions depending on the score.

Postprocedure Checks

1. If arterial puncture, apply direct pressure for up to five minutes until bleeding has stopped (applying gauze and tape once satisfied).

2. Observe for haematoma formation, infection, catheter misplacement.

3. Observe the hand colour (if radial) and if there is evidence of blanching or poor filling, consider relocating the catheter.

Pearls and Pitfalls

- For weak and thready pulse, the Seldinger technique is usually more successful.
- Proper positioning and splinting can be the difference between first-pass success or failure.
- Practise both with and without ultrasound guidance to build upon ultrasound needling technique.

Circulation: Central Venous Access Via Central Venous Catheter

Areas commonly used for central venous catheter (CVC) insertion are the internal jugular vein, subclavian vein and femoral vein (brachial vein for midline access). Indications and contraindications can be found in Table 8.5. Risks associated with all locations include inadvertent arterial puncture, infection (more so in the femoral region) and haematoma. Risks associated with internal jugular and subclavian access

TABLE 8.5 Indications and contraindications for central venous access.

Indications	Contraindications
• Haemodynamic monitoring (central venous pressure)	• Uncorrected coagulopathy
• Infusion of drugs which cannot be given peripherally	• Thrombocytopenia
• Parenteral feeding	• Anatomical distortion
• Rapid fluid resuscitation	• Vasculitis
• Poor peripheral access (such as intravenous drug users, chemotherapy or oedematous patient)	• Cellulitis
• Transvenous pacing	• Superior vena cava syndrome
• Plasmapheresis	• Patient refusal

include cardiac arrhythmia, pneumothorax and stenosis. Consideration must also be given to what type of catheter is inserted (including number of lumens). All needles used for central venous access are non-sharp safe, therefore care must be taken not to sustain a needle stick injury.

CLINICAL INVESTIGATIONS: COAGULATION SCREEN

Coagulation screen should be reviewed prior to the procedure and corrected if indicated and time permits. Figure 8.9 details how the functionality of the patient's coagulation cascade is measured using tests of enzymatic coagulation.

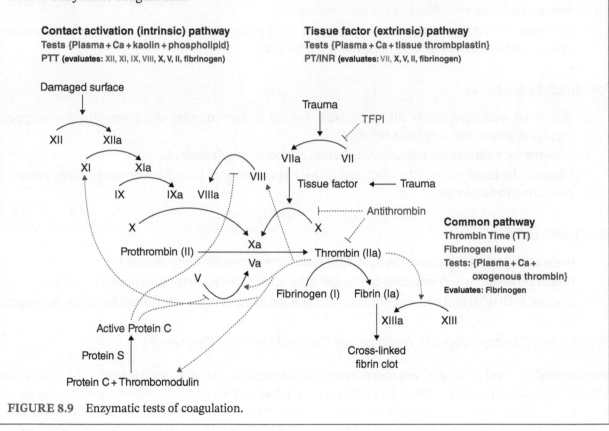

Contact activation (intrinsic) pathway
Tests {Plasma + Ca + kaolin + phospholipid}
PTT (evaluates: XII, XI, IX, VIII, X, V, II, fibrinogen)

Tissue factor (extrinsic) pathway
Tests {Plasma + Ca + tissue thrombplastin}
PT/INR (evaluates: VII, X, V, II, fibrinogen)

Common pathway
Thrombin Time (TT)
Fibrinogen level
Tests: {Plasma + Ca + oxogenous thrombin}
Evaluates: Fibrinogen

FIGURE 8.9   Enzymatic tests of coagulation.

Technique

1. Expose (maintaining dignity) and position the patient and attach monitoring (if subclavian or internal jugular, ECG monitoring is imperative).
2. Assess preferred location with ultrasound, assessing structures and vessel size.
3. Conduct asepsis.
4. Prepare sterile field and ask assistant to pass in all equipment in a sterile manner.
5. Flush all lumens of the central venous catheter with normal saline.
6. Clean the insertion site with the chlorhexidine sticks in a circular motion, starting at the insertion site and moving outward.

7. Apply sterile drapes and prepare ultrasound.

8. Assess the neck or groin with ultrasound (scanning up and down looking for where the vein is most lateral to the artery) and inject local anaesthetic, working through each layer.

9. With the introducer needle attached to a syringe, guide the needle at a 30° angle, inserting the needle proximal to the probe (holding probe in non-dominant hand).

10. Keeping a continuous eye on the ultrasound screen, direct the needle into the vein, aspirating whilst inserting until flashback is achieved.

11. Releasing the ultrasound probe, stabilise and anchor the needle and detach the syringe from the needle (blood should flow steadily and not spurt).

12. Insert the guidewire (if internal jugular or subclavian, the assistant should be asked to observe the ECG rhythm, informing the operator of any ectopic beats or arrhythmias: if present, the operator should retract the guidewire until the ECG normalises). The wire should pass freely and without resistance.

13. Remove the introducer needle, leaving the guidewire in situ.

14. Scan the guidewire, tracing the wire from the skin down to the vessel and beyond, ensuring that the wire is situated in the vein (a compressible vessel) before dilating the vessel.

15. Load the dilator onto the wire.

16. Make a nick in the skin with the scalpel.

17. Dilate over the guidewire into the vessel, keeping hold of the guidewire so as not to lose it intra-vascularly (repeat dilation if inserting a Vascath® which has two sizes of dilators).

18. Insert the central venous catheter (again, feeding the guidewire back until it can be held before advancing the catheter).

19. Remove the guidewire and confirm its removal with your assistant.

20. If taking blood culture and/or blood for gas analysis, do this now.

21. Aspirate and flush each lumen with sodium chloride.

22. Suture the central venous catheter in situ (ideally in four locations to prevent migration).

23. Apply dressing.

24. Transduce the line and assess waveform and pressure.

25. Conduct chest X-ray if internal jugular or subclavian.

Pharmacological Considerations

Chlorhexidine preparation is available with or without tint and contains the active ingredients chlorhexidine gluconate and isopropyl alcohol. It works by disrupting cell membranes of bacteria and has action on a wide range of gram-negative and gram-positive bacteria, as well as some viruses and fungi. There is little if any absorption through the skin. It can have effects on the skin up to 48 hours after application.

Pearls and Pitfalls

- Positioning and good ultrasound skills are key.
- Monitor ECG for arrhythmias when inserting the guidewire.

- Confirm the wire is in the vein before dilating (do not dilate until you are certain that the wire is in the vein).
- Holding the guidewire whilst keeping traction on the skin will prevent the guidewire from kinking.
- During internal jugular or subclavian insertion, ensure the assistant is watching the cardiac monitor and is competent to interpret arrhythmias.
- Exclude pneumothorax with chest X-ray after the procedure.
- If there is inadvertent insertion into the artery, leave the line in situ while seeking advice from vascular/cardiovascular surgeons.

Circulation: Intraosseous Needle Insertion

Intraosseous (IO) needle insertion involves advancement of a needle through the subcutaneous tissue, through the periosteum and into the medullary canal which contains the bone marrow. Common areas for insertion include the humeral head, distal femur and both the proximal and distal tibia. Care must be taken when placing these devices, which is carried out using landmark techniques. Multiple education videos on the EZ-IO® device can be found here: www.teleflex.com/usa/en/clinical-resources/ez-io/index. The indications and contraindications for IO insertion can be found in Table 8.6.

Preprocedure Considerations

- Can peripheral or central access be gained in a timely manner?
- Practitioners must be familiar with the IO kit available (manual or power-driven devices).
- All equipment for insertion must be available.

Pearls and Pitfalls

- Select the appropriate needle.
- Clear identification is required for all limbs that have had IO placed (colourful wristband included in IO kit). Note that 48 hours is the minimum time before reattempts can be made in the same location.
- Remove the IO as early as possible once peripheral or central access has been obtained.
- Attach a 50 ml syringe to the needle to assist in its removal.

TABLE 8.6   Indications and contraindications for IO insertion.

Indications	Contraindications
• During resuscitation when peripheral vascular access is unobtainable (mostly in cardiac arrest)	• Proximal fractures to the insertion site • Previous IO attempts in same bone • Previous surgery at insertion site (knee replacement, sternotomy) • Osteogenesis imperfecta • Osteoporosis • Underlying infection • Inability to identify landmarks • Acute burns

Disability: Lumbar Puncture

Lumbar puncture (LP) is performed to collect cerebrospinal fluid for diagnostic testing to rule in/out diseases of the central nervous system such as infection or subarachnoid haemorrhage. Other indications and contraindications can be found in Table 8.7. Knowledge of the anatomy of the lumbar spine is essential for safe performance of an LP (Figure 8.10).

Patient assessment prior to LP must include medication review, paying particular attention to anticoagulant drugs, blood results, particularly coagulation and platelets, and patient anatomy. LP can be performed with the patient sitting, but most commonly is done in the lateral position. Patients need to be able to or be assisted to flex their lumbar spine to facilitate maximal opening of intervertebral spaces (Byrne 2010).

Ask the patient to lie on their left side with their head on a pillow, put their chin on their chest and draw their knees up as far as they can, and push out their lower back (curl up) (Figure 8.11). Sedated and ventilated patients will require three staff to achieve this position. Having the patient close to the edge of the bed/trolley will make it easier for the practitioner and avoid overreaching.

TABLE 8.7   Indications and contraindications of LP.

Indications	Contraindications
• Suspected CNS infection • Subarachnoid haemorrhage • Assessment/diagnosis of neurological diseases such as GBS/MS • Assessment of CSF opening pressures • Removal of CSF, for example in idiopathic intracranial hypertension	• If consent/assent not given • Clotting abnormality • Raised intracranial pressure (a CT head and neurological assessment should be performed prior to LP) • Local infection at insertion site

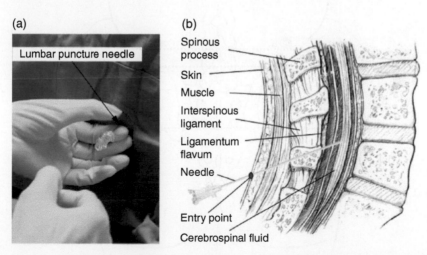

FIGURE 8.10   Essential anatomy of the lumbar spine in relation to performance of an LP. The LP is usually performed 'blind' by the practitioner with the patient in either the sitting or lateral position. Figure (a): a typical setup and approach to performing a lumbar puncture in the sitting or lateral position. Figure (b): The needle penetrates the ligamentum flavum, entering the epidural space where the fluid is located. *Source:* Li et al. (2021) A novel manipulator with needle insertion forces feedback for robot-assisted lumbar puncture. International Journal of Medical Robotics 17, e2226.

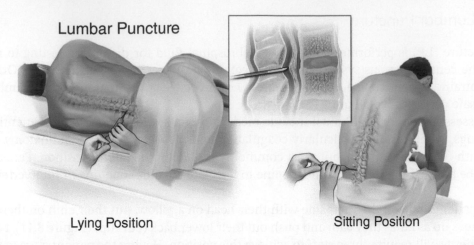

Lumbar Puncture

Lying Position   Sitting Position

FIGURE 8.11   Common positions for lumbar puncture procedure. *Source*: Blausen Medical/Creative Commons Licence.

Technique

1. Palpate the spine at L3–4 and identify landmarks. The most important landmark is the intercristal line (Tuffier's line) located between the top of the iliac crests and lumbar spine midline (Figure 8.12), which is accurate in 95% of the population (Doherty and Forbes 2014).
2. Scrub for procedure.
3. Sterilise the skin using the chlorhexidine spray.
4. Apply drapes so that L3–4 can be identified.
5. Inject lidocaine to cause a subcutaneous wheal. Give it time to work.

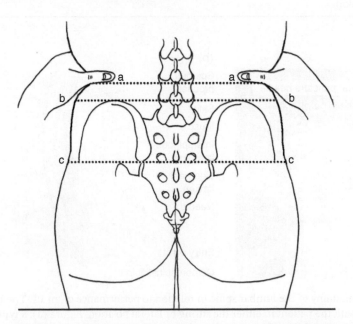

FIGURE 8.12   The palpated intercristal line (a), the imaged intercristal line (b) and the palpated posterior superior iliac spine line (c). *Source*: Chakraverty et al. (2007) Which spinal levels are identified by palpation of the iliac crests and the posterior superior iliac spines? Journal of Anatomy 210, 232–236.

6. With the non-dominant hand, grip the spinous process of L3 between thumb and middle finger to anchor skin and allow easier identification of midline.

7. Insert introducer at 90° to the skin in the midline. The bevel should be facing laterally to part dural fibres rather than cutting them (can reduce risk of postdural headache).

8. Advance the needle through the ligaments and you will feel a pop or 'give' at around 4–6 cm (depending on the body habitus of the patient).

9. Withdraw stylet; CSF should flow freely. Narrow gauge needles can take longer for CSF to be seen (Byrne 2010).

10. Once CSF is obtained, connect the manometer to record the opening pressure. The meniscus of the CSF may oscillate with respiration; this is normal (Doherty and Forbes 2014).

11. Collect 10 drops of CSF in each bottle labelled in order, then the grey blood bottle.

12. The stylet should be replaced before the needle is withdrawn.

13. A simple sterile dressing should be applied to the site.

14. Patients can mobilise as soon as they are comfortable to do so.

15. Ensure samples are correctly labelled and sent to the laboratory as an urgent sample.

Pearls and Pitfalls

- If you hit bone, reassess the patient's position and landmarks for the midline. If this fails, try L4 –5 (do not attempt L2–3 as there is arisk of damaging the spinal cord).
- Some patients, particularly obese patients, may require an image-guided procedure and a clinician experienced in this should be asked for help.
- Samples are precious; they must be correctly labelled and should be transferred to the lab via a porter rather than a pod system.
- Biochemistry and microbiology should be informed about the samples before the procedure.

CLINICAL INVESTIGATION: CEREBROSPINAL FLUID PROFILE

After obtaining the CSF sample from an LP, the results obtained will be analysed to differentiate common aetiologies of central nervous system disorders (Figure 8.13).

	Appearance	Opening Pressure mmHg	WBC (cell/μL)	Protein (mg/dl)	Glucose (mg/dL)
Normal	Clear	90-180	< 8	15-45	50-80
Bacterial Meningitis	Turbid	Elevated	>1000-2000	>200	<40
Viral Meningitis	Clear	Normal	<300; Lymphocytic predominance	<200	Normal
Fungal Meningitis	Clear	Normal-elevated	<500	>200	Normal - Low

FIGURE 8.13   CSF interpretation (Hersi et al. 2022). *Source*: Hersi et al. 2022/StatPearls Publishing LLC/ CC BY 4.0.

Exposure: Nasogastric Tube Insertion

Nasogastric tube (NGT) placement is a commonly performed procedure across all clinical settings. The indications and contraindications for NGT insertion are explored in Table 8.8.

Selection of the appropriate NG tube is essential. Large-diameter tubes have the advantages of easier aspiration and irrigation with less chance of blockage. However, large size may result in discomfort and irritation, and these tubes may not always be licensed for feeding. Small-diameter tubes are better tolerated in terms of patient comfort, less interference with eating and drinking, decreased risk of reflux, and early return of swallowing mechanism. Conversely, the disadvantage is a high chance of obstruction so regular irrigation/flushing is required. Soft, flexible, light and small feeding tubes are preferred for administration of nutrition or giving medication. These tubes must meet the latest ENFit (ISO 80369-3) connector. The practitioner may wish to consider administration of local anaesthesia spray/nebulisation to the patient five minutes before the procedure as this may increase patient comfort.

Technique – Awake Patient

1. Position the patient in the sitting position with neck gently flexed to align the oesophagus and ease the NGT insertion.
2. Measurements for insertion of appropriate length of NGT must be undertaken. NEX (nose, ear, xiphisternum) measurement is recommended prior to the insertion of an NGT.
3. Apply adequate lubricant.
4. Insert the tube gently through the selected nostril. As the tube reaches the nasopharynx, the patient might have 'gag reflex'. The patient is then advised to swallow the tube. Depending on the patient's condition and local operating procedures, a small amount of sterile water can be provided to aid swallowing.
5. If the measured length is reached smoothly, the tube has reached the oesophagus and then stomach.
6. Fix the NGT in place using appropriate devices, ensuring there is no risk of pressure damage to the nose.
7. Fixation with a bridle could be considered based on clinical need.
8. Documentation and position confirmation should be completed as per local policy before use.

TABLE 8.8   Indications and contraindications for nasogastric tube insertion (Gurjar (2015).

Indications	Contraindications
Diagnostic	*Absolute*
• Evaluation of radiographic material for computed tomography-based diagnosis	• Severe facial trauma
• Assessment of gastric pH	• Recent nasal surgery
• Gastric bleeding	• Suspected basal skull fracture
• Gastric lavage	
	Relative
Therapeutic	• Anticoagulant/coagulopathy
• Enteral feeding	• Oesophageal varices
• Administration of medicine	• Oesophageal stricture
	• Recent oesophageal surgery or known trauma such as Boerhaave syndrome
Preventive measures	• Nasopharyngeal tumour
• To reduce nausea, vomiting	
• To reduce gastric distension	

Technique - Unconscious/Anaesthetised/Intubated Patient

1. These patients are in supine position, but the head–neck position remains the same as that of the awake patient.
2. Apply adequate lubricant.
3. The blind end of the NGT is passed through one of the nostrils and generally reaches the oropharynx uneventfully.
4. Once into the oropharynx, it can either proceed smoothly through the oesophagus to reach the stomach or it can go to the trachea.
5. Fix the NGT in place using appropriate devices, ensuring there is no risk of pressure damage to the nose.
6. Fixation with a bridle could be considered based on clinical need.
7. Documentation and position confirmation should be completed as per local policy before use.

Postprocedure Checks

This should be undertaken in accordance with local policy, with an awareness that an NGT placed incorrectly, going undetected and delivering food, liquid or medication into the lungs is a well-recognised never event in the NHS. An inappropriately placed NGT has caused morbidity and mortality.

A National Patient Safety alert 'Reducing the harm caused by misplaced nasogastric tubes in adults, children and infants' (2011) stated that a gastric aspirate with a pH of 1–5.5 or an X-ray are the only acceptable methods for confirming initial placement of a NGT, confirming the NGT tip below the left diaphragm. The 'whoosh test' should not be used to confirm position.

The documentation should be clear about the length of the NGT at the naris and this should be confirmed before any medication or feeding is given through the NGT.

Learning Events: Complications of NGT Insertion

Numerous complications are described in the literature. They may include:

- throat (mild irritation, trauma, bleeding)
- oesophageal injury
- intrathoracic placement
- intracranial placement in head injury/major facial injury
- feeding in an unconfirmed tube may lead to tracheobronchial aspiration which increases morbidity and mortality
- accidental removal of NGT. This can be minimised with a NGT bridle.

Pearls and Pitfalls

- Insertion – patients may desaturate when oxygen is removed for a NGT insertion. Therefore, they may require preoxygenation before attempting the procedure.
- Insertion – in case of respiratory distress during the procedure, such as coughing or choking, this is a sign of tracheal irritation so withdraw the tube and consider trying again.

- Insertion – neck positioning, particularly flexion, may assist insertion of a NGT.
- Insertion – resistance may be felt at the nasopharynx; at this point do not use any force; withdraw the tube and manipulate it again gently. If still not able to pass the tube, try the other nostril.
- Postprocedural checks – change in pH due to drugs (H2 blocker, proton pump inhibitor) may decrease the pH; a chest X-ray must be used to confirm position.
- Postprocedural checks – error in interpretation of chest radiograph placement of the NGT. Follow local procedures for checking.
- Maintenance – rechecking of tube position; confirm the position before every feed/after shifting or mobilisation of patient/patient complaining of discomfort. If in doubt, do not use and recheck the position.
- Maintenance – the NGT should be routinely checked and flushed frequently (before and after feeding or medication) to prevent blocking.

LEARNING FROM PATIENT SAFETY EVENTS

Undertaking any procedural skill has the potential for an associated patient safety event. If such an event occurs, it must be documented, in accordance with the duty of candour incumbent on the practitioner in accordance with local procedures and reflection by the clinician. A new national NHS Learn from Patient Safety Events service is in the final stages of development as a central service for the recording and analysis of patient safety events that occur in healthcare and is anticipated for launch in 2023. Organisations, staff and patients will be able to record the details of patient safety events, contributing to a NHS-wide data source to support learning and improvement.

CONCLUSION

Clinical procedures are an integral part of the advanced practitioner role and as such come with responsibility to achieve and maintain competence and ensure patient safety. Advanced practitioners must be aware of the legal and ethical issues relating to procedures, particularly consent processes. Communication, preparation and patient positioning are all key factors in ensuring successful, high-quality procedures. Advice on how to undertake core procedural skills has been provided in an airway, breathing, circulation, disability and exposure format.

Take Home Points

- Consent is essential to all procedures.
- Patient positioning and preparation are key to success, as is having a skilled and competent assistant who can pre-alert to potential problems/monitor patient.
- Understand the anatomy and physiology and equipment range for the procedure being undertaken.
- Understand human factors relevant to undertaking procedures.
- Work within your own competence and legal and ethical frameworks.

REFERENCES

Byrne, M. (2010). Sampling: lumbar puncture. In: *ABC of Practical Procedures* (ed. T. Nutbeam and R. Daniels). Oxford: Blackwell Publishing.

Catchpole (2010). Cited in Department of Health Human Factors Reference Group, Interim Report, 1 March 2012. www.england.nhs.uk/wp-content/uploads/2013/11/DH-rep.pdf

Chakraverty, R., Pynset, P., Isaacs, K. (2007) 'Which spinal levels are identified by palpation of the iliac crests and the posterior superior iliac spines?'. Journal of Anatomy, 210 (2), pp. 232–236.

Dennhey, L. and White, S. (2012). Consent, assent and the importance of risk stratification. *British Journal of Anaesthesia* 109: 40–46.

Department of Health (2009). Reference guide to consent to examination or treatment. www.gov.uk/government/publications/reference-guide-to-consent-for-examination-or-treatment-second-edition

Difficult Airway Society (2015). Difficult Airway Society 2015 guidelines for management of unanticipated difficult intubations in adults. https://das.uk.com/guidelines/das_intubations_guidelines

Doherty, C.M. and Forbes, R.B. (2014). Diagnostic lumbar puncture. *Ulster Medical Journal* 83: 93–102.

Faculty of Intensive Care Medicine (2015). Curriculum for Training for Advanced Critical Care Practitioners. www.ficm.ac.uk/sites/fcm/files/documents/2022-12/ACCP%20Curriculum%20Part%210%20-%20Handbook%20v1%202019%20Revusion.pdf

Farmer, L. (2017). Informed consent: ethical and legal considerations for advanced practice nurses. *Journal for Nurse Practitioners* 13 (2): 124–130.

Gurjar, M. (2015). *Manual of ICU Procedures*. New Delhi: Jaypee Brothers Medical Publishers.

Health Education England (2017). Multi-professional framework for advanced clinical practice in England. www.hee.nhs.uk/sites/default/files/docuemtns/HEE%20ACP%20Framework.pdf

Health Education England (2020a). Surgical Advanced Clinical Practitioner (SACP) Curriculum and Assessment Framework. www.iscp.ac.uk/media/1141/sacp_curriculum_dec20_accessible-1.pdf

Health Education England (2020b). Core capabilities for Advanced Clinical Practice (Nurses) Working in General Practice/Primary care in England. https://www.hee.nhs/uk/sites/default/files/documents/ACP%20%Primary%Care%20Nurse%20Fwk%202020.pdf

Health Education England (2021). Advancing Practice: Signpost for Continuing Professional Development. https://advanced-practice.hee.nhs.uk/signpost-for-continuing-professional-development/

Health Education England (2022a). Advanced Clinical Practice in Older People Curriculum Framework. https://healtheducationengland.sharepoint.com/sites/APWC/Shared%20Documents/Forms/AllItems.aspx?id=%2Fsites%2FAPWC%2FShared%20Documents%2FCredentials%2FCredentials%20Endorsement%20Documents%2FAdvanced%20clinical%20practice%20older%20people%20curriculum%20framework%20%20%2Epdf&parent=%2Fsites%2FAPWC%2FShared%20Documents%2FCredentials%2FCredentials%20Endorsement%20Documents&p=true&ga=1

Health Education England (2022b). Advanced Clinical Practice in Acute Medicine Curriculum Framework. https://healtheducationengland.sharepoint.com/sites/APWC/Shared%20Documents/Forms/AllItems.aspx?id=%2Fsites%2FAPWC%2FShared%20Documents%2FCredentials%2FCredentials%20Endorsement%20Documents%2FAdvanced%20clinical%20practice%20in%20acute%20medicine%20curriculum%20framework%2Epdf&parent=%2Fsites%2FAPWC%2FShared%20Documents%2FCredentials%2FCredentials%20Endorsement%20Documents&p=true&ga=1

Hersi, K., Gonzalez, F.J., and Kondamudi, N.P. (2022). Meningitis. StatPearls, Treasure Island, FL. www.ncbi. nlm.nih.gov/books/NBK459360/

Hughes, S.J. and Mardell, A. (2009). Intraoperative care – patient positioning for surgery. In: *Oxford Handbook of Perioperative Practice*. Oxford: Oxford University Press.

Huang, A. S., Sarver, A., Widing, A., Hajduk, J., Jagannathan, N. (2020) 'The design of the perfect pediatric supraglottic airway device'. Pediatric Anesthesia, 30 (3), pp. 280–287.

Lister, S., Hofland, J., and Grafton, H. (2021). *The Royal Marsden Manual of Clinical Nursing Procedures, Professional Edition*, 10e. Oxford: Wiley Blackwell.

Li, H., Wang, Y., Li, Y., Zhang, J. 'A novel manipulator with needle insertion forces feedback for robot-assisted lumbar puncture'. The International Journal of Medical Robotics and Computer Assisted Surgery, 17 (2), pp. 1–11.

Lloyd, G (2019). RCEM Learning. Chest Drain Insertion in Adult Trauma. www.rcemlearning.co.uk/ reference/chest-drain-insertion-in-adult-trauma/#1572952397747-627848bf-1c9b

Mengistu, D.A., Tolera, S.T., and Dummu, Y.M. (2021, 2021). Worldwide prevalence of occupational exposure to needle stick injury among healthcare workers: a systematic review and meta-analysis. *Canadian Journal of Infectious Diseases and Medical Microbiology* 1: 1–10.

Munshey, F., Parra, D. A., McDonnell, C., Matava, C. (2020) 'Ultrasound-guided techniques for peripheral intravenous placement in children with difficult venous access'. Pediatric Anesthesia, 30 (2), pp. 108–115.

NHS England (2015). National Safety Standards for Invasive Procedures (NatSSIPs). www.england.nhs.uk/ wp-content/uploads/2015/09/natssips-safety-standards.pdf

NHS National Patient Safety Agency (2011). Patient Safety Alert. Reducing the harm caused by misplaced nasogastric feeding tubes in adults, children and infants. London: NPSA.

NICE (2018). Decision making and mental capacity guidance. NG108. https://nice.org.uk

Nutbeam, T. and Daniels, R. (2010). Introduction – chapter 1. In: *ABC of Practical Procedures* (ed. T. Nutbeam and R. Daniels), 1–2. Oxford: Wiley-Blackwell.

Oxford Medical Education (2021). Chest drain/Pleural drain insertion. https://oxfordmedicaleducation.com/clinical-skills/procedures/intercostal-drain/

Powell, R., Scott, N.W., Manyande, A. et al. (2016). Psychological preparation and postoperative outcomes for adults undergoing surgery under general anaesthesia. *Cochrane Database of Systematic Reviews* (5): CD008646.

Rahman, N.M., Hunt, I., and Gleeson, F. (2018). *ABC of Pleural Diseases*. Chichester: Wiley.

Royal College of Emergency Medicine (2022). Emergency Medicine Advanced Clinical Practitioner Curriculum 2022 Adult. https://rcem,ac,uk/wp-content/uploads/2022/09/ACP_Curiculum_Adult_Final_060922.pdf

Thomas, R. K., Taylor, C. J., Richards, A. E., and Thomas, D. E. (2015) 'Performing Venepuncture (Chapter 11)' IN Thomas, R. K. (Ed) Practical Medical Procedures at a Glance. Oxford: John Wiley & Sons Ltd

Torp, K.D. and Simon, L.V. (2022). Lidocaine Toxicity. www.ncbi.nlm.nih.gov/books/NBK482479/

UK Government (2010). Equality Act 2010. www.legislation.gov.uk/ukpga/2010/15/contents

Yousuf, A. and Rahman, N.M. (2018). Chest drain insertion. In: *ABC of Pleural Diseases* (ed. I. Hunt, N.M. Rahman, N.A. Maskell, and F.V. Gleeson), 56–59. Oxford: Wiley.

FURTHER READING

Burgess, A., van Diggele, C., Roberts, C. et al. (2020). Tips for teaching procedural skills. *BMC Medical Education* 20 (Suppl 2): 458. https://doi.org/10.1186/s12909-020-02284-1.

Jevon, P. and Joshi, R. (2021). *Procedural Skills*. Wiley Blackwell.

SELF-ASSESSMENT QUESTIONS

1. What are the principles of obtaining consent?
2. What are the contraindications to the insertion of a nasopharyngeal airway?
3. What are the contraindications to the insertion of a central venous catheter (CVC)?
4. What is the maximum recommended dose of lidocaine for local anaesthesia in ml/kg?

GLOSSARY

Activated prothrombin time (aPTT)   A measure of the functionality of the intrinsic and common pathways of the coagulation cascade.

Capnography and end-tidal carbon dioxide (EtCO$_2$)   Provides a numerical value for ETCO$_2$. ETCO$_2$ is the level of carbon dioxide that is released at the end of an exhaled breath. ETCO$_2$ levels reflect the adequacy with which carbon dioxide (CO$_2$) is carried in the blood back to the lungs and exhaled.

Chlorhexidine   A disinfectant and antiseptic that is used for skin disinfection before surgery or other invasive procedure. It may also be used to sterilise surgical instruments.

Coagulation screen   A group of tests used for haemostatic assessment. The screen consists of the prothrombin time, INR, APTT, APTT ratio and derived fibrinogen.

Fibrinogen   Produced in the liver and circulates in the bloodstream. It becomes activated during tissue and vascular injury and is converted enzymatically by thrombin to fibrin and then to a fibrin-based blood clot.

Mental Capacity Act 2005   Designed to protect and empower people who may lack the mental capacity to make their own decisions about their care and treatment. It applies to people aged 16 and over.

Prothrombin time   Measures the time taken (in seconds) for the blood to clot following addition of an activating enzyme known as thromboplastin.

Psychomotor   Relating to the origination of movement in conscious mental activity.

Supraglottic airway   A group of airway devices that can be inserted into the pharynx to allow ventilation, oxygenation and administration of anaesthetic gases, without the need for endotracheal intubation.

Ultrasonography   A non-invasive imaging test. An ultrasound picture is called a sonogram. Ultrasound uses high-frequency sound waves to create real-time pictures or videos of internal organs or other soft tissues, such as blood vessels.

CHAPTER 9

Clinical History Taking and Physical Examination

Sadie Diamond-Fox, Rebecca Connolly, Alexandra Gatehouse, and John Wilkinson

> **Aim**
> The aim of this chapter is to provide a deeper understanding of history taking and physical examination (HTPE), alongside the underpinning process and theories, to ensure a comprehensive and effective clinical consultation is performed.

LEARNING OUTCOMES

After reading this chapter the reader will have a comprehensive knowledge of:

1. The multitude of consultation models that may be used to elicit a detailed medical history for diverse populations (including neurodiverse, non-verbal and LGBTQIA+ populations)
2. Evidence-based physical examination techniques
3. Evidence-based physical findings and their relation to common pathology
4. The psychosocial considerations required to elicit an evidence-based diagnosis via the principles of HTPE.

INTRODUCTION

Once deemed the reserve of doctors, 'the medical interview' has since transitioned across professional boundaries and is now a key part of the advanced practitioner (AP) role. Much of the literature surrounding this topic focuses on a purely medical model; however, the AP's use of consultation and clinical assessment of complex patient caseloads with undifferentiated and undiagnosed diseases is

The Advanced Practitioner: A Framework for Practice, First Edition. Edited by Ian Peate,
Sadie Diamond-Fox, and Barry Hill.
© 2024 John Wiley & Sons Ltd. Published 2024 by John Wiley & Sons Ltd.

now a regular feature in healthcare practice. This chapter explores how knowledge of the fundamental principles surrounding AP–patient communications, along with the use of appropriate consultation frameworks and examination skills, can provide a deeper insight and enhance the existing skills of the AP.

Multi-Professional Framework for Advanced Clinical Practice (MPFfACP)

1.4 Work in partnership with individuals, families and carers, using a range of assessment methods as appropriate

1.6 Use expertise and decision-making skills to inform clinical reasoning approaches when dealing with differentiated and undifferentiated individual presentations and complex situations, synthesising information from multiple sources to make appropriate, evidence-based judgements and/or diagnoses

2.1 Support systems and infrastructure for delegated roles

(HEE 2017)

Accreditation Considerations – Advanced Critical Care Practitioners (ACCP)

This chapter maps to the following areas of the Faculty of Intensive Care Medicine Curriculum (FICM) for ACCP training:

2.2 History taking and examination

3.1 History taking

3.2 Clinical examination

4.2 Interpretation of clinical data and investigations in the assessment and management of critical care patients

(FICM 2015)

Accreditation Considerations – ACPs in Emergency Care (ACP-EC)

This chapter maps to the following areas of the Royal College of Emergency Medicine (RCEM) curriculum for training ACP-EC:

SLO 1 Care for physiologically stable adult patients presenting to acute care across the full range of complexity

SLO 2 Support the ED team by answering clinical questions and making safe decisions

SLO3 Identify sick adult patients, be able to resuscitate and stabilise and know when it is appropriate to stop

SLO4 Care for acutely injured adult patients across the full range of complexity

(RCEM 2022)

THE CONSULTATION AS A DIAGNOSTIC TOOL

The knowledge obtained about the patient through a comprehensive history and physical examination informs the diagnostic reasoning and in turn the treatment options and clinical decisions. The process of conducting a patient consultation and performing a subsequent clinical assessment has historically been termed 'the most powerful and sensitive and most versatile instrument available to the physician' (Engel and Morgan 1973). Despite the rapid growth of healthcare technology, this remains the case today. A skilled practitioner has the potential to make a significant contribution to several fundamental outcomes, including patient satisfaction, patient concordance with prescribed therapies and interventions, and overall diagnostic accuracy. This can ultimately have measurable changes in health or quality of life that result from safe patient care. Evidence suggests that, by conducting a high-quality medical history alone, 60–80% of the relevant information to form a diagnosis can be ascertained (Peterson et al. 1992; Roshan and Rao 2000). The overall aim is to identify symptoms and physical manifestations that represent a final common pathway of a wide range of pathologies, which may be highly suggestive or even pathognomonic of one such pathology, or multiple concurrent pathologies.

Various established consultation models exist to give structure to the consultation, with the aim of effectively, efficiently and accurately collecting the required information from the patient while continuing to build rapport with them.

Communication

Communication with patients is key to all aspects of clinical practice. Seminal NHS frameworks and policy drivers place effective communication at the core of providing a person-centred approach in health and care. Communication skills are consequently core strands of AP training and ongoing professional development. Effective communication with patients can lead to improvement in both treatment quality and safety metrics; conversely, poor communication has been highlighted as one of the main concerns that lead to complaints to the Parliamentary and Health Service Ombudsman.

In order to develop effective clinician–patient relationships, we must consider some of the fundamental principles of effective/therapeutic communication within the healthcare setting, such as patient health literacy, cultural understanding and language barriers. However, there are other aspects that could potentially have an impact, such as those that have triggered the initial consultation.

The Cone Technique

This established aid, described in the Three Function Approach to the Medical Interview (Bird and Cohen-Cole 1990), guides the practitioner in using open to gradually more closed questions (Figure 9.1). This aims to collect information:

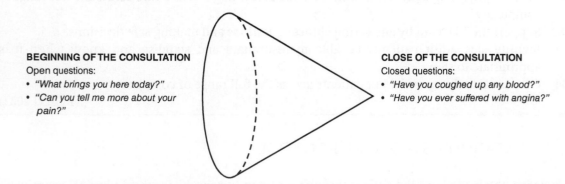

BEGINNING OF THE CONSULTATION
Open questions:
- *"What brings you here today?"*
- *"Can you tell me more about your pain?"*

CLOSE OF THE CONSULTATION
Closed questions:
- *"Have you coughed up any blood?"*
- *"Have you ever suffered with angina?"*

FIGURE 9.1   A pictorial representation of the open to closed cone described in the Three Function Approach to the Medical Interview. *Source*: Bird and Cohen-Cole (1990).

- Thoroughly, reducing the risk of missing pertinent information using open questions
- Efficiently, using closed questions
- While allowing the patient time to express the elements of their presentation which are significant to them.

When moving to closed questions, there are a variety of mnemonics available to assist with the gathering of pertinent details and as a mental aid to ensure completeness of information. Examples of commonly used mnemonics are detailed in Chapter 24.

Ideas, Concerns and Expectations (*ICE*)

While the consultation's primary aim is to collect information to formulate a differential diagnosis and management plan, additional objectives are to build rapport, explore concerns, improve patient satisfaction, review the patient's agenda and promote shared decision making. Considering the acronym ICE throughout the consultation helps to achieve these objectives.

Triggers to Consultation

The primary trigger for a consultation can be extremely varied. Considering the trigger for consultation can be a powerful tool in setting up and directing the consultation appropriately. Triggers may include:

- interpersonal crisis
- interference with social or personal relations
- sanctioning or pressure from family or friends
- interference with work or physical activity
- reaching the limit of tolerance with symptoms.

CONSULTATION MODELS

To maximise the efficiency and efficacy of the consultation, several models or frameworks have been proposed over the decades. These can be task oriented, clinician centred, behaviour centred and patient centred. Although most models have been developed for use within the primary care/GP setting, they are arguably also applicable to secondary care and tertiary care settings, with adaptation as necessary.

All consultation frameworks share the common task of obtaining a medical history; however, Mehay et al. (2012) classify them as differing in three ways.

- *Concept versus implementation*: conceptual frameworks have clear aims but lack integration of the process of implementation into practice. The more modern-day frameworks (2003 and onwards) include both aspects.
- *Clinician versus patient centredness*: frameworks vary in their degree of focus on the consultation's agenda, process and outcome in respect of the practitioner's perspective (biomedical/disease framework) versus the patient's perspective (illness framework). Although disease and illness

usually co-exist, the same disease can lead to markedly different experiences of illness in different patient populations.

- *Task-oriented versus behavioural focus*: the degree to which frameworks focus on the tasks to be achieved in the consultation versus the range of behaviours required in the consultation.

Mehay et al. (2012) also propose a simple diagram which details the degree to which a selection of existing frameworks differ, in terms of their focus on the three aforementioned classifications. Figure 9.2 has been adapted from this original work to include more recent consultation frameworks.

Consultation frameworks promote a thorough and safe approach to the information gathering, information processing and subsequent outputs of the patient–practitioner consultation. Practitioners may differ as to which framework they use and how they adapt it into their own practice, which will largely depend on the nature of the encounter.

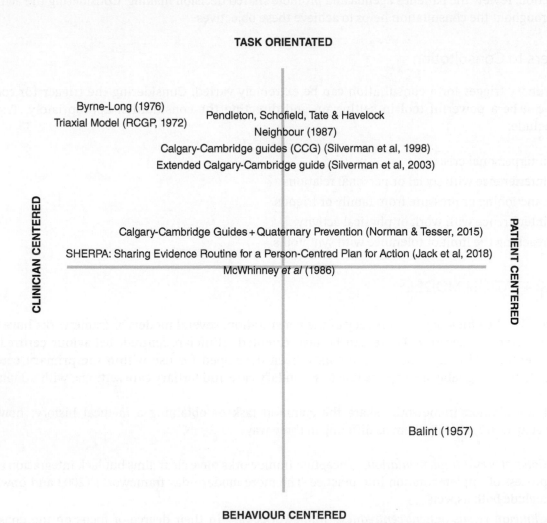

TASK ORIENTATED

Byrne-Long (1976)
Triaxial Model (RCGP, 1972)

Pendleton, Schofield, Tate & Havelock

Neighbour (1987)

Calgary-Cambridge guides (CCG) (Silverman et al, 1998)

Extended Calgary-Cambridge guide (Silverman et al, 2003)

CLINICIAN CENTERED   **PATIENT CENTERED**

Calgary-Cambridge Guides + Quaternary Prevention (Norman & Tesser, 2015)

SHERPA: Sharing Evidence Routine for a Person-Centred Plan for Action (Jack et al, 2018)

McWhinney *et al* (1986)

Balint (1957)

BEHAVIOUR CENTERED

FIGURE 9.2   Consultation models and their differing emphasis on four common domains. *Source*: Adapted from Mehay et al. (2012). Reproduced with kind permission.

Calgary-Cambridge Guide to the Medical Interview

The Calgary-Cambridge Guides (CCG) and the enhanced CCG (eCCG) (Kurtz and Silverman 1996; Kurtz et al. 2005) have become the dominant models used for teaching consultation skills in advanced practice and medical training programmes, and for subsequent use within the clinical arena. The CCG and eCCG are evidence-based frameworks that enable the AP to tailor the medical consultation by improving 71 communication skills and behaviours (Figure 9.3).

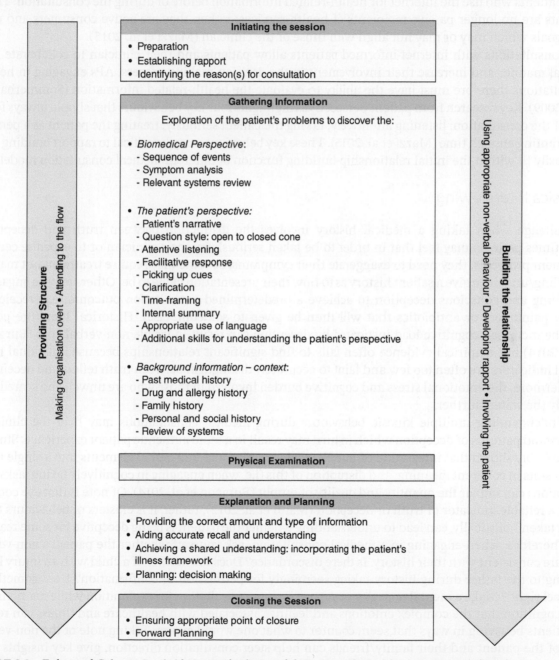

FIGURE 9.3   Enhanced Calgary-Cambridge consultation model. *Source*: Adapted from Kurtz et al. (2003).

Patient Perspective of Consultation

The AP–patient therapeutic relationship is one of the most unique and privileged relations a person can have with another human being (Bahadori et al. 2020) and can be critical in treatment success. However, despite good intentions, consultations can sometimes overlook patients with the patient perspective seldom considered. As such, the success of a medical consultation is a joint responsibility of both the patient and the clinician (Bensing et al. 2011). This can pose specific challenges as APs are now faced with patients who use the internet for health-related information before or during the consultation. Thus, patients are no longer passive recipients of health services; rather, they are active consumers and may have goals which may or may not align with those of the clinician (Mazzi et al. 2015).

Consultations with internet-informed patients allow patients and their clinician to collaborate in a mutual manner and increase their involvement in the decision-making process. APs engaging in health consultations therefore must have the ability to evaluate the health-related information (Sommerhalder et al. 2009). Key research from patient perspectives highlights four key behaviours that should always form part of the consultation: listening attentively; taking the patient seriously; treating the patient as a person; and granting enough time (Mazzi et al. 2015). These key behaviours may be critical to rapport building and can easily fit within the initial relationship-building function of different medical consultation models.

Kinesics Interviewing

A challenge when taking a medical history involves the distinction between truth and deception. Sometimes patients may feel that in order to be taken seriously by their clinician or to expedite certain treatment protocols, they need to exaggerate their symptoms, or some may require treatment but may be unwilling/unable to give a salient history as to how their presentation came to be. Others may be engaging in willing and conscious deception to achieve a predetermined consultation outcome (e.g. receipt of strong painkillers or antibiotics that will then be given to someone else). Historical literature posits that the increased cognitive load instigated by deception can result in visible non-verbal cues (Burgoon et al. 2014) but empirical evidence often fails to find significant relationships because individual non-verbal indicators are often too few and faint to accurately distinguish between truth tellers and deceivers. Furthermore, the emotional stress and cognitive burden involved in those who are unwell and scared can muddy the waters further.

Understanding multiple kinesic behaviours during medical consultations may help the clinician understand patterns of deception which in turn may result in a more authentic patient experience. Studies have reliably shown that integration of interdependent verbal and non-verbal elements into a single message results in coherent meaning, and disruption of this (i.e. when engaging in cognitively taxing tasks like deception) can impair the quantity and quality of output (Burgoon et al. 2014). Of note is that eye contact is not a reliable indicator of truth or deception (Mann et al. 2012); rather, it is clusters of behaviours that, when taken holistically, can lead to understanding whether the patient is being deceptive for some reason.

Therefore, when engaging in a medical consultation, ask yourself whether the patient's non-verbal cues are consistent with their history. Is there discordance? Does the mother of a child with an injury keep looking to the father during history taking seemingly for permission or confirmation? Does something 'not feel right'? Make a mental note as you engage in your consultation for exploration while maintaining metacognition that the complex emotions and feelings associated with healthcare and illness can result in patients behaving in ways that seem counter to what one would expect. Taking note of the non-verbal cues of the patient and their family/friends can help steer consultation direction, give key insights into the patient's cognitive status, and help the clinician in achieving effective therapeutic care.

ASPECTS OF OBTAINING A MEDICAL HISTORY

As mentioned, obtaining a medical history is embedded within the background information section of the eCCG (Figure 9.3). A comprehensive history commonly consists of several components, each of which has a variety of mnemonics that can aid the practitioner to elicit salient information at each stage (Table 9.1) (Hocking et al. 1998; Rothman and Kulkarni 2008; Talley and O'Connor 2017; Innes and Dover 2018; Bickley 2020).

RED FLAGS – PATHOLOGICAL CONSIDERATIONS

Red flags are specific attributes derived from a patient's history and/or physical examination that raise suspicion of a potentially life-threatening disease process. Common red flags in the context of HTPE include:

- progressing chest pain
- unilateral leg swelling
- unintentional weight loss.

TABLE 9.1   Components of an adult health history and associated mnemonics.

Components of the Adult Health History	Data	Mnemonics	
Identifying data/ personal information	• Demographic data • Source of history (patient/carer/ medical records) • Source of referral (if appropriate)		
Presenting complaint (PC)/ Principle symptoms (PS) (may be multiple)	• Major symptoms • Duration • Record each symptom using the patient's own terminology	**O** **P** **E** **R**	Onset of complaint Progress of complaint Exacerbating factors Relieving factors
History of presenting complaint (HPC)/ History of presenting illness (HPI)/ Present illness (PI)	• Each presenting symptom should be explored in detail • Pulls in relevant portions of the ROS section • May include relevant medications, allergies or social influences (alcohol, smoking, etc.) which may impact upon the PC • Events should be presented in chronological order	**A** **T** **E** **3** <u>OR</u> **S** **W** **I** **P** **E** <u>OR</u> (FOR PAIN) **S** **O**	Associated symptoms Timing Episodes of being symptom free Relevant systemic and general inquiry can be added here Start – When did it start? Worse – What is making it worse? Improve – What makes it improve? Pace – When does it occur? Evaluate – What is working? Site Onset

(Continued)

TABLE 9.1   (Continued)

Components of the Adult Health History	Data	Mnemonics	
		C	Character frequency
		R	Radiation
		A	Associations
		T	Time course
		E	Exacerbating/relieving factors
		S	Severity
Past medical history (PMH)	• List childhood illnesses • List adult illnesses (medical, surgical, obstetric/gynae and psychiatric) complete with date of initial diagnosis	Common illnesses with associated morbidity and mortality:	
		M	Myocardial infarction
		J	Jaundice
		T	Tuberculosis
		H	Hypertension
		R	Rheumatic fever
		E	Epilepsy
		A	Asthma
		D	Diabetes
		S	Stroke
		CS	Cancer (and associated treatments)
Drug history (DH)	• Allergies <u>and</u> severity – ask specifically for PMH of Stevens–Johnson syndrome	**D**	Doctor – medications prescribed by a registered healthcare professional
		R	Recreational – tobacco, alcohol, illicit drugs, anabolic steroids
		U	User – over-the-counter purchases (inc. alternative and homoeopathic medicine)
		G	Gynaecological – contraceptives or hormone replacement
		S	Sensitivities – allergies and sensitivities to medications, including severity
Family history (FH)	• May be represented in diagram format • Outlines age and health, or age and cause of death, siblings, parents, grandparents • Consider a genetic cause or contribution to a patient's condition	**FAMILY:**	Multiple affected siblings or individuals in multiple generations (lack does NOT rule out genetic causes)
		G	Group of congenital anomalies – ≥2 may indicate presence of genetic-related syndrome
		E	Extreme/exceptional presentation – early-onset cardiovascular disease, severe reactions to infections/metabolic stress, etc.
		N	Neuro – developmental delay or degeneration
		E	Extreme/exceptional pathology – phaeochromocytoma, acoustic neuroma, medullary thyroid cancer, multiple colon polyps, neurofibromas, etc.
		S	Surprising lab results – in an otherwise apparently healthy individual

TABLE 9.1   (Continued)

Components of the Adult Health History	Data	Mnemonics	
Social history (SH)	• Occupation and education • Overseas travel • Immunisations • Family of origin • Current household • Personal interests – hobbies, etc. • Lifestyle – activities of daily living, smoking, alcohol consumption, etc.	**W** **H** **A** **C** **S**	What do you do? Note chemical, dust, animal, paint and disease exposure How do you do it? Are you concerned about any exposure or experience? Co-workers or others exposed? Satisfied with your job?
Review of symptoms (ROS)	• Review of common symptoms associated with each body system, taking particular note of any red flag symptoms	**M** **U** **N** **C** **H** **E** **B** **A** **R** **S**	**Musculockeletal** – bone and joint pain/ muscular pain **Urinary** – volume of urine passed/ frequency/colour/dysuria/urgency/ incontinence **Neurological** – vision/headache/motor of sensory disturbance/ loss of consciousness/ confusion **Cardiovascular** – chest pain/dyspnoea/ syncope/orthopnoea **Hepato** – jaundice/itching/increased abdominal **Endocrine** – fatigue/polyuria/polydipsia/ weight loss/weight gain/hair loss **Blood** (and oncology) – fever/bleeding/ lumps/bumps/sweating/previous clots **Alimentary** – appetite/nausea/vomiting/ indigestion/dysphagia/weight loss/ abdominal pain/bowel habit **Respiratory** – dyspnoea/cough/sputum/ wheeze/haemoptysis/chest pain **Skin (and hair)** – hair loss/growths/skin eruptions/rashes/lesions/ulcers

History Taking in Special Circumstances: Time-Critical Situations

The traditional history-taking format meets many challenges in the time-critical situation, and the nature of these dynamic situations often means that a quick, focused history is required. The mnemonic 'AMPLE', originally developed for use in the context of trauma (Zemaitis et al. 2020), may be applied to quickly obtain pertinent information.

- A = allergies
- M = medications
- P = past medical history

- L = last meal (timing)
- E = events related to presentation

Pharmacological Principles

Some of the information elicited from conducting an in-depth HTPE may influence prescribing decisions, particularly where renal and liver disease is concerned. These disease process will often impact upon the drug metabolism.

The British National Formulary (BNF) provides useful information in the following respective chapters:

- `https://bnf.nice.org.uk/medicines-guidance/prescribing-in-renal-impairment`
- `https://bnf.nice.org.uk/medicines-guidance/prescribing-in-hepatic-impairment`
- `https://bnf.nice.org.uk/medicines-guidance/prescribing-in-pregnancy`

History Taking for Neurodiverse and Non-verbal Populations

Neurodiverse populations challenge historical paradigms where to be neurodiverse was seen in terms of deficits focusing on impairments and limitations, or of people who are broken and need to be fixed. Neurodiversity is now rightly celebrated and rethought through the lens of human diversity with individuals possessing a complex combination of cognitive strengths and challenges. For example, difficulties in understanding social nuances, filtering competing sensory stimuli, and planning the tasks of daily living may be coupled with strengths in detailed thinking, memory and complex pattern analysis (Nicolaidis 2012) (see Table 9.2).

Thus, setting in history taking may help obtain salient information to assist treatment. Ensure the consultation setting is low stimulation, with as little change to the patient's routine as possible. Ask direct and simple questions that can easily be understood and are not open to interpretation.

Fields of Practice – Mental Health

An effective history, as in most specialties, is integral to help determine a possible aetiology, determine appropriate investigations and form a clinical impression/diagnosis (Kumar and Clark 2016). However, the psychiatric history differs from a standard medical assessment slightly due to having a greater emphasis on the history component.

Furthermore, a large element of the examination is undertaken during the history component rather than as a discrete set of procedures afterwards (Davidson 2018). As such, obtaining a collateral history may be necessary and while a history may be taken from the patient alone, information from their friends, family or other healthcare professionals may offer additional important keys in establishing a clinical impression.

TABLE 9.2 Specific challenges in taking a history in neurodiverse populations.

Verbal and non-verbal considerations	• May have difficulty with pragmatic language • May have difficulty expressing wants and needs • May not offer clarification when misunderstood • May speak with unusual volume, rhythm and pitch • May have difficulty understanding nuances of sarcasm, idioms and humour • Will often fail to make eye contact and understanding facial expressions or body language
Social interactions	May have difficulty initiating conversations May not respond when called by name or addressed directly May not take an interest in the feelings or preferences of others May not respond to praise May have an aversion to physical contact
Ritualised behaviour	May have excessive resistance to change or unplanned events May be inflexible in thinking

History Taking for Ethnic Minority Populations

Effective history taking and physical examination involves understanding the specific cultural nuances that exist with different patient populations and how different cultures consume and treat healthcare. This can sometimes lead to discordance in expectations or frustrations between clinicians, the patient and the patient's wider network of friends and family.

Patients who do not speak English present a challenge due to the increased linguistic barrier which can result in miscommunication and misinterpretation of expressing empathy or eliciting patients' feelings and expectations (Alnahdi et al. 2021). It is recommended in these situations that telephone or in-person interpretation services are used, rather than a friend or family. This is to safeguard the clinician and ensure that the information given to the clinician and patient is a direct translation and not a facsimile provided by someone who is not an independent participant in the medical consultation.

History Taking for LGBTQIA+ Populations

Added challenges in history taking for LGBTQIA+ populations involve stigma. Stigma has many definitions but all generally include a process of othering, blaming and shaming (Poteat et al. 2013), and may be broadly conceptualised into three domains: *enacted* (such as overt actions like hate crimes), *anticipated* (concerns about possible future discrimination) and *internalised* (acceptance of stigma against someone as part of one's own doxastic self-schema) (Herek et al. 2015). Within the healthcare setting, internalised stigma by healthcare professionals may influence their care of LGBTQIA+ patients (Parameshwaran et al. 2017).

LGBTQIA+ people in the UK experience high levels of all three domains of stigma. Trans women (i.e. those individuals who were assigned male at birth but who through hormones and surgery live and present as female) in particular are disproportionately affected by health disparities that pervade multiple health outcomes (Rodríguez Madera et al. 2019) and there is persuasive evidence that negative attitudes are held by health professionals towards those who are socially stigmatised (Díaz et al. 2008; van Boekel et al. 2013). This idea is supported by Poteat et al. (2013) who report that a 2012 literature review relating to nurses' attitudes towards LGBT patients evidenced widespread negative attitudes in all articles studied.

Stigma is so damaging due to what researchers have called the 'stigma-sickness slope' (Winter et al. 2016) in which early stigma leads to a litany of negative experiences, such as discrimination and marginalisation, which then predisposes an individual to sickness and ultimately to an early death (Pinkston and Schierberl Scherr 2020).

Furthermore, for some clinicians, their personal socioreligious norms, attitudes and experiences may have implications for the care given to LGBTQIA+ people (Scott et al. 2021). The diversity of workforce within the NHS is undoubtedly one of its greatest strengths: racial, religious and cultural concordance between patient and clinician bodies contributes to a more effective therapeutic relationship and improved healthcare (Jetty et al. 2021) – put simply, we relate better to those with similar values and cultural frameworks. However, this diversity of religious and cultural expression may also present unique challenges for patients who are 'othered'; Judeo-Christian beliefs have been associated with 'deleterious anti-LGBT stigma and discrimination' (Scott et al. 2021) and religion-based sexual, heretical and/or moral deviance has been associated with LGBTQIA+ communities in many cultures (Wylie et al. 2016; Widiastuti 2018). Thus, when clinicians from these cultures work in a clinician–patient relationship, they may bring with them (consciously or not) certain stigmas that may potentiate negative treatment of LGBTQIA+ people.

Therefore, key to history taking for patient populations that have been historically discriminated against or stigmatised is a collaborative and understanding approach – one that understands the challenges that are faced and a clinician who is willing to attempt to dismantle barriers and work in collaboration with the patient.

Field of Practice – Paediatrics

The Paediatric Assessment Triangle can be used as a tool to evaluate a child's clinical status and need for rapid intervention (adapted from Ma et al. 2021).

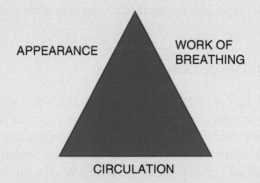

Appearance   The **TICLS** mnemonic can be used here:

T (Tone) – how is the patient's tone? Is the patient floppy or obtunded?

I (Interactivity) – is the patient interacting with their environment or caregiver?

C (Consolability) – can the child be consoled by their caregivers?

L (Look/gaze) – is the patient tracking things appropriately with their eyes, or are they non-focused and/or dysconjugate?

S (Speech) – is there stridor? Hoarse cry? Barking cough? Absent sound?

Work of breathing   Abnormal airway sounds: snoring, muffled/hoarse speech, stridor, grunting, wheezing
Abnormal positioning: sniffing position, tripoding, prefers seated posture
Retractions: supraclavicular, intercostal, substernal, head bobbing
Flaring: flaring of the nares on inspiration
Circulation   Pallor: white/pale skin or mucous membranes
Mottling: patchy skin discolouration due to variable vasoconstriction
Cyanosis: blue discolouration of the skin or mucous membranes

---

ORANGE FLAGS – PSYCHOLOGICAL CONSIDERATIONS

It is essential to establish a therapeutic alliance as this forms the groundwork of history taking because initially the patient will be making a decision as to your trustworthiness (Carlat 2017) and as a corollary, instituting a therapeutic relationship is one of the key aims of the psychiatric interview. This is followed by eliciting the symptoms, history and background information at the same time as examining the patient's mental state by means of the Mental State Examination (MSE), and concluding by providing information, reassurance and advice to them.

GREEN FLAGS – SOCIAL CONSIDERATIONS

Physical manifestations of disease can arise as a result of social, behavioural and cultural factors. These factors have clear implications and links for health and disease outcomes. The AP should ensure that the social history is given due care and attention within the consultation.

CLINICAL ASSESSMENT – ASPECTS OF PHYSICAL EXAMINATION

Introduction

The physical examination should always begin with an introduction to the patient, application of relevant infection control procedures and donning of personal protective equipment (PPE), where necessary. Patient positioning and comfort are paramount, as is adequate exposure. The pneumonic 'WIIPPPE' may be used to guide the practitioner in this element of the process (Oxford Medical Education 2021).

- **W**ash your hands – don appropriate PPE.
- **I**ntroduce yourself – name, professional role and focus of encounter/examination.
- **I**dentity of patient – confirm name and add one further element of demographic date (e.g. date of birth, address, NHS number, etc.).
- **P**ermission – gain consent to perform examination and explain your intentions/technique.
- **P**ain – is the patient currently in any pain or distress? If so, tend to this as a matter of urgency before proceeding with the examination.

- **Position at 45°** – this is the default positioning until any specific examination techniques are required, such as for abdominal examination.
- **Privacy** – aim to conduct the consultation in a location where privacy, dignity and confidentiality are maintained.
- **Expose chest to waist** – if further exposure is required, ensure dignity is promoted at all times.

General Inspection

A great deal of information can be gleaned from observing the patient's environment and their general demeanour. The practitioner should first assess whether there are any time-critical presentations that need to be attended to. The full physical examination approauch may not be appropriate in this case, and these situations lend themselves to an ABCDE (airway, breathing, circulation, disability and exposure) approach (Resuscitation Council UK 2015).

Where time-critical presentations are not present, the practitioner should glean information from any available clinical data present (e.g. monitoring systems, documented observation trends, etc.), observe for any adjuncts (e.g. wheelchairs, GTN spray, inhalers, infusions, etc.) and presence of any syndromic or dysmorphic features (e.g. macrocephaly, hypertelorism, etc.).

Vital Signs

It may be necessary and pertinent to assess vital signs early within the clinical examination process. Abnormal physiology may indicate a deteriorating patient, in which case initial management precedes definitive clinical diagnosis. In the UK, the National Early Warning Score (NEWS2) was introduced in 2012 and updated in 2017, providing a validated standardised system for assessing patients before hospital or in hospital, identifying acute illness and severity and therefore urgency of response required (Royal College of Physicians 2017).

The six physiological parameters are:

- respiration rate
- oxygen saturations
- systolic blood pressure
- heart rate
- level of consciousness or new confusion
- temperature.

Scores are assigned to physiological observations, allowing tracking and triggering of patients and a subsequent clinical response, graded by urgency and seniority, according to derangement on one or several parameters (Figure 9.4). Other observations or clinical investigations may include urine output, blood glucose and assessment of pain. Without early recognition and intervention, those high-risk patients may deteriorate further, leading to cardiac arrest and significant morbidity and mortality.

In patients who are generally well or stable, vital signs may remain a necessity but a more measured approach may be adopted for clinical examination.

Physiological parameter	Score						
	3	2	1	0	1	2	3
Respiration rate (per minute)	≤8		9–11	12–20		21–24	≥25
SpO$_2$ Scale 1 (%)	≤91	92–93	94–95	≥96			
SpO$_2$ Scale 2 (%)	≤83	84–85	86–87	88–92 ≥93 on air	93–94 on oxygen	95–96 on oxygen	≥97 on oxygen
Air or oxygen?		Oxygen		Air			
Systolic blood pressure (mmHg)	≤90	91–100	101–110	111–219			≥220
Pulse (per minute)	≤40		41–50	51–90	91–110	111–130	≥131
Consciousness				Alert			CVPU
Temperature (°C)	≤35.0		35.1–36.0	36.1–38.0	38.1–39.0	≥39.1	

FIGURE 9.4   The NEWS2 scoring chart. *Source*: Adapted from Royal College of Physicians (2017).

Physical Examination Techniques

After completing the introduction, general observation and vital signs components of the physical examination, a well-conducted, thorough physical examination requires a systematic approach; however, it does not always require a full examination for each body system (see Figure 9.5). Salient points from the initial consultation stage may guide the clinician as to the focus of a general examination.

Four techniques are applied in varying degrees throughout the physical examination.

- *Inspection* – utilising the senses of smell, touch and sight, the practitioner should observe for presence of abnormalities. These may include masses or bruising and/or fetor.
- *Palpation* – using various parts of the hand (dependent upon the examination), the practitioner should feel for size, consistency, texture, location and tenderness of underlying organs or masses.
- *Percussion* – a method for assessing the underlying structures. Percussion is utilised in thoracic and abdominal examinations to determine one of four percussion notes; resonant, hyperresonant, stony dull or dull.
- *Auscultation* - utilising a stethoscope, the practitioner will listen to heart and breath sounds and abnormalities causing turbulent flow within vascular structures such as bruits.

HANDS AND NAILS

The hands and nails should be examined for colour, temperature, deformity and skin changes, all of which may indicate specific disease processes. Clinical findings in the hands and nails as well as their associated disease and pathological processes can be found in Table 9.3.

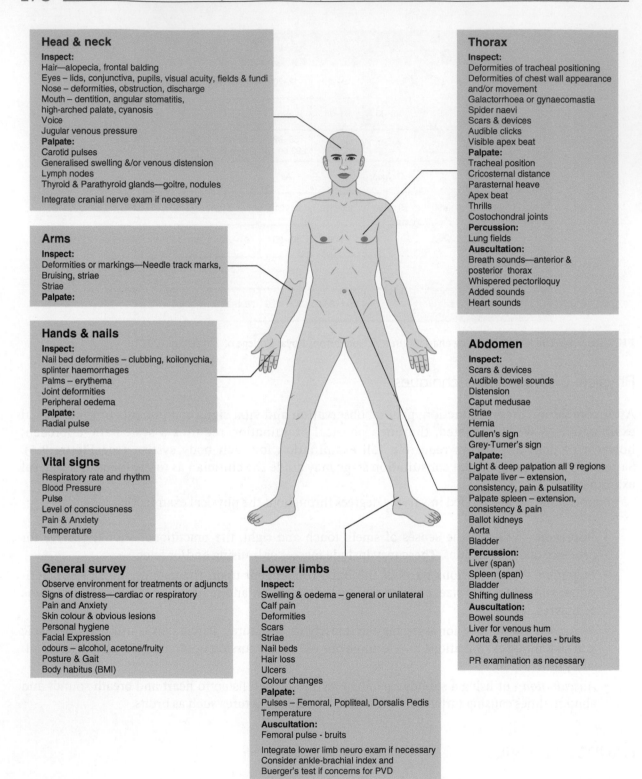

Head & neck
Inspect:
Hair—alopecia, frontal balding
Eyes – lids, conjunctiva, pupils, visual acuity, fields & fundi
Nose – deformities, obstruction, discharge
Mouth – dentition, angular stomatitis,
high-arched palate, cyanosis
Voice
Jugular venous pressure
Palpate:
Carotid pulses
Generalised swelling &/or venous distension
Lymph nodes
Thyroid & Parathyroid glands—goitre, nodules

Integrate cranial nerve exam if necessary

Arms
Inspect:
Deformities or markings—Needle track marks,
Bruising, striae
Striae
Palpate:

Hands & nails
Inspect:
Nail bed deformities – clubbing, koilonychia,
splinter haemorrhages
Palms – erythema
Joint deformities
Peripheral oedema
Palpate:
Radial pulse

Vital signs
Respiratory rate and rhythm
Blood Pressure
Pulse
Level of consciousness
Pain & Anxiety
Temperature

General survey
Observe environment for treatments or adjuncts
Signs of distress—cardiac or respiratory
Pain and Anxiety
Skin colour & obvious lesions
Personal hygiene
Facial Expression
odours – alcohol, acetone/fruity
Posture & Gait
Body habitus (BMI)

Lower limbs
Inspect:
Swelling & oedema – general or unilateral
Calf pain
Deformities
Scars
Striae
Nail beds
Hair loss
Ulcers
Colour changes
Palpate:
Pulses – Femoral, Popliteal, Dorsalis Pedis
Temperature
Auscultation:
Femoral pulse - bruits

Integrate lower limb neuro exam if necessary
Consider ankle-brachial index and
Buerger's test if concerns for PVD

Thorax
Inspect:
Deformities of tracheal positioning
Deformities of chest wall appearance
and/or movement
Galactorrhoea or gynaecomastia
Spider naevi
Scars & devices
Audible clicks
Visible apex beat
Palpate:
Tracheal position
Cricosternal distance
Parasternal heave
Apex beat
Thrills
Costochondral joints
Percussion:
Lung fields
Auscultation:
Breath sounds—anterior &
posterior thorax
Whispered pectoriloquy
Added sounds
Heart sounds

Abdomen
Inspect:
Scars & devices
Audible bowel sounds
Distension
Caput medusae
Striae
Hernia
Cullen's sign
Grey-Turner's sign
Palpate:
Light & deep palpation all 9 regions
Palpate liver – extension,
consistency, pain & pulsatility
Palpate spleen – extension,
consistency & pain
Ballot kidneys
Aorta
Bladder
Percussion:
Liver (span)
Spleen (span)
Bladder
Shifting dullness
Auscultation:
Bowel sounds
Liver for venous hum
Aorta & renal arteries - bruits

PR examination as necessary

FIGURE 9.5   Example physical examination content.

TABLE 9.3 Clinical findings of the hands and nails and their associated pathological processes.

Finding	Associated Diseases	Pathological Process
Hands		
Osler's nodes	Infective bacterial endocarditis Systemic lupus erythematosus (SLE)	• Deposition of immune complexes in the dermis secondary to microemboli
Janeway lesions	Infective bacterial endocarditis	• Deposition of immune complexes in the dermis secondary to microemboli
Dupuytren contractures	Familial Diabetes Epilepsy Alcohol excess Smoking	• Contractures of the palmar fascia secondary to fibroblast proliferation and collagen deposition
Ulnar deviation of the metacarpophalangeal joints	Rheumatoid arthritis	• Autoantibodies (rheumatoid factors and anticitrullinated peptide antibodies) cause complement activation resulting in chronic joint inflammation, cartilage and bone errosion
Muscle wasting	Carpal tunnel syndrome T1 nerve damage – trauma, herniated disc, radiculopathy, diabetes mellitus, neoplasm	• Idiopathic with median nerve neuropathy secondary to chronically increased pressure within the carpal tunnel • Compression or avulsion of the nerve root
Cyanosis	Heart or lung disease Shock – hypovolaemic, cardiogenic Hypothermia	• Deoxygenated haemoglobin in the small vessels of the peripheries
Palmar erythema	Chronic liver disease, rheumatoid arthritis, thyrotoxicosis, sarcoidosis, pregnancy	• Dilation of the palmar capillaries as a result of increased circulating oestrogen due to hepatic dysfunction or pregnancy
Asterixis	Hepatic encephalopathy, respiratory disease causing carbon dioxide retention, renal failure	• Inability to maintain position due to dysregulation of innervation of muscles via the diencephalic motor centre
Burrows – finger webs, palms	Scabies	• Mites burrow in the epidermis
Nails		
Clubbing	COPD Lung cancer Pulmonary fibrosis Infective endocarditis Congenital heart disease Liver cirrhosis Inflammatory bowel disease Thyrotoxicosis	• Increased release of platelet-derived growth factor (PDGF) and vascular endothelial growth factor (VEGF) from peripheral megakaryocytes leads to increased vascularity, permeability and ultimately connective tissue changes • The release of both PDGF and VEGF is thought to be enhanced by hypoxia
Beau's lines	Acute illness Nutritional deficiency	• Reduced activity of the nail matrix

(Continued)

TABLE 9.3   (Continued)

Finding	Associated Diseases	Pathological Process
Leuconychia: • Terry's nails • Muehrcke's lines • Lindsay's nails • Mees lines	Hypoalbunimaemia: • Liver disease • Chronic renal failure • Protein-losing enteropathies – ulcerative colitis, Crohn's disease Heavy metal poisoning Chemotherapy	• Overgrowth of connective tissue leading to changes in nail bed vascularity • Local oedema causing compression of vascular structures in the nail bed
Koilonychia	Severe iron deficiency B12 deficiency Diabetes	• Reduced blood flow causing disruption of the subungual connective tissue
Splinter haemorrhages	Infective endocarditis Vasculitis Trauma	• Platelet microthrombi within nail bed capillaries • Damage to the nail bed capillaries
Onycholysis	Psoriasis Thyrotoxicosis Vascular insufficiency Infection Trauma	• Compromise or disruption of the hyponychium altering nail plate attachment
Pitting	Psoriasis Alopecia Lichen planus	• Inflammation of the proximal nail matrix
Onychomysis	Fungal nail infection secondary to immunosuppression	• Nail bed hyperkeratosis damaging the nail matrix
Nail fold erythema and telangiectasia	SLE Systemic sclerosis Dermatomyositis	• Dilated capillaries associated with erythema at the nail fold
Melanonychia	Melanoma	
Yellow nail	Chronic bronchitis Pleural effusion Diabetes Thyroid disease Lymphoedema	• Abnormality in the lymphatic flow associated with nail plate hyperkeratosis

Case Study

Tony is a 42 year old who has been admitted to hospital with new-onset increasing shortness of breath. They are currently being monitored in the emergency department. The symptoms started a week ago and over the last 24 hours have worsened and associated with rigors, night sweats and aching limbs. Past medical history includes intravenous drug use; they last injected nine months ago. An advanced care practitioner finds the following on assessment.

Assessment

Airway – patent, the patient is speaking in full sentences.

Breathing – oxygen saturations of 95% on 2l nasal cannulae, respiratory rate 18, auscultation reveals fine bibasal inspiratory crepitations.

Circulation – heart rate 105, sinus rhythm, blood pressure 110/56 mmHg, warm peripherally with a capillary refill time of three seconds, calves are soft and non-tender, mild pedal oedema, auscultation reveals an early diastolic murmur, splinter haemorrhages are present in four finger nails and six toe nails with clubbing, conjunctival haemorrhage.

Disability – patient is alert on the AVPU scale, pupils are size 3, equal and reactive to light, blood glucose is 8, temperature is 38.1 °C.

Exposure – long-standing chronic ulcer in the left groin, the dressing is clean. One 22 g cannula in the right anticubital fossa. Tony passed urine approximately four hours ago.

Advanced care practitioner actions

- Request a chest X-ray and transthoracic echocardiogram.
- Perform 12-lead electrocrdiography.
- Take admission bloods including full blood count, CRP, U+Es, coagulation screen, arterial blood gas and blood culture.
- Swab the chronic ulcer.
- Start intravenous antibiotics according to local antimicrobial guidelines.

Diagnosis

- Bacterial endocarditis with evidence of heart failure.
- The blood culture was positive for *Staphylococcus aureus*.
- The transthoracic echocardiogram demonstrated a vegetation on the aortic valve.
- Full blood count and CRP were both raised at 23.4 and 256 respectively.
- The arterial blood gas was pH 7.34 pCO$_2$ 5.6 pO$_2$ 9.6 HCO$_3$ 22 BXS – 3.4
- Tony was admitted to the medical ward for ongoing management.

Upper Limbs

The upper limb neurological examination constitutes general inspection, tone, power, deep tendon reflexes, sensation and co-ordination. The presence of specific signs may indicate an upper (brain or spinal cord) or lower (peripheral nervous system) motor neuron lesion.

Arterial peripheral pulses of the upper limb (radial or brachial) should be examined for rate, rhythm, volume and character. Bruits on auscultation over an artery may indicate stenosis of the vessel. Abnormal findings may be pathological and these are detailed in Table 9.4.

Head and Neck

The head and neck should be examined for appearance, deformity, asymmetry and skin changes. In addition, palpation, auscultation and percussion may reveal abnormal clinical findings indicating specific disease processes. It is beyond the scope of this chapter to discuss in detail examination of the ears, nose and throat. Clinical findings of the head and neck, as well as their associated disease and pathological processes, can be found in Table 9.5.

TABLE 9.4 Arterial pulse examination, abnormal findings and common pathological causes.

Arterial Pulse Examination	Abnormal Finding	Pathological Cause
Rate and rhythm	Bradycardia	Hypothyroidism Arrhythmia: • Sick sinus syndrome • Heart block Medications
	Tachycardia	Hyperthyroidism Sepsis Pain Arrhythmia: • Atrial fibrillation or flutter • Ventricular or supraventricular tachycardia Medications
Volume	Low	Hypovolaemia Left ventricular failure Peripheral arterial disease
	High	Hypertension Thyrotoxicosis Aortic regurgitation
Character	Collapsing	Aortic regurgitation
	Slow-rising	Aortic stenosis
	Pulsus bisferiens	Severe aortic stenosis Aortic stenosis and aortic regurgitation
	Pulsus alternans	Severe heart failure
	Pulsus paradoxus	Cardiac tamponade Constrictive pericarditis

Assessment for the presence of the carotid pulse tends to occur more commonly in cardiac arrest. The cranial nerves should be assessed as part of the neurological examination, disorders of which may affect vision, hearing, balance, swallow, phonation, tongue movements, facial sensation and motor function due to a vast number of disease processes. It is beyond the scope of this chapter to detail their abnormal findings and associated pathological processes.

Fields of Practice – Learning Disabilities

People with learning disabilities have increased prevalence of multimorbidity at a younger age associated with poorer physical and mental health and consequently premature mortality (RCGP 2017). Annual health checks were explicitly recommended to facilitate prompt detection and management of health conditions for anyone over the age of 14 on their general practitioner's learning disability register (NICE 2016). This resulted in increased investigations, recognition and management of co-morbid conditions, medication reviews and specialist referrals in primary and secondary care (Buszewicz et al. 2014).

TABLE 9.5   Clinical findings of the head and neck and their associated pathological processes.

Finding	Associated Disease	Pathological Process
Face		
Central cyanosis	Heart failure Hypoxaemia	• Deoxygenated haemoglobin in the small vessels of the peripheries
Xanthelasma	Hypercholesterolaemia Thyroid dysfunction Diabetes mellitus	• Accumulation of lipids within the foam cells of the skin
Arcus senilis	Hypercholesterolaemia	• Deposition of lipids between the cornea and sclera
Malar flush	Mitral valve stenosis	• Retention of carbon dioxide resulting in vasodilation
Malar rash	SLE Polycythaemia	• Chronic inflammation due to autoantibodies
Scleral icterus	Haemolytic anaemia, hepatitis, alcoholic liver disease, autoimmune disorders, malignancy of the liver, gall bladder or pancreas, gallstones Drugs	• High levels of serum bilirubin secondary to unconjugated bilirubin as a result of excessive red blood cell breakdown or dysfunction of the hepatic cells, or conjugated bilirubin due to obstruction of the biliary tract
Ptosis (blepharoptosis)	Multiple sclerosis Horner' syndrome Myasthenia gravis Ocular myopathy Trauma	• Defective innervation or neuromuscular junction, myopathy, aponeurosis or trauma of the levator muscle of the upper eyelid
Altered facial appearance	Cushing disease Acromegaly Hypothyroidism Polycycstic ovary syndrome Hyperthyoidism Parkinson disease Myotonic dystrophy	• Particular facial appearances are associated with certain pathological disease processes
Unilateral facial weakness	Lower motor neuron: • Bell's palsy • Ramsay Hunt syndrome • Malignancy – acoustic neuroma Upper motor neuron: • Stroke • Traumatic brain injury • Spinal cord injury • Multiple sclerosis • Huntington disease	• Inflammation causing oedema or a tumour causing compression of the facial nerve secondary to viral infection
Tongue		
Leucoplakia	Keratotic precancer	• Mutation of tumour suppression gene leading to uncontrolled cell growth
Atrophic glossitis	Iron or B12 deficiency	• Unknown

(Continued)

TABLE 9.5　(Continued)

Finding	Associated Disease	Pathological Process
Angular stomatitis	Iron deficiency anaemia Chronic atrophic candidiasis	• Immunocompromise leading to opportunistic infection
Macroglossia	Hypothyroidism Amyloidosis Down syndrome	• Lack of degradation of subcutaneous mucopolysaccharides leading to accumulation • Amyloid protein deposition in the tongue • Lingual muscular hypertrophy or glandular hyperplasia resulting in overgrowth of tissue
Wasting and fasciculations	Motor neuron disease	• Wasting – degeneration of motor neurons • Fasciculations – spontaneous depolarisation of motor neurons
Neck		
Swelling	Thyroglossal cyst Thyroid or laryngeal cancer Carotid aneurysm	• Formation of fibrous cyst due to a persistent thyroglossal duct • Carotid aneurysm – weakening of the vessel wall due to trauma, atherosclerosis, infection, fibromuscular dysplasia, arteritis
Palpable lymph nodes: • Parotid • Submandibular • Cervical chain	Infection – viral or bacterial Malignancy Mumps	• Cellular proliferation leading to enlarged lymph nodes • Replication of the mumps virus within the parotid gland
Neck stiffness	Meningitis	• Inflammation of the cervical nerve roots and meninges causes muscle spasm
Raised jugular venous pressure (JVP)	Heart failure Acute pulmonary embolism Cor pulmonale Superior vena cava obstruction	• Fluid overload and/or pump failure • Sudden increase in right ventricular afterload leading to right ventricular dysfunction and failure • Pulmonary hypertension leading to right ventricular failure
Cannon waves (JVP) on inspiration	Complete heart block Junctional rhythm Supraventricular or ventricular tachycardia	• Atrial contraction against a closed tricuspid valve due to atrioventricular dissociation
Kussmaul's sign	Cardiac tamponade Constrictive pericarditis Severe right ventricular failure	• Decreased diastolic filling of the right ventricle due to poorly compliant myocardium or pericardium • Fibrosis of the pericardium resulting in raised diastolic pressure

Thorax

The thorax should be examined for appearance, integrity, deformity, asymmetry and skin changes. In addition, palpation, auscultation and percussion may reveal abnormal clinical findings indicating specific disease processes. Certain scars signify previous surgery such as a median sternotomy (coronary artery bypass grafting, valve replacement, heart transplant), thoracotomy (lobectomy, pneumonectomy, oesophagectomy) or infraclavicular (pacemaker, implantable cardioverter defibrillator). Dilated superficial veins over the thorax in addition to distended neck veins may indicate obstruction of the superior vena cava. Clinical findings of the thorax, as well as their associated disease and pathological processes, can be found in Table 9.6.

Specific clinical investigations of the thorax may include chest X-ray, echocardiography, arterial blood gas, lung function tests, thoracic ultrasound, computed tomography, bronchoscopy, lung biopsy and percutaneous needle aspiration.

CLINICAL INVESTIGATIONS

A classic feature of asthma is airflow resistance in expiration. Diagnosis, severity and/or the presence of an exacerbation of asthma may be determined by use of sequential peak expiratory flow (PEFR) (BT/SIGN 2019). This is a simple non-invasive measure of the highest flow achieved on forced expiration from a position of maximal inspiration, expressed in terms of litres per minute (Miller et al. 2005).

TABLE 9.6   Clinical findings of the thorax and their associated pathological processes.

Finding	Associated Diseases	Pathological Process
Thorax shape or integrity:		
• 'Barrel'	Severe COPD, cystic fibrosis, arthritis	• Chronic hyperinflation of the lungs due to obstructed airflow
• Kyphoscoliosis	Poliomyelitis, spinal tuberculosis, osteoporosis, osteoarthritis, neuromuscular diseases	• Develops due to the underlying pathology of the disease process
• Pectus carinatum	Severe, poorly controlled asthma prepuberty Osteomalacia or rickets	• Lung hyperinflation with excessive diaphragmatic contraction while the thorax is pliable
• Pectus excavatum	Congenital abnormality	
• Flail segment	Traumatic rib fractures	• Three or more sequential ribs fractured in two or more places
• Costal cartilage tenderness	Costochondritis due to infection or trauma	• Inflammation of the costochondral cartilage
Chest expansion:		
• Decrease unilaterally	Pleural effusion, pneumothorax, lung or lobar collapse	• Accumulation of fluid between the parietal and visceral pleura preventing airflow due to cardiopulmonary disease, malignancy or systemic inflammation

(Continued)

TABLE 9.6   (Continued)

Finding	Associated Diseases	Pathological Process
		• Accumulation of air between the parietal and visceral pleural preventing airflow which may be associated with certain respiratory diseases, iatrogenic or traumatic
• Decrease bilaterally	COPD, lung fibrosis	• Lobar or lung collapse caused by plugging of sputum, foreign body or intrinsic or extrinsic malignancy or granulomatous diseases preventing airflow
		• Destruction of lung parenchyma or reduced lung compliance decreasing airflow
Breathing pattern:		
• Excessive accessory muscle use	Severe COPD, pneumonia	• Occurs due to impaired ventilatory demands, increased negative intrathoracic pressure and lung volume
• Paradoxical	Spinal cord injury, neurological diseases, traumatic phrenic nerve damage	• Diaphragmatic dysfunction due to denervation or direct trauma preventing contraction on inspiration
Tracheal deviation:		
• Away	Pleural effusion Tension pneumothorax	• Volume expansion due to fluid or air pushes the trachea away
• Towards	Collapse of lung or upper lobe Pneumonectomy	• Volume loss due to atelectasis or overinflation of remaining lung
Gynaecomastia	Liver disease, thyrotoxicosis, adrenal malignancy, drugs	• If associated with loss of hair and testicular atrophy. Due to increased circulating oestrogen as a result of hepatic dysfunction
Stridor	Partial upper airway obstruction – epiglottitis, tumour, anaphylaxis, vocal cord oedema, foreign body	• Increased airflow turbulence due to partial obstruction
Displacement of cardiac apex beat	Left ventricular hypertrophy Pectus excavatum Kyphoscoliosis	• Hypertension, aortic stenosis increase afterload leading to hypertrophy • Anatomical deformity
Parasternal heave	Right ventricular hypertrophy	• Pulmonary hypertension results in right ventricular hypertrophy due to increased vascular resistance
Percussion:		
• Dull	Consolidation	• Alveoli filled with inflammatory cellular exudate, pus or pulmonary oedema results in poorly aerated lung parenchyma, decreasing transmission of sound
• Stony dull	Pleural effusion, haemothorax	• Fluid in the pleural space decreases transmission of sound
• Hyperresonant	Pneumothorax	• Presence of air in the pleural space increases transmission of sound

TABLE 9.6 (Continued)

Finding	Associated Diseases	Pathological Process
Auscultation: *Lung*		
• Decreased air entry	Pleural effusion, pneumothorax, lobar collapse	• Poorly aerated lung and reduced airflow due to intrinsic or extrinsic factors
• Bronchial breath sounds	Consolidation	• Alveoli filled with inflammatory cellular exudate, pus or pulmonary oedema
• Crackles: – Early – Mid/late	Bronchiolitis Pulmonary oedema, pulmonary fibrosis, bronchiectasis, pneumonia	• Peripheral airways opening on inspiration • Air moving through secretions or fluid in the airways • Abrupt opening of the alveoli and distal airways on inspiration
• Pleural rub	Pneumonia, pulmonary embolism, pulmonary infarction	• Inflammation of the parietal and visceral pleura
• Wheeze	Asthma, COPD, bronchiolitis, anaphylaxis, tracheobronchomalacia	• Turbulent airflow caused by airway narrowing resulting in oscillation of the airway walls
Heart • Sounds – Quiet (first and second)	Low cardiac output, prolonged P-R interval, aortic or mitral regurgitation, poor left ventricular function, aortic stenosis	• First heart sound pathology is related to the closing of the tricuspid and mitral valves on ventricular contraction. Second heart sound pathology is related to the closing of the aortic and pulmonary valves at the end of ventricular contraction
– Loud (first and second)	Increased cardiac output, short P-R interval, mitral stenosis, hypertension – systemic or pulmonary	
– Variable	Atrial fibrillation, complete heart block	• Splitting occurs due to pathological causes of delayed right or left ventricular contraction
– Splitting	Bundle branch block, aortic or pulmonary stenosis, atrial or septal defect, pulmonary hypertension, hypertrophic cardiomyopathy, ventricular pacing	• Ventricular filling following opening of the tricuspid and mitral valves
–Third	Left ventricular failure, mitral regurgitation	• Atrial contraction against non-compliant ventricle
– Fourth	Left ventricular hypertrophy	
• Added sounds – Opening snap – Ejection click	Mitral stenosis Aortic or pulmonary stenosis, mitral valve prolapsed, metallic valve	• Sudden opening of a stenosed valve
– Pericardial rub	Pericarditis, myocardial infarction	• Inflammation of the pericardial sac
• Murmurs – Systolic	Atrial or septal defect, aortic or pulmonary stenosis, mitral or tricuspid regurgitation, leaking valve prosthesis or prolapsed, pregnancy, sepsis, severe anaemia	• Turbulent blood flow due to an abnormal valve, obstructed outflow, septal defect or increased blood flow velocity across a normal valve. Timing, duration, character, pitch, location, intensity and radiation will determine specific pathology
–Diastolic – Continuous	Aortic regurgitation, mitral stenosis Patent ductus arteriosus	

(Continued)

TABLE 9.6   (Continued)

Finding	Associated Diseases	Pathological Process
Skin: • Lesions • Lumps • Subcutaneous emphysema • Spider naevi	Malignancy Lipoma Pneumothorax, ruptured oesophagus, severe acute asthma	• Ruptured alveoli or mediastinal air travels to the vascular interstitium via fascial planes into the subcutaneous tissues of the head and neck • Dilation of the palmar capillaries as a result of increased circulating oestrogen due to hepatic dysfunction or pregnancy

Abdomen

The abdomen should be examined for appearance, deformity, asymmetry and skin changes. In addition, palpation, auscultation and percussion may reveal abnormal clinical findings indicating specific disease processes. Clinical findings of the abdomen as well as their associated disease and pathological processes can be found in Table 9.7.

TABLE 9.7   Clinical findings of the abdomen and their associated pathological processes.

Finding	Associated Diseases	Pathological Process
Involuntary guarding	Perforated bowel	• Inflammation of the parietal peritoneum
Tenderness – general and rebound	Cholecystitis, peptic ulcer, diverticulitis, appendicitis, ileitis, peritonitis	• Location of tenderness may be specific to the underlying pathological process
Palpable mass	Malignancy, aortic aneurysm	• Loss of structural integrity of the aorta due to inflammation, smooth muscle apoptosis, proteolysis and deposition of collagen
Organomegaly: • Liver	Chronic liver diease, malignancy, right heart failure, haematological disease, amyloidosis, sarcoidosis	• Occurs as a result of the underlying pathological process
• Splenomegaly	Haematological disease, infection, SLE, amyloidosis, sarcoidosis, rheumatoid arthritis	
• Enlarged kidneys	Autosomal dominant polycystic kidney disease, hydronephrosis, acute pyelonephritis	
Palpable bladder	Acute urinary retention	• Bladder outflow obstruction, impaired contraction, loss of innervations (sensory or motor)
Murphy's sign	Acute cholecystitis	• Obstruction of biliary outflow causing inflammation

TABLE 9.7   (Continued)

Finding	Associated Diseases	Pathological Process
Rovsing's sign	Acute appendicitis	• Obstruction of the appendiceal lumen causing inflammation
Iliopsoas	Appendicitis, abscess – iliopsoas or perinephric, Crohn's, pyelonephritis, vertebral osteomyelitis	• Primary or secondary infection
Grey Turner and Cullen signs	Pancreatitis, aortic or ectopic pregnancy rupture	• Intra-abdominal bleeding causing superficial bruising
Ascites: • Shifting dullness • Fluid thrill	Liver disease, intra-abdominal malignancy or tuberculosis, right heart failure, hypoproteinaemia, pancreatitis	• Abnormal hydrostatic and osmotic pressures between the intravascular and extravascular space
Auscultation: • Absent bowel sounds	Paralytic ileus, peritonitis	• Autonomic and enteric nervous system dysfunction and inflammatory mediators
• Succussion splash	Pyloric stenosis	• Delayed gastric emptying
Hernia	Inguinal, umbilical, incisional	• Protrusion of bowel or omentum due to increased abdominal pressure
Rectal examination: • Hard, asymmetrical irregular prostate	Prostate cancer	
• Faeces	Constipation	
Caput medusae	Portal hypertension	• Recanalisation and dilation of the umbilical veins due to increased pressure in the portal vein

---

CLINICAL INVESTIGATIONS – URINALYSIS

Substance present	Interpretation
Blood	• Haematuria (renal – glomerulonephritis, pyelonephritis, tumour, infarction, polycystic kidney disease), haemaglobinuria (haemolysis of intravascular origin), myoglobinuria (rhabdomyolysis)
Protein	• Test ranges from + to ++++ • Only sensitive to albumin • Causes of proteinuria include renal disease, particularly glomerular in nature, non-renal causes include fever, exercise, burns, congestive cardiac failure, postoperative, blood transfusion and acute alcohol abuse
Ketones	• Specifically tests acetoacetic acid and not other ketones • Presence occurs in diabetic ketoacidosis, starvation and low-carbohydrate diets
Glucose	• Small amounts may be present in the urine • May indicate diabetes mellitus or the inability of the renal tubules to reabsorb glucose
Leucocytes	• Presence may indicate urinary infection, inflammation, carcinoma

Nitrites	• Presence may indicate gram-negative bacteria
pH	• Normally acidic
	• Treatment of specific conditions such as myoglobinuria or urinary calculi may include urinary alkinisation
	• Renal tubular acidosis should be suspected if urine is never acidic
	• Infection, e.g. *Proteus mirabilis* may cause alkaline urine
Bile and urobilinogen	• Presence may indicate hepatobiliary disease or haemolysis

Examination Scenarios – Rectal Examination

Rectal examination is an important part of the gastrointestinal examination. An explanation should be given, consent sought and a chaperone offered. The patient should be examined in the left lateral position with the hips and knees flexed. The perineal skin should be examined wearing gloves. The rectum should be examined with a lubricated forefinger, applying steady gentle pressure to the anal sphincter. Tone may be assessed by asking the patient to voluntarily contract the anal muscles. The rectum should then be systematically palpated, making a record of any mucosal abnormality, masses, presence of faeces, blood or mucus. The cervix and prostate should be identified and anomalies noted in female and male patients respectively.

Lower Limbs

The lower limb neurological examination constitutes general inspection, tone, power, deep tendon reflexes, sensation and co-ordination. The presence of specific signs may indicate an upper (brain or spinal cord) or lower (peripheral nervous system) motor neuron lesion.

Arterial peripheral pulses of the lower limb (femoral, popliteal, tibialis posterior, dorsalis pedis) should be examined. Abnormal findings may be pathological and include peripheral vascular disease or trauma, compartment syndrome, an aortic aneurysm or shock.

Skin changes may indicate systemic diseases, including:

- erythema nodosum – acute sarcoidosis and tuberculosis
- xanthomata of the patella or Achilles tendon – hyperlipidaemia
- rash – eczema, dermatitis, psoriasis, cellulitis or vasculitis
- foot ulcer – diabetes mellitus.

Bilateral or unilateral lower limb oedema may be attributed to lymphoedema, heart failure, nephritic syndrome or deep vein thrombosis.

CLOSING THE CONSULTATION

Closing the consultation should include forward planning and agreement of the next steps, provision of appropriate safety netting, a brief summary of the consultation and time for additional queries.

CONCLUSION

Consultation and clinical assessment are fundamental skills of the AP role, the process of which is complex and requires an array of underpinning knowledge in physiology, pathophysiology and theories of effective communication within the healthcare setting. There are multiple frameworks to guide this process, not all of which will be suitable for the vast array of specialist areas in which APs practise.

Take Home Points
- Best practice suggests that advanced practitioners must utilise a consultation model to strengthen their assessment detailing a holistic medical history for diverse populations.
- Evidence-based physical examination techniques are imperative to enable safe practice.
- An understanding of physiology and altered pathophysiology is essential within advancing practice.
- Proficiency must be obtained and continuous when undertaking history taking and physical examination (HTPE) skills at the level of advanced practice.

REFERENCES

Alnahdi, M.A., Alhaider, A., Bahanan, F. et al. (2021). The impact of the English medical curriculum on medical history taking from Arabic speaking patients by medical students. *Journal of Family Medicine and Primary Care* 10 (3): 1425–1430.

Bahadori, M., Yaghoubi, M., Haghgoshyie, E. et al. (2020). Patients' and physicians' perspectives and experiences on the quality of medical consultations: a qualitative study. *International Journal of Evidence-Based Healthcare* 18 (2): 247–255.

Bensing, J.M., Deveugele, M., Moretti, F. et al. (2011). How to make the medical consultation more successful from a patient's perspective? Tips for doctors and patients from lay people in the United Kingdom, Italy, Belgium and the Netherlands. *Patient Education and Counseling* 84 (3): 287–293.

Bickley, L.S. (2020). *Bates' Guide To Physical Examination and History Taking*, 13e. Philadelphia: Wolters Kluwer Health.

Bird, J. and Cohen-Cole, S.A. (1990). The three-function model of the medical interview. An educational device. *Advances in Psychosomatic Medicine* 20: 65–88.

van Boekel, L.C., Brouwers, E., van Weeghel, J., and Garretsen, H. (2013). Stigma among health professionals towards patients with substance use disorders and its consequences for healthcare delivery: systematic review. *Drug and Alcohol Dependence* 131 (1–2): 23–35.

British Thoracic Society and Scottish Intercollegiate Guidelines Network (2019). British Guideline on the management of asthma: A national clinical guideline. www.brit-thoracic.org.uk/quality-improvement/guidelines/asthma

Burgoon, J.K., Schuetzler, R., Wilson, and D. (2014). Kinesic patterning in deceptive and truthful interactions. *Journal of Nonverbal Behavior* 39 (1): 1–24.

Buszewicz, M., Welch, C., Horsfall, L. et al. (2014). Assessment of an incentivised scheme to provide annual health checks in primary care for adults with intellectual disability: a longitudinal cohort study. *Lancet Psychiatry.* 1 (7): 522–530.

Carlat, D.J. (2017). *The Psychiatric Interview*. New York: Wolters Kluwer.

Davidson, S. (2018). *Davidson's Principles and Practice of Medicine*, 23e (ed. S.H. Ralston et al.). Amsterdam: Elsevier B.V.

Díaz, N.V., Rivera, S.M., and Bou, F.C. (2008). AIDS stigma combinations in a sample of Puerto Rican health professionals: qualitative and quantitative evidence. *Puerto Rico Health Sciences Journal* 27 (2): 147–157.

Engel, G.E. and Morgan, W.L. (1973). *Interviewing and Patient Care*. Philadelphia: Saunders.

Faculty of Intensive Care Medicine (2015). Curriculum for Training for Advanced Critical Care Practitioners. www.ficm.ac.uk/sites/fcm/files/documents/2022-12/ACCP%20Curriculum%20Part%210%20-%20Handbook%20v1%202019%20Revusion.pdf

Health Education England (2017). Multi-professional framework for advanced clinical practice in England. www.hee.nhs.uk/sites/default/files/docuemtns/HEE%20ACP%Framework.pdf

Herek, G.M., Gillis, J.R., and Cogan, J.C. (2015). Internalized stigma among sexual minority adults: insights from a social psychological perspective. *Stigma and Health* 1 (S): 18–34.

Hocking, G., Kalyanaraman, R., and deMello, W.F. (1998). Better drug history taking: an assessment of the DRUGS mnemonic. *Journal of the Royal Society of Medicine* 91 (6): 305–306.

Innes, J.A. and Dover, A.R. (2018). *Macleod's Clinical Examination*, 14e. London: Elsevier.

Jetty, A., Jabbarpour, Y., Pollack, J. et al. (2021). Patient–physician racial concordance associated with improved healthcare use and lower healthcare expenditures in minority populations. *Journal of Racial and Ethnic Health Disparities* 9 (1): 68–81.

Kumar, P. and Clark, M.L. (2016). *Kumar and Clark's Clinical Medicine*, 9e. Amsterdam: Elsevier B.V.

Kurtz, S.M. and Silverman, J.D. (1996). The Calgary-Cambridge referenced observation guides: an aid to defining the curriculum and organizing the teaching in communication training programmes. *Medical Education* 30: 83–89.

Kurtz, S., Silverman, J., Benson, J., and Draper, J. (2003). Marrying content and process in clinical method teaching. Enhancing the Calgary–Cambridge Guides. *Academic Medicine* 78 (8): 802–809.

Kurtz, S.M., Silverman, J., and Draper, J. (2005). *Teaching and Learning Communication Skills in Medicine*, 2e. Oxford: Radcliffe Medical Press.

Ma, X., Liu, Y., Du, M. et al. (2021). The accuracy of the pediatric assessment triangle in assessing triage of critically ill patients in emergency pediatric department. *International Emergency Nursing* 58: 101041.

Mann, S., Vrij, A., Leal, S. et al. (2012). Windows to the soul? Deliberate eye contact as a cue to deceit. *Journal of Nonverbal Behavior* 36 (3): 205–215.

Mazzi, M.A., Rimondini, M., Boerma, W. et al. (2015). How patients would like to improve medical consultations: insights from a multicentre European study. *Patient Education and Counseling* 99 (1): 51–60.

Mehay, R., Beaumont, R., Draper, J. et al. (2012). Revisiting models of consultation. In: *The Essential Handbook for GP Training and Education* (ed. R. Mehay). Ohio: CRC Press.

Miller, M.R., Hankinson, J., Brusasco, V. et al. (2005). Standardisation of spirometry. *European Respiratory Journal* 26: 319–338.

NICE (2016). Mental health problems in people with learning disabilities: prevention, assessment and management. NG54. www.nice.org.uk/guidance/ng54

Nicolaidis, C. (2012). What can physicians learn from the neurodiversity movement? *AMA Journal of Ethics* 14 (6): 503–510.

Oxford Medical Education (2021). Cardiovascular Examination. https://oxfordmedicaleducation.com/clinical-examinations/cardiovascular-examination

Parameshwaran, V., Cockbain, B., Hillyard, M. et al. (2017). Is the lack of specific lesbian, gay, bisexual, transgender and queer/questioning (LGBTQ) health care education in medical school a cause for concern? Evidence from a survey of knowledge and practice among UK medical students. *Journal of Homosexuality* 64 (3): 367–381.

Peterson, M.C., Holbrook, J.H., von Vales, D. et al. (1992). Contributions of the history, physical examination, and laboratory investigation in the medical diagnosis. *Western Medical Journal* 156: 163–165.

Pinkston, M.M. and Schierberl Scherr, A.E. (2020). "Being diagnosed with HIV was the icing on the cake of my life": a case study of fostering resiliency through flexible interventions along the stigma-sickness slope. *Psychotherapy* 57 (1): 50–57. https://doi.org/10.1037/pst0000255.

Poteat, T., German, D., and Kerrigan, D. (2013, 1982). Managing uncertainty: a grounded theory of stigma in transgender health care encounters. *Social Science & Medicine* 84: 22–29.

Resuscitation Council UK (2015). The ABCDE Approach. www.resus.org.uk/library/2015-resuscitation-guidelines/abcde-approach

Rodríguez Madera, S.L., Diaz, N., Padilla, M. et al. (2019). "Just like any other patient": transgender stigma among physicians in Puerto Rico. *Journal of Health Care for the Poor and Underserved* 30 (4): 1518–1542.

Roshan, M. and Rao, A.P. (2000). A study on relative contributions of the history, physical examination and investigations in making medical diagnosis. *Journal of the Association of Physicians India* 48 (8): 771–775.

Rothman, A. and Kulkarni, K. (2008). PasTest Online Revision for Medical Students. www.revise4finals.co.uk/medicine/mnemonics/index.php

Royal College of Emergency Medicine (2022). Emergency Medicine Advanced Clinical Practitioner Curriculum 2022 Adult. https://rcem,ac,uk/wp-content/uploads/2022/09/ACP_Curriculum_Adult_Final_060922.pdf

Royal College of General Practitioners (2017). Step-by-step guide to health checks for people with a learning disability. www.rcgp.org.uk/clinical-and-research/resources/toolkits/health-check-toolkit.aspx

Royal College of Physicians (2017). National Early Warning Score (NEWS) 2: Standardising the assessment of acute-illness severity in the NHS. Updated report of a working party. www.rcplondon.ac.uk/projects/outputs/national-early-warning-score-news-2

Scott, D., Pereira, N., Harrison, S. et al. (2021). "In the Bible Belt:" the role of religion in HIV care and prevention for transgender people in the United States south. *Health and Place* 70: 102613–102613.

Sommerhalder, K., Abraham, A., Zufferey, M. et al. (2009). Internet information and medical consultations: experiences from patients' and physicians' perspectives. *Patient Education and Counseling* 77 (2): 266–271.

Talley, N. and O'Connor, S. (2017). *Talley and O'Connor's Clinical Examination*, 8e. London: Elsevier.

Widiastuti, R.S.K. (2018). Research method for exploring discourse on the rights for religion for transgender. *Esensia : Jurnal Ilmu-Ilmu Ushuluddin* 18 (1): 105–122.

Winter, S., Diamond, M., Green, J. et al. (2016). Transgender people: health at the margins of society. *Lancet* 388 (10042): 390–400.

Wylie, K., Knudson, G., Khan, S. et al. (2016). Serving transgender people: clinical care considerations and service delivery models in transgender health. *Lancet* 388 (10042): 401–411.

Zemaitis, M.R., Planas, J.H., and Wassem, M. (2020). Trauma Secondary Survey. *Stat Pearls*. www.ncbi.nlm.nih.gov/books/NBK441902/.

FURTHER READING

McGee, S. (2017). *Evidence-Based Physical Diagnosis*, 5e. Philadelphia: Elsevier.

Talley, N.N. and O'Connor, S. (2021). *Talley and O'Connor's Clinical Examination: 2-Volume Set: A Systematic Guide to Physical Diagnosis*. Philadelphia: Elsevier.

SELF-ASSESSMENT QUESTIONS

1. As a trainee AP, what are your learning needs in relation to clinical history taking and physical examination?
2. How will you identify your HTPE needs for supervision and what documents and guidance will support this?
3. How will you evaluate and assess your HTPE skills to prove your competency and capability in practice?
4. How can you ensure that you continue to develop your ability to refine your HTPE practice?

GLOSSARY

Caput medusae   A cluster of engorged veins surrounding the navel.

Cullen's sign   Superficial oedema with bruising in the subcutaneous fatty tissue around the periumbilical region due to retroperitoneal or intraabdominal bleeding.

Grey Turner's sign   Bruising of the flanks due to retroperitoneal or intraabdominal bleeding.

Iliopsoas   A large compound muscle of the inner hip composed of the iliacus and psoas major muscles.

Kinesics   The study of the way in which certain body movements and gestures serve as a form of non-verbal communication.

Murphy's sign   A manoeuvre performed during abdominal examination which is useful for differentiating pain in the right upper quadrant. Typically, it is positive in cholecystitis but negative in choledocholithiasis, pyelonephritis and ascending cholangitis.

Organomegaly   The general term for enlargement of an organ (or organs).

Paradoxical breathing   Breathing movements in which the chest wall moves in on inspiration and out on expiration, in reverse of the normal movements.

Rovsing's sign   A right lower quadrant pain elicited by pressure applied on the left lower quadrant which is indicative of acute appendicitis.

Xanthomas   Lesions on the skin containing cholesterol and fats.

CHAPTER 10

Clinical Decision Making and Diagnostic Reasoning

Helen Francis-Wenger and Colin Roberts

Aim

The aim of this chapter is to facilitate an approach to clinical decision making and reasoning through a process of exploring critical thinking and analytical skills when applied to clinical scenarios.

LEARNING OUTCOMES

The learning outcomes of the chapter will enable the reader to:

1. understand and apply a toolkit of thought processes and approaches that advanced practitioners can use to nurture, foster and develop clinical skills to become sound, confident, decisive clinicians
2. enhance their application of evidence-based practice and the value of reading through citation and references to clinical decision making
3. build upon their existing ability to utilise a formulaic approach that can be reproduced to provide best-quality patient care
4. enable an appreciation of lifelong learning in practice, exploring the dynamic recognition that underpins curiosity and reflexive attention to advanced practitioners' learning needs.

INTRODUCTION

Clinical decision making is the process of combining our experience, intuition, knowledge, wisdom, clinical skills and problem-solving ability to help an unwell and worried human through the process of diagnosis (or not) and management of their health-related condition or symptoms. When entering the realms of advanced practice, this seems intimidating and unwieldy. Yet, when broken down, this is a skill

The Advanced Practitioner: A Framework for Practice, First Edition. Edited by Ian Peate,
Sadie Diamond-Fox, and Barry Hill.

we often possess unconsciously. Through years of experience in our individual fields, we already have embedded unconscious pattern recognition and can utilise considerable skills in communication and formulation to recognise various conditions and their severity.

Multi-Professional Framework for Advanced Clinical Practice (HEE 2017)

1.1   Practise in compliance with their respective code of professional conduct and within their scope of practice, being responsible and accountable for their decisions, actions, and omissions at this level of practice.

1.2   Demonstrate a critical understanding of their broadened level of responsibility and autonomy and the limits of own competence and professional scope of practice, including when working with complexity, risk, uncertainty, and incomplete information.

1.3   Act on professional judgement about when to seek help, demonstrating critical reflection on own practice, self- awareness, emotional intelligence, and openness to change.

1.4   Work in partnership with individuals, families, and carers, using a range of assessment methods as appropriate (e.g. of history-taking; holistic assessment; identifying risk factors; mental health assessments; requesting, undertaking and/or interpreting diagnostic tests; and conducting health needs assessments).

1.5   Demonstrate effective communication skills, supporting people in making decisions, planning care, or seeking to make positive changes, using Health Education England's framework to promote person-centred approaches in health and care

1.6   Use expertise and decision-making skills to inform clinical reasoning approaches when dealing with differentiated and undifferentiated individual presentations and complex situations, synthesising information from multiple sources to make appropriate, evidence-based judgements, and/or diagnoses.

1.7   Initiate, evaluate and modify a range of interventions which may include prescribing medicines, therapies, lifestyle advice, and care.

1.8   Exercise professional judgement to manage risk appropriately, especially where there may be complex and unpredictable events and supporting teams to do likewise to ensure safety of individuals, families, and carers.

1.9   Work collaboratively with an appropriate range of multi-agency and inter-professional resources, developing, maintaining, and evaluating links to manage risk and issues across organisations and settings.

1.10   Act as a clinical role model/advocate for developing and delivering care that is responsive to changing requirements, informed by an understanding of local population health needs, agencies, and networks.

1.11   Evidence the underpinning subject-specific competencies i.e. knowledge, skills, and behaviours relevant to the role setting and scope, and demonstrate application of the capabilities to these, in an approach that is appropriate to the individual role, setting, and scope.

2.3   Evaluate own practice, and participate in multi-disciplinary service and team evaluation, demonstrating the impact of advanced clinical practice on service function and effectiveness, and quality (i.e. outcomes of care, experience, and safety).

2.4   Actively engage in peer review to inform own and other's practice, formulating and implementing strategies to act on learning and make improvements.

3.1   Critically assess and address own learning needs, negotiating a personal development plan that reflects the breadth of ongoing professional development across the four pillars of advanced clinical practice.

3.2   Engage in self-directed learning, critically reflecting to maximise clinical skills and knowledge, as well as own potential to lead and develop both care and services.

4.2   Evaluate and audit own and others' clinical practice, selecting and applying valid, reliable methods, then acting on the findings.

Accreditation Considerations

- Association of Advanced Practice Educators (UK). https://aape.org.uk
- Royal College of Emergency Medicine (RCEM) Curriculum (Adult and Paediatrics). https://rcem.ac.uk/wp-content/uploads/2021/10/EC_ACP_Curriculum_2017_Adult_and_Paediatric-for_publication-Last_Edit_14-03-2019.pdf
- Royal College of General Practitioners (RCGP) Core Capabilities Framework for Advanced Clinical Practice. https://skillsforhealth.org.uk/wp-content/uploads/2020/11/ACP-Primary-Care-Nurse-Fwk-2020.pdf
- Royal College of Nursing Standards for Advanced Level Nursing. www.rcn.org.uk/-/media/royal-college-of-nursing/documents/publications/2018/july/pdf-007038.pdf?la=en
- Royal Pharmaceutical Society (RPS) Competency Framework for all Prescribers. https://www.rpharms.com/Portals/0/RPS%20document%20library/Open%20access/Professional%20standards/Prescribing%20competency%20framework/prescribing-competency-framework.pdf
- Society of Radiographers (SoR). www.sor.org/learning-advice/career-development/practice-level-information/advanced-practitioners
- Faculty of Intensive Care Medicine (FICM) ACCP Curriculum. www.ficm.ac.uk/consultation-on-updated-ficm-accp-curriculum www.ficm.ac.uk/careersworkforce accps/accp-curriculum
- Numbers Needed to Treat (NNT). www.theNNT.com

CLINICAL REASONING AND CLINICAL DECISION MAKING

The terms 'clinical reasoning' and 'clinical decision making' are often used interchangeably and synonymously. Higgs and Jensen (2019) provide clear definitions of both. Clinical reasoning involves the overall process of 'thinking' in clinical practice and clinical decision making is then applied to determine and emphasise the outcomes of the clinical encounter, with these decisions based upon the 'thinking'. Consequently, the authors will use these terms interchangeably to demonstrate that both 'thinking' and 'decision' must take place synonymously when in clinical practice.

The Roberts & Francis-Wenger model (Figure 10.1) has been created by the authors, illustrating the journey of a decision maker, and the factors and steps involved in clinical reasoning and decision making. Clinical reasoning is central, pivotal and essential in clinical practice and is often challenging to understand and apply. Higgs and Jensen (2019) described a three-factor approach to all patients in the clinical setting.

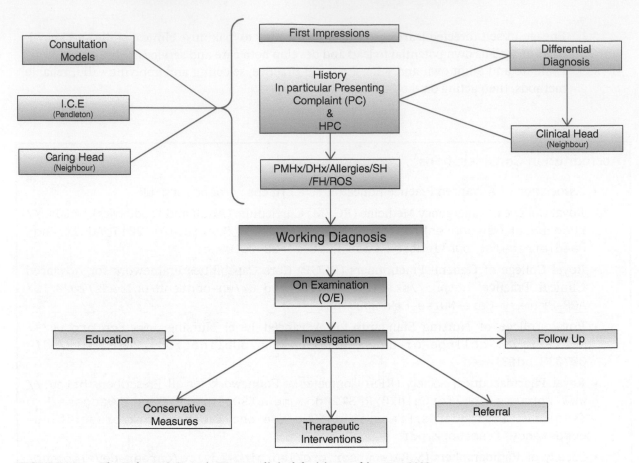

FIGURE 10.1   The Roberts & Francis-Wenger clinical decision-making tree 2022.

- *Wise action* – based on a specific context, taking the best judged action.
- *Professional action* – ensuring we adopt and include ethical, accountable and self-regulatory decisions and conduct.
- *Person-centred action* – demonstrating and upholding respect for, and collaboration with, clients, carers and colleagues.

Clinical reasoning can be complex and multifaceted and frequently leads to uncertainty. Developing advanced skills in autonomous diagnostic practice demands the acknowledgement, acceptance and tolerance of uncertainty. Such is the complexity in contemporary clinical practice that there cannot ever be a single method to manage a case. Our ability to manage uncertainty evolves over time as we gain both generic and role-specific experience. Exposure to clinical scenarios and developing trust in ourselves as clinicians occur as we build upon this experience. When managing these complexities, the clinician must be prepared to adopt a high tolerance of ambiguity and undertake reflexive understanding, practice artistry and collaboration. Herein lie some of the issues and concerns faced by clinicians on a case-by-case basis.

A natural conclusion is to ask, 'Why can I not learn one way to manage a presentation such as a sore throat or a patient with chest pain?'. Our clinical practice is founded on a dynamic, multifactorial,

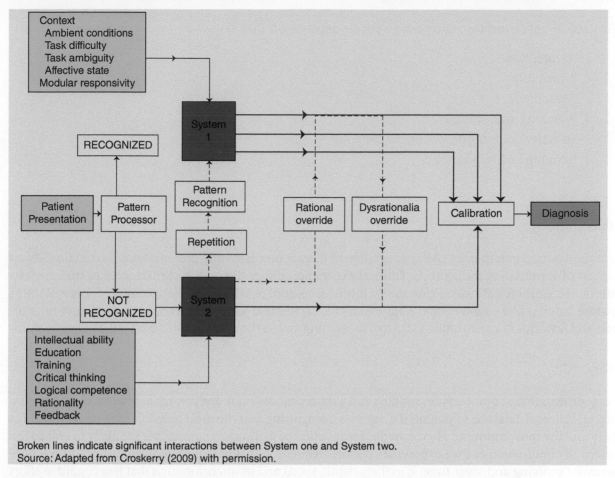

Broken lines indicate significant interactions between System one and System two.
Source: Adapted from Croskerry (2009) with permission.

FIGURE 10.2   Schematic model for diagnostic decision making. *Source*: Adapted from `https://bpspubs.` `onlinelibrary.wiley.com/doi/pdfdirect/10.1111/j.1365-2125.2012.04366.x?download=true.`

human interaction. Therefore, the diagnostic and clinical aspect is one set of factors to consider but no two human beings are the same, present the same way, tell their story the same way, demonstrate their concerns in the same way and, indeed, do not react the same way to treatments and our management plans. Figure 10.2. demonstrates the Croskerry (2009) schematic decision-making process that can facilitate the decision maker's journey.

Wilkinson et al. (2017) suggests techniques to adopt for diagnosis. Despite the diagnosis being the ultimate goal, we must be aware that it may not be achieved. This is common and acceptable. Managing the multitude of factors at play in the consultation while attempting to define a diagnosis is paramount to patient satisfaction. Patients are often content that we have addressed their concerns; they have been 'heard' and we have ruled out the most sinister diagnoses from the story given to us. Many methods can be adopted in attempting to arrive at a diagnosis (Box 10.1). The clinician's dissatisfaction on failing to arrive at a definitive diagnosis can be tempered by the acknowledgement that this perceived 'failure' is common. Sharing uncertainty and the application of alternative approaches is good practice and patient centred.

Box 10.1   Methods of Diagnosis (Wilkinson et al. 2017)

- Recognition
- Probability
- Reasoning
- Watching and waiting
- Selective doubting/tolerating uncertainty
- Iteration and reiteration

Recognition

For the advanced practitioner (AP), recognition of disease processes and presentations is often the default method of formulating a diagnosis. Clinical experience, either direct or vicarious, creates unconscious pattern recognition pathways, essentially intuitive responses where the symptoms and presentations become familiar like an old friend. Kahneman's (2012) seminal work details the human reliance on intuition and how this is an essential, valid tool in learning and in the evolution of advanced diagnostic skills.

Probability

Using probability in our decision making is fundamental. We look for commonality based on our own personal clinical database of potential diagnoses, recognising that the most probable diagnosis is the most likely and the most common. Hence, in our formulation of working diagnoses, we are likely to embed the pattern of commonality as we experience it more frequently. This personal algorithmic approach is continuously evolving and, over time, it gathers depth, speed and momentum such that less cognitive effort is required to establish common diagnoses followed by the recognition of rarity developing.

Reasoning

Diagnosing by reasoning interrogates a range of potential differential diagnoses, examining and excluding them until the diagnosis becomes evident. The success of this approach depends on adequate clinical experience with prolonged exposure to a range of symptoms and conditions. Without adequate experience, supervision in practice and case discussion, the potential to miss significant diagnoses is clear. Although this method remains credible and useful, the unsupervised clinician may miss significant diagnoses through lack of experience or knowledge (they don't know what they don't know) or become trapped in exhaustive reasoning. Here, time, effort and resources are used to eliminate every single potential diagnosis. Consultation times are prolonged, tests are exhaustive and ultimate decision making is delayed due to clinican uncertainty and fear of missing vital steps in the process.

Watching and Waiting

A useful adjunct to reasoning is that of watching and waiting – a valid and useful tool that takes courage and conviction, steeped in rapport building in the consultation and a reliance on trust in the therapeutic relationship. The benefits are clear with a shared responsibility for the outcome, where safety netting and follow-up is the notable primary intervention. Naturally, this is situational and depends on the client group and clinical setting. In primary care, this is frequently used as a management tool as the patient 'belongs' to the patient community served by the organisation, whereas in the emergency department this is less effective and the application places more onus on the patient to seek help elsewhere in cases where symptoms do not resolve.

Selective Doubting

Patients expect clinicians to be professional, confident and certain. This, however, is not always the case and we could ask about the relevance of this in the diagnostic process. Frequently, clinicians rely heavily on clinical signs and investigative tests to reach a diagnosis, but this scientific method dictates that when testing a hypothesis, the clinical examination, or the investigations we request, cannot be absolute. This ties in with decision-making theories that have evolved over time, such as the hypothetico-deductive approach (Elstein et al. 1978), that facilitate the management of clinical complexity. Wilkinson et al. (2017) temper this by suggesting that when establishing a diagnosis becomes difficult, the initial cognitive step is to doubt the clinical signs, and the clinician will then move to doubt the investigations. The reality is, the 'game' of medicine is unplayable if you doubt everything: so, doubt selectively.

Iteration and Reiteration

An alternative approach to arriving at a diagnosis is the iteration and reiteration of presenting symptoms. Within the fundamental dynamic history-taking exercise, we are using the human desire to tell and retell stories to establish understanding and 'hear' the patient. Here, our humanity is central to managing the relationship, while our clinical acumen constantly sifts the information presented, driving further questioning as we iterate and reiterate elements of the story. The process of sifting allows our cognitive mind to rule out potential diagnoses and develop others. Considering the complexity of the processes at play gives insight into the inherent difficulties in honing these skills; recognising what they are and where our individual strengths and weaknesses lie. The ultimate goal, however, is that we can enhance patient care through good, sound, clinical decision making.

Considering the AP in contemporary multidisciplinary teams, we can see that newfound knowledge and skills, which were traditionally associated with the medical degree, alongside contemporary training in the origins of the individual, create a 'value-added' role rather than a role substitute. The word 'substitution' has no place in advanced practice (Council of Deans 2021). Those training and working at an advanced level must be aware of their competence and capability. This insight is critical at the outset, recognising that the humanity and instinctive empathy brought by the practitioner are critical to the role while accepting that it will take years to acquire the knowledge, skills and experience to work at this level. It is easy to fail to recognise that in medical colleagues, those formative years and experience have already been traversed in a highly supervised fashion.

THINKING, GROWING AND EVOLVING

The concepts of how we learn are inherently complex. The 'real world' of healthcare, peppered by inherent pressure and stresses, can force learning through error or perceived failure. Considering the complexity of the decision-making process, and adding the influences of dynamic environmental, human and systemic factors (to name a few), it is inevitable that errors will occur. To learn from an error or mistake is paramount while we aim to avoid the negativity and scapegoating that too frequently surround this subject in healthcare settings.

The role of clinical governance in healthcare is pivotal, seeking to provide the reasons behind errors, driving understanding of root causes, creating impetus for changes in procedures and processes and supporting learning. However, before the admission of error becomes routine in healthcare, all clinicians need to trust the system that evaluates their practice to be supportive. There have been many public high-profile cases of condemnation, leading to staff feeling insecure in the system. However, safety and security in reporting must be the fundamental goal.

The phenomenological and seminal work of Benner (1984) defines the route of the practitioner from novice to expert, through a series of stages. Some argue that this transition occurs naturally throughout our careers as we change jobs or develop into roles encompassing advanced practice. In the development of advanced roles, it is imperative to recognise several factors.

- The concept of 'skills currency' in defining and developing new roles.
- Defining where the clinician sits on the skills continuum is a hard judgement to make for both the individual and the organisation when new roles are developed.
- In role development, a deep and unambiguous understanding of the role, its standards and the assumed responsibility will allow a more accurate appraisal of the status of the clinician appointed.

It is common for the AP to deem themselves a novice and remain in this mindset when the opposite is true. Progression through the continuum from novice to expert should be fluid and allow transition from expert in our base careers and original disciplines, through to a novice AP with transitioning steps, steeped in training, experience and exposure towards becoming a proficient and expert AP. Intuition can be brought into this identification and used to distinguish the novice from the expert when drawing comparisons to this continuum.

Moving through the Benner continuum, we hold less risk as we become unconsciously competent (Figure 10.3), i.e. we automatically know what we know through tried and tested methods. So, in

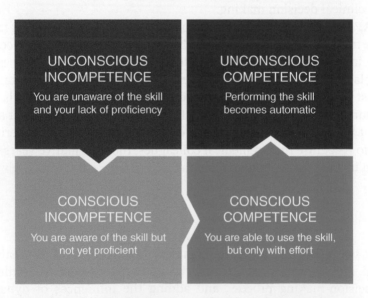

FIGURE 10.3   The four stages of competence. *Source*: https://onlinelibrary.wiley.com.

progressing to become an 'expert', it can be deduced that we present less risk to our organisations. However, as we transition into advanced practice, we are practising in new realms, and some may argue that this level of practice is akin to our medical colleagues. Therefore, aligning to medicine, we are reduced to being a novice again, therefore, arguably, increasing the risk. This fluctuating continuum must be acknowledged and embraced so that we maintain high levels of safety and adequate risk management in our organisations and for ourselves.

In the acquisition of advanced clinical skills, the aim is to enhance patient care. Brook and Rushforth (2011) believe that as a novice, we hold more risk within our role as related to the cognitive continuum (Standing 2008; Hammond 1978). We can further delineate this with the stepping stones required to achieve expert status. This is well described by the conscious competence model (Figure 10.3), of which there have been several adaptations over time due to its relevance and applicability to all learners. There is a caveat here that the cognitive continuum may allow the focus of our work to deviate from theoretical divisions and suggest that our concentration should be on the practicalities of improving practice (Harbison 2001). Over time, there has been contemplation over the incorporation of the laws in intuitive judgement. Failures in these judgements have led to curricula to include normative approaches to the concept of clinical judgement. In addition, the humanist stance ensures that ethics and communication skills are also included.

DECISION-MAKING THEORIES

Normative, Prescriptive and Descriptive Interactions

Theories surrounding thought development influencing decision making are steeped in history. The emphasis has always been on developing a process where information is utilised, assessing a series of alternatives and based on that evaluation, selecting an action and a direction of travel. The concepts of judgement and decision are finely intertwined and delineated between judgement as the 'assessment' of alternatives and decisions denoting the choice between these alternatives. There are three overarching judgement concepts that have evolved over time and most subsequent theories fall into one of these categories.

Bell et al. (1998) drew together the two traditionally defined distinct perspectives within the theory of decision making. These were descriptive and normative interactions. Their seminal work studied how we make decisions, and stemmed from a range of various interdisciplinary studies and contributions from the worlds of statistics, mathematics, economics, psychology, operations research, management science and other domains, resulting in these two perspectives.

Descriptive Approach

As we begin to consider thought evolution, the 'descriptive approach' is pivotal. Many theorists suggest that the processing of information by clinicians is the most influential descriptive theory. It encompasses how individuals make judgements and use these to reach decisions. It is deemed to be heavily orientated towards the process and is unique in that it takes into consideration the actual 'real-world' elements that have a significant influence on us. Moving into the realms of this theory is the goal towards autonomy and is only limited by the capacity of the human memory.

Normative Approach

The 'normative approach' is concerned with how people 'should' make decisions to obey and comply with certain rules, laws, principles or axioms that reflect our beliefs surrounding logical, rational behaviour. The focus is on being able to make rational and logical decisions that employ statistics, focused on the quality of judgements and decisions and with a clear focus on the outcome. This is evident in practice as the use of risk assessments, probability scores, risk stratification and decision trees that intrinsically use data from research allows us to formulate decisions on the management of our decisions.

Prescriptive Approach

The 'prescriptive approach' is drawn from those who facilitate people to make better decisions by using evidence, empirically influencing decisions. It is an approach that examines 'how' people make decisions and judgements and facilitates the most appropriate choice through exploration of the process involved. When applying this theory, the overall aim is to improve the judgements and decisions taken by the individual and the development of tools that can facilitate these decisions. Some examples in practice are the development and use of clinical guidelines which take the decision maker through a series of steps to reach the ultimate decision. This offers a unique safety net for an organisation to facilitate a standardised approach to healthcare, ensuring that similar decisions are prescribed and adhered to according to the presentations. This is an extremely useful tool to support novice decision makers to learn, practise and evolve in a safe manner while promoting the ultimate goal of full autonomy and freedom of thought to arrive at decisions independently. Prescriptive decision making is useful in allowing for adaptation to the nuances of human interactions which is paramount in healthcare and allows for evolution into effective and efficient decision makers in the long run.

INTUITION

Pioneering studies have tried to quantify the role of intuition in the decision-making process and have explored the concept that the traditional 'gut feeling' is often central to clinicians' thinking and often seen as being just as important as formalised reasoning. Yet this is difficult to quantify and certainly cannot be taught as it is often associated with experience.

Kahneman (2012) proposed that intuition was nothing more or less than recognition, reiterating the importance of experience when approaching clinical decision making with reasoned thought. However, Adair (2022) introduced the concept of the depth mind principle – an alternative subsection of thinking alongside the subconscious and unconscious. Deemed as fundamental, the depth mind is believed to organise thoughts in a non-chaotic manner, filtering into the scientific and creative elements of our being. Associated with this organising of previous experience and learning, Adair suggests that this is the source of intuition – the all-important 'sixth sense' that has been inherently challenging to quantify.

Considering the many tasks we undertake daily – even washing the dishes – deep in our unconscious and subconscious minds, thoughts connect and draw links to past experiences, memories, feelings, cues, clues and hints to previous solutions. Creative thinking and arriving at decisions cannot be forced. Utilising the depth mind concept, it is suggested that stepping away from struggling to find the solution and letting your subconscious work its magic enables the identification of solutions. Have you ever woken in the night with the solution to your problem? This is the depth mind at work, processing the data and organising your memory banks for the next time you face a similar decision, so that the information is ready to hand to formulate an educated intuition.

HYPOTHETICO-DEDUCTIVE REASONING

(Adapted from Elstein et al. 1978 and Elstein and Bordage 1988)

One major theory that underpins this style of information processing is the hypothetico-deductive approach. As we move towards the 'sharp end' of decision making, the authors have provided an amalgamated diagram of several models to demonstrate the complexities involved (Figure 10.4).

Cue Acquisition Stage

The focus here involves gathering preliminary information (cues) about a certain situation. These cues are gleaned from a variety of different means, some of which, at times, we may not be aware of. Quantitative and qualitative streams of information can enter the consultation in verbal, non-verbal and situational forms, based on what you see (observations) and what you hear (are told), and will inherently be affected by prior knowledge and experience. Gathering this information allows us to determine the needs of the specific situation but can go awry if not approached in a coherent and logical manner. Ensuring that cues are not missed in the initial consultation is imperative to avoid the mismatch between the agendas of the patient and the clinician. Therefore, the overarching aim here is to obtain an accurate picture of the patient's presenting condition.

Hypothesis Generation

Based on all the information obtained in the initial stage, the focus shifts to generating tentative explanations in conjunction with additional cues held in the short-term memory to generate a working hypothesis – often called a working diagnosis. It is imperative to remember that here, it is based on the clinical working knowledge and the generation of one or more hypotheses that can be tested. At times, though, it is not always feasible or viable to wait for tests to confirm or refute this and so we need to rely on a certain level of experience and knowledge. The issues here will be concerned with the generation of the wrong hypothesis and will therefore require the clinician to be adept at shifting the focus to an alternative hypothesis.

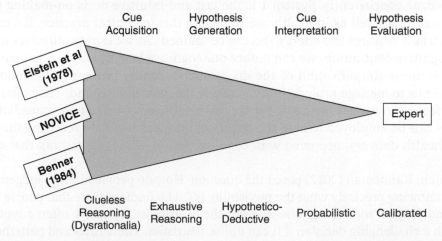

FIGURE 10.4 Heading to the 'sharp end' of advanced practice. *Source*: Benner (1984) and Elstein et al. (1978). Adapted by Roberts and Francis-Wenger (2022).

Cue Interpretation

This stage involves the accurate utilisation of good judgement and careful selection of and attention to the cues previously acquired. This activity requires robust clinical reasoning to confirm or refute the hypothesis that has been developed. This element relies on skills related to sensory memory, long- and short-term memory and individual ability to recall coding strategies based on experiential learning and pattern recognition. This stage is peppered with dangers – falsely interpreting the hypotheses is something to be wary of in every encounter, as is the temptation to jump to conclusions. We must also avoid applying stereotypes, being mindful of biases and prejudices.

Hypothesis Evaluation

This stage gets us to the 'sharp' end (Figure 10.4) of the process in our decision-making journey and is the determination of the value of the data collated and interpreted. This decision represents the selection of the hypothesis which is favoured by most of the evidence available and facilitates this final evaluation of the situation.

THE COGNITIVE PROCESS

The concept of decision making has psychology at its core. An understanding of *how* we think is critical when developing new skills as this provides insight into how *we* work and the influences that derail or support the decision-making process.

Kahneman (2012) addresses the idea that to be a good clinician and diagnostician, you need to be able to recollect a large set of diseases, presentations and subsequent management strategies. The posit here is that learning medicine is steeped in learning the 'language' of medicine and deeper understanding of the judgements required. Two different thought processes were identified – thinking fast (System 1) and thinking slow (System 2). System 1 functions fast, unconsciously and automatically with little or no effort and often with no sense of voluntary control. It is important to note that these processes do not represent two separate parts of the brain that work independently; they are processes that occur concurrently. System 1 is the fast and intuitive decision-making thoughts that can be seen in nature as well as in healthcare. Likening this to clinical practice, it can often be our default approach as it requires less energy and can be 'trained'. As we expose ourselves to clinical situations in our cognitive continuum, we can reduce our cognitive load by employing heuristics, mental shortcuts, which allow simplification of the diagnostic reasoning process (Ritter and Witte 2019). Heuristics enable us to manage probabilities to answer the question in hand. They often employ suboptimal, imperfect or irrational methods, yet are often sufficient to reach an immediate, short-term goal. Heuristics can be employed to ease the cognitive load and facilitate reaching that end-goal. In contemporary health delivery, peppered with cognitive biases, this is something that we all employ at some stage.

In his research, Kahneman (2012) posed the question 'How do people manage judgements on probability without knowing precisely what the probability is?'. The findings were that people simplified the task in hand and judged 'something' else and not the probability. System 1 often adopts this process when faced with a challenging decision if it can utilise heuristics. These rules and patterns are based on evolved and learned capacities and make use of prior knowledge and regularities that are often tacit in nature. Therefore, they have an inherent tendency to reproduce known solutions and judgements by, for example, relying only on past events to anticipate future events (Schirrmeister et al. 2020). Kahneman (2012) suggests that System 1 thinking is insensitive to the quality and quantity of the information being processed and that it gives rise to impressions and intuitions often referred to as 'What You See Is All There Is' (WYSIATI).

While System 1 is highly effective in some situations, there are times when our cognitive processing must be slower and more deliberate, especially when dealing with increasingly complex clinical situations. According to Kahneman (2012), System 2 is controlled operations thinking. It allocates focused attention to the demands of the mental activity taking place and is often linked with the subjective experience of choice and concentration. System 2 will often influence the formulations of cognitive processing that contribute to our System 1 thinking. System 1 is often considered as lazy and will often automatically endorse many intuitive beliefs but when our System 1 thinking is overwhelmed or exhausted, it calls upon our System 2 processing centre to step in and help.

BIASES

Without doubt, healthcare decisions are not easy, with no one right answer, and it can appear that there are only different degrees of 'wrong'. This cognitive dissonance is a mental conflict occurring when our beliefs/assumptions are contradicted by the gathering of new information (Syed 2015). The resolution of this unease often employs several defensive actions: avoiding the new information; persuading oneself that there is no conflict; reconciling the differences; or resorting to manoeuvres that preserve the perceived stability. Techniques of managing cognitive dissonance are something that we must be aware of in our day-to-day work, ensuring that we are focused and aware of all factors that may affect, impede or, indeed, improve the quality of our decision-making skills.

How the brain works has been at the centre of psychologists' work for many years. In the world of clinical practice and with a focus on advanced practice, these cognitive mechanisms are often referred to as heuristics and biases. They have a very profound effect on personal development and being aware of cognitive mechanisms is extremely important.

Our ability to rationalise information and make decisions can also be affected by cognitive biases that in general describe deviations from the norm or systematic errors relating to perception, memory, cognition and judgement (Haselton et al. 2015). Biases are often thought to be substantially unconscious and often result from the use of heuristics.

It serves healthcare well to draw comparisons with the aviation industry where error can be catastrophic. Within aviation, error is categorically seen as 'normal', leading to monitoring for patterns whilst supporting individuals using a constructive approach. To 'not report' is the failure. Within aviation, the core concept is to embrace errors to facilitate the generation of ideas and innovations to find solutions before incidents occur.

Kapur et al. (2015) draw pertinent links between the two industries and state some fundamental differences that can affect the decision-making process. One pillar of governance in the NHS relates to clinical effectiveness and risk management. This premise assists in the evaluation of practices and organisational processes, policies and procedures. Yet, a substantial difference between the two industries is that some high-profile clinical errors in the UK have led to human factor experts influencing the investigation of serious incidents. Drawing demonstrable links between the two outwardly appearing, vastly different, environments, the healthcare system in the UK and across the world is becoming more accepting of learning from adverse events. Syed (2015) draws these conclusions together under the umbrella of allowing ourselves to succeed but only if we learn from our mistakes. Kapur et al. (2015) documented several safety-related cultural attributes that distinguish aviation from healthcare. The following three are the most relevant for comparison.

1. Blame-free culture in aviation in relation to reporting and owning up to incidents. Syed (2015) suggests that historically in healthcare, data on incidents allude to details that explain why incidents occurred rather than 'how' the errors were manifested. Whereas, in contrast, pilots are actively encouraged to be open and honest about errors and near misses. The key difference is that failure is not seen as an indictment of the individual but rather a precious learning opportunity.

2. Competing demands and target setting in healthcare, such as economic, financial and safety factors, often make the news headlines. Setting targets within aviation is relatively infrequent whereas in healthcare, targets are interpreted as measures of success which add a multidimensional pressure felt across the entire system.

3. Safety permeates all levels of the business of airlines, from the ground crew to the pilots to the air traffic controllers. However, within healthcare, contentiously, safety is still regarded as the priority of some and not the obligation of all.

These good practices observed in the aviation industry must be emulated in advanced practice roles. There should be no differences between the two industries as safety-related attributes should be central and integral to all roles in healthcare, even before entering the realms of autonomy.

Healthcare should be deemed a safety-critical industry akin to the aviation industry. Human factors (HF) training and the need to recognise/manage the implications of how being 'human' can lead to variations in healthcare are imperative in systems and systems thinking. Assessing the impact of HFs and providing related psychological training and the assurance of staff well-being should be seen as imperative and integral to NHS staff workplans with bespoke and specific HF/patient safety psychologists in post. Cognitive bias avoidance training has started to become mandatory in many organisations as a core element of cognitive decision making is often identified in adverse incidents. Therefore, an assumption could be that if all these elements are addressed in training, the potential for reducing diagnostic errors is improved.

Another factor that can have an impact on all levels of healthcare, but more specifically here, around clinical reasoning, is the current state of mind of the practitioner. Of course as humans, we are affected by emotions, fatigue, compassion fatigue, burnout and physical conditions that compound why and how we make decisions differently at different times of the day or night. Being aware is paramount and there are many tools (Box 10.2) that can help identify and address these throughout the course of a day. This is analogous to the aviation industry and should any of these emotions or feelings be identified, then the subject is advised (if safe to do so) to stop the task in hand, address the 'feeling' and return later to the task to address this cognitive dissonance.

Box 10.2   HALT: An Assistive Tool to Address Cognitive Dissonance

H – Hungry
A – Angry
L – Lonely
T – Tired

An additional consideration is the tangible impact that imposter syndrome (IS) can have on our self 'trust' as clinicians. IS is a common phenomenon amongst all clinicians. It can be interpreted both positively and negatively, but often becomes a hindrance to the clinician when they start doubting their ability to function, leading to loss of confidence and feelings of inadequacies. This phenomenon is steeped in anxiety and self-doubt. As we gain exposure to clinical scenarios, we should inherently develop a sense of 'ourselves'. IS is often associated with high-pressure environments, especially in healthcare, and with comparing oneself to another colleague. When considering the impact on clinical reasoning, the concepts of self-doubt and managing clinical uncertainty return to the fore. Therefore, a balance must be achieved between doubting everything, including your own ability, and 'playing' the 'game' of medicine, so, we reiterate, doubt selectively!

The Dunning–Kruger effect (Dunning 2011) is another pertinent concept to be aware of in advanced practice. Here, incompetence and metacognitive defects can lead to an overestimation of an individual's abilities and performance. People in this group find it challenging to recognise genuine levels of competence when applied to themselves or (objectively) in more competent peers. Gaining insight into one's own limitations and inadequacies is also a challenge by social comparison demonstrating an inability to 'see' their own deficits in relation to their peer's performance. The presence of this in advanced practice must be recognised and challenged to counterbalance the effect of IS, thus creating a balanced, objective practitioner. Figure 10.5 shows the actual overestimation of individuals involved in the study conducted by Muller et al. (2020). Participants who performed in the first quartile showed the most overestimation; therefore, clinicians need to be mindful as the gap between their actual abilities and their perception can be vast, thus creating the potential for error and compromise of safety.

All these factors are pivotal in the continued expansion, prevalence and evolution of advanced practice roles. Encompassing, utilising and facilitating the four fundamental pillars of advanced practice are essential. Interpersonal skills and insight are equally important in ensuring that advanced practice is a sustainable development in the future workforce planning and longevity of the NHS.

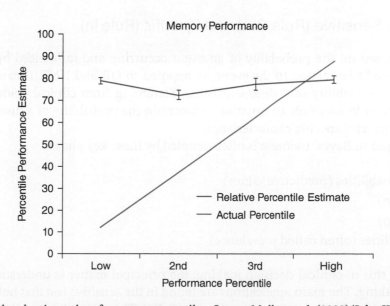

FIGURE 10.5   Actual and estimated performance percentiles. *Source*: Muller et al. (2020)/John Wiley & Sons.

ASSISTIVE TOOLS AND CONCEPTS: RISK ASSESSMENTS/PROBABILITY SCORES/ RISK STRATIFICATION

Odds Ratios

Managing risk and arriving at a diagnosis is not a skill that can be learned or taught overnight. Japp and Robertson (2018) believe a sensible approach is to consider two contrasting approaches: pattern recognition and probability analysis. Many of the theoretical concepts mentioned earlier are concerned with the honing of experience, identifying personal thought processes, factors affecting them and tools to help develop personal knowledge and skills. Pattern recognition is imperative to help the novice decision maker formulate the most commonly encountered and clinically important situations. Therefore, the prevalence and availability of probability analysis, decision-making 'tools' and stratification tools to manage risk have been exponential, to assist our decision-making abilities.

Odds ratios (ORs) measure the association between an exposure and an outcome (LITFL 2020). They allow interpretation of the chances of an outcome occurring based on a particular exposure versus the absence of that exposure. At times, this is a difficult concept to comprehend but to clarify, 'odds' are different from 'probability'. Odds is the ratio of the probability that the event of interest occurs versus the probability that it does not.

The importance of these to decision making and reasoning is that ORs allow for comparison between the strength of association between groups. They are commonly utilised in high-level research such as meta-analysis to be able to influence guidelines and risk stratification scores/tools.

Numbers Needed to Treat

Numbers needed to treat (NNT) is a statistical formula that represents the number of patients that would need to be treated to prevent one additional bad outcome. NNT (2022) develop their explanation with the caveat that the concept is statistical in nature but intuitive, for we know that not everyone is helped by interventions.

Bayes' Theorem: Sensitive (Rule Out) and Specific (Rule In)

Bayes' theorem is based on the probability of an event occurring and influenced by prior knowledge of conditions that might be related to the event, as opposed to OR and NNT. It can be used to objectively determine the probability of a disease existing. Stemming from clinical epidemiology, this is a mathematical approach to establish an equation to ascertain the probability of a disease process occurring in specific groups with specific characteristics.

The language used in Bayes' theorem is often denoted by these key phases.

- Posterior probabilities (predictive values)
- Sensitivity (Sn)
- Specificity (Sp)
- Prior probabilities (often called prevalence)

When applying this to clinical decision making, the principal matter is understanding how a 'test' informs decision making. The main applications are found in the sensitive test that helps rule out disease (SnOUT) and the specific test that helps rule in disease (SpIN). The main goal here is to rule in or rule out the presence of a disease with a level of certainty that provides confidence. The better the diagnostic test, the more confidence and certainty will prevail, leading to a diagnosis and hence the evolution of tools to assist in providing the assurance and confidence in decision making.

Risk Stratification

Derived from the mathematical approach, in recent years many risk stratification tools have evolved to assist us in identifying probability, alongside ensuring safety and helping us identify the correct management. Professional web resources such as MDCalc (2022) provide information on clinical scores, equations, algorithms, risk assessments and diagnostic criteria to aid assessment and diagnosis. These are steeped in research, bolstered by the contemporaneous evidence available. Many risk stratification scores use a combination of objective and subjective data to assign a level of risk and therefore, we can systematically use this information to make clinical decisions and management plans for all patients while maintaining safety.

CONCLUSION

Clinical decision making underpins everything that we do in the world of advanced practice and healthcare. It can be influenced by many factors that we need to be mindful of. Having a toolkit of resources to rely on, including personal traits, personal strategies and mental flexibility backed up by validated risk assessment algorithms, will allow us to face every decision with a consistent approach. To progress from novice to expert takes time alongside knowledge, patience and acceptance. Being inherently self-aware is imperative in order to minimise error and biases. To achieve this, we must balance our emotional and instinctive responses with the cognitive analysis described here to ensure our decision making is most appropriate to deal with the uncertainty of day-to-day life in healthcare.

Take Home Points

- Clinical decision making and diagnostic reasoning skills develop with knowledge and experience. Working together while becoming proficient in such skills is best practice.
- Best practice suggests that advanced practitioners must be proficient in their use of clinical decision making and diagnostic reasoning and must work within their scope of practice.
- Utilisation and understanding of theoretical underpinnings and evidence-based literature are imperative to enable safe advanced-level practice and patient care.
- The concept of decision making has psychology at its core and the way that clinicians think and work impacts on the decision-making process.

REFERENCES

Adair, J. (2022). *Decision Making and Problem Solving: Breakthrough Barriers and Banish Uncertainty at Work*, 5e. London: Kogan Page.

Bell, D.E., Raiffa, H., and Tversky, A. (1998). Descriptive, normative and prescriptive interactions in decision making. In: *Decision Making – Descriptive, Normative, and Prescriptive Interactions* (ed. D. Bell, H. Raiffa, and A. Tversky), 9–30. Cambridge: Cambridge University Press.

Benner, P. (1984). *From Novice to Expert. Excellence and Power in Clinical Nursing Practice*. Menlo Park: Addison-Wesley Publishing Co.

Brook, S. and Rushforth, H. (2011). Why is the regulation of advanced practice essential? *British Journal of Nursing* 20 (16): 996–1000.

Council of Deans of Health (2021). Advanced Clinical Practice Education in England. `https://coun cilofdeans.org.uk/wp-content/uploads/2018/11/081118-FINAL-ACP-REPORT.pdf`

Croskerry, P. (2009). A universal model of diagnostic reasoning. *Academic Medicine* 84 (8): 1022–1028.

Dunning, D. (2011). The Dunning–Kruger effect: on being ignorant of one's own ignorance. *Advances in Experimental Social Psychology* 44: 247–296.

Elstein, A.S. and Bordage, G. (1988). Psychology of clinical reasoning. In: *Professional Judgment: A Reader in Clinical Decision Making* (ed. J. Dowie and A. Elstein), 109–129. Cambridge: Cambridge University Press.

Elstein, A.S., Shulman, L.S., and Sprafka, S.A. (1978). *Medical Problem Solving. An Analysis of Clinical Reasoning*. Cambridge, MA: Harvard University Press.

Hammond, K.R. (1978). Toward increasing competence of thought in public policy formation. In: *Judgement and Decision in Public Policy Formation* (ed. K.R. Hammond), 11–32. Boulder, CO: Westview Press.

Harbison, J. (2001). Clinical decision making in nursing; theoretical perspectives and their relevance to practice. *Journal of Advanced Nursing* 68 (7): 1469–1481.

Haselton, M.G., Nettel, D., and Murray, D.R. (2015). The evolution of cognitive bias. In: *The Handbook of Evolutionary Psychology* (ed. D.M. Buss). Hoboken, NJ: John Wiley and Sons Inc.

Health Education England (2017). Multi-professional Framework for Advanced Clinical Practice in England. `www.hee.nhs.uk/sites/default/files/documents/multi-professional framework foradvanc edclinicalpracticeinengland.pdf`

Higgs, J. and Jensen, G.M. (2019). Understanding clinical reasoning. In: *Clinical Reasoning in the Health Professions*, 4e (ed. J. Higgs, G.M. Jensen, S. Loftus, and N. Christensen), 3–11. London: Elsevier.

Japp, A. and Robertson, C. (2018). *Macleod's Clinical Diagnosis*, 2e. London: Elsevier.

Kahneman, D. (2012). *Thinking, Fast and Slow*. London: Penguin Books.

Kapur, N., Parand, A., and Sevdalis, N. (2015). Aviation and healthcare: a comparative review with implications for patient safety. *Journal of the Royal Society of Medicine Open* 7 (1): 1–10.

Life in the Fast Lane (2020). `https://litfl.com/odds-ratio/`

MDCalc (2022). `https://www.mdcalc.com`

Muller, A., Sirianni, L.A., and Addante, R.J. (2020). Neural correlates of the Dunning-Kruger effect. *European Journal of Neuroscience* 53 (2): 460–484.

Numbers Needed to Treat (2022). `www.thennt.com/`

Ritter, B.J. and Witte, M.J. (2019). Clinical reasoning in nursing. In: *Clinical Reasoning in the Health Professions*, 4e (ed. J. Higgs, G.M. Jensen, S. Loftus, and N. Christensen), 235–245. London: Elsevier.

Schirrmeister, E., Göhring, A., and Warnke, P. (2020). Psychological biases and heuristics in the context of foresight and scenario processes. *Futures and Foresight Science* 2 (2): 1–18. `https://onlinelibrary. wiley.com/doi/epdf/10.1002/ffo2.31`.

Standing, M. (2008). Clinical judgement and decision-making in nursing – nine models of practice in a revised cognitive continuum. *Journal of Advanced Nursing* 62 (1): 124–134.

Syed, M. (2015). *Black Box Thinking*. London: John Murray.

Wilkinson, I.B., Raine, T., Wiles, K. et al. (2017). *Oxford Handbook of Clinical Medicine*. Oxford: Oxford University Press.

FURTHER READING

Adair, J. (2022). *Decision Making and Problem Solving: Breakthrough Barriers and Banish Uncertainty at Work*, 5e. London: Kogan Page.

Bickley, L. (2020). *Bates' Guide to Physical Examination and History Taking.*, 12e. New York: Wolters Kluwer.

SELF-ASSESSMENT QUESTIONS

1. As a trainee AP, what are your learning needs in relation to clinical decision making and diagnostic reasoning?
2. How will you identify your clinical decision making and diagnostic reasoning needs for supervision and what documents and guidance will support this?
3. How will you evaluate and assess your clinical decision making and diagnostic reasoning skills to prove your competency and capability in practice?
4. How can you ensure that you continue to develop your ability to refine your clinical decision making and diagnostic reasoning practice?

GLOSSARY

Clinical reasoning   A complex cognitive process that uses formal and informal thinking strategies to gather and analyse patient information, evaluate the significance of this information and weigh alternative actions.

Decision-making theory   A balance of experience, awareness, knowledge and information gathering, using appropriate assessment tools, multiple professional practitioners and evidence-based practice, which guides the clinician. Good decisions equate to safe care provision. Good, effective clinical decision making requires a combination of experience and skills.

Hypothetico-deductive reasoning   Information from the patient is gathered and used to construct a hypothesis, which is then tested out, or a further hypothesis is constructed. The hypotheses should be confirmed by responses to treatment; thus, the process involves repeated reassessment.

Intuitive knowledge   Intuitive knowledge, that is, automatically knowing by intuition, is considered an integral part of human decision making and also a phase of clinical reasoning.

Probability   In clinical decision making, clinical estimation of probability strongly affects a clinician's belief as to whether or not a patient has a disease, and this belief in turn determines actions: to rule out, to treat or to do more tests.

CHAPTER 11

Diagnostic Interpretation

Colin Roberts, Christine Eade, and Helen Francis-Wenger

Aim

The aim of this chapter is to enhance understanding around diagnostic test interpretation for clinicians working at an advanced level of practice. A key focus is to provide practitioners with the necessary knowledge and skills to correctly interpret diagnostic tests and feel confident to request and interpret basic radiological investigations.

LEARNING OUTCOMES

After reading this chapter the reader will be able to:

1. develop a systematic approach to ordering and interpreting laboratory tests
2. understand normal physiology and apply pathophysiology within the systems tested
3. understand and apply the rationale for ordering lab tests in testing hypotheses
4. interpret the results in the context of the disease process by recognising patterns of disease through testing to inform patient management.

INTRODUCTION

This chapter will focus on the common tests advanced clinical practitioners request and interpret. The aim is to develop a routine approach to this difficult, often neglected area. Tests are a challenging area to master. This chapter is not exhaustive and will focus on common scenarios and a logical approach.

The Advanced Practitioner: A Framework for Practice, First Edition. Edited by Ian Peate,
Sadie Diamond-Fox, and Barry Hill.
© 2024 John Wiley & Sons Ltd. Published 2024 by John Wiley & Sons Ltd.

Multi-Professional Framework for Advanced Clinical Practice (HEE 2017)

1.1 Practise in compliance with their respective code of professional conduct and within their scope of practice, being responsible and accountable for their decisions, actions, and omissions at this level of practice.

1.2 Demonstrate a critical understanding of their broadened level of responsibility and autonomy and the limits of own competence and professional scope of practice, including when working with complexity, risk, uncertainty, and incomplete information.

1.3 Act on professional judgement about when to seek help, demonstrating critical reflection on own practice, self- awareness, emotional intelligence, and openness to change.

1.4 Work in partnership with individuals, families, and carer's, using a range of assessment methods as appropriate (e.g. of history-taking; holistic assessment; identifying risk factors; mental health assessments; requesting, undertaking and/or interpreting diagnostic tests; and conducting health needs assessments).

1.5 Demonstrate effective communication skills, supporting people in making decisions, planning care, or seeking to make positive changes, using Health Education England's framework to promote person-centred approaches in health and care

1.6 Use expertise and decision-making skills to inform clinical reasoning approaches when dealing with differentiated and undifferentiated individual presentations and complex situations, synthesising information from multiple sources to make appropriate, evidence-based judgements and/or diagnoses.

1.7 Initiate, evaluate and modify a range of interventions which may include prescribing medicines, therapies, lifestyle advice and care.

1.8 Exercise professional judgement to manage risk appropriately, especially where there may be complex and unpredictable events and supporting teams to do likewise to ensure safety of individuals, families, and carer's.

1.9 Work collaboratively with an appropriate range of multi-agency and inter-professional resources, developing, maintaining, and evaluating links to manage risk and issues across organisations and settings.

1.10 Act as a clinical role model/advocate for developing and delivering care that is responsive to changing requirements, informed by an understanding of local population health needs, agencies, and networks.

1.11 Evidence the underpinning subject-specific competencies i.e. knowledge, skills and behaviours relevant to the role setting and scope, and demonstrate application of the capabilities to these, in an approach that is appropriate to the individual role, setting and scope.

2.3 Evaluate own practice, and participate in multi-disciplinary service and team evaluation, demonstrating the impact of advanced clinical practice on service function and effectiveness, and quality (i.e. outcomes of care, experience, and safety).

2.4 Actively engage in peer review to inform own and other's practice, formulating and implementing strategies to act on learning and make improvements.

3.1 Critically assess and address own learning needs, negotiating a personal development plan that reflects the breadth of ongoing professional development across the four pillars of advanced clinical practice.

3.2 Engage in self-directed learning, critically reflecting to maximise clinical skills and knowledge, as well as own potential to lead and develop both care and services.

4.2 Evaluate and audit own and others' clinical practice, selecting and applying valid, reliable methods, then acting on the findings.

Accreditation Considerations

- Royal College of Emergency Medicine (RCEM) Curriculum (Adult and Paediatrics). https://rcem.ac.uk/wp-content/uploads/2021/10/EC_ACP_Curriculum_2017_Adult_and_Paediatric-for_publication-Last_Edit_14-03-2019.pdf
- Royal College of General Practitioners (RCGP) Core Capabilities Framework for Advanced Clinical Practice. https://skillsforhealth.org.uk/wp-content/uploads/2020/11/ACP-Primary-Care-Nurse-Fwk-2020.pdf
- Royal College of Nursing Standards for Advanced Level Nursing. www.rcn.org.uk/-/media/royal-college-of-nursing/documents/publications/2018/july/pdf-007038.pdf?la=en
- Royal College of Radiologists. Clinical Radiology Standards. www.rcr.ac.uk/clinical-radiology/being-consultant/publications/standards
- Royal Pharmaceutical Society (RPS). Competency Framework for all Prescribers. www.rpharms.com/Portals/0/RPS%20document%20library/Open%20access/Professional%20standards/Prescribing%20competency%20framework/prescribing-competency-framework.pdf
- Society of Radiographers (SoR). www.sor.org/learning-advice/career-development/practice-level-information/advanced-practitioners
- Faculty of Intensive Care Medicine (FICM). ACCP Curriculum. www.ficm.ac.uk/consultation-on-updated-ficm-accp-curriculum
- Numbers Needed to Treat (NNT). www.theNNT.com

PRINCIPLES TO FOLLOW

In clinical practice, advanced practitioners arrive at a differential diagnosis using pre-encounter information, first impressions and history taking. This directs a focused clinical examination and the ordering of investigations in testing the diagnostic hypothesis. We use tests to confirm or refute our potential diagnoses, as, when building a clinical impression, we have many potential outcomes. Should the test confirm our diagnosis, we move on to management of the problem. If it does not, or the results are unexpected, we are forced to revisit the patient and the problem. The development of this skill demands concentration, time and support.

Principles of Ordering and Interpretation

When ordering tests, the rationale behind your request is critical and you have responsibility for those results. Ask yourself, 'Could I justify this test in this patient?'.

For example: You come across a CRP result late in the day. It is elevated at 60 and the requesting practitioner has left. The notes state 'not unwell but concerned, check bloods and review with results'. The response to this depends on a range of factors but the interpretation of test results is either the role of the requesting practitioner or they record their rationale clearly in the clinical record. If you are clear about why you are ordering a test, both in your own practice and in your note keeping, then the skill of interpretation will follow.

Negative test results are both common and helpful and, in logically testing your hypothesis, they can rule out certain diagnoses. We often worry about missing rare diagnoses in patients and this can drive scattergun testing, exhaustively investigating with little rationale behind the approach. Apply the adage that 'common things are common. . .'. as testing for rarity leads to unnecessary and expensive requests.

Reference Ranges

To give context for borderline results, we need to understand the reference range. To develop a reference range for haemoglobin in adult males, primary studies take place. For example, 100 adult males who are healthy and well have measurements taken of haemoglobin levels. This creates a range (lowest to highest), and we apply a 95% confidence level, i.e. we are confident that this is an accurate range from bottom to top for 95% of results. This range will exclude the bottom 2.5% and the top 2.5%. They are now 'out of range' but are clearly not unwell or abnormal. Hence, awareness is required to avoid misjudgement, potentially an overreaction to a result.

Patient and Clinician Factors to Consider When Interpreting Results: Context

The origin and intention of the test are interpreted alongside previous results and the patient's history, looking for patterns acutely or over time. Learning the skill of ordering and interpretation needs time and exposure to this role in a structured, protected and supervised way, using colleagues to guide you through the uncertainty. Experience allows us to embed a robust routine to ensure we become calibrated to this critical element of the role.

Case Study

George is 64 years old. He attends with long-term fatigue, weight gain and low mood. He is normally fit and well, but these symptoms have developed over time. He now falls asleep after work and never feels refreshed when he wakes. He is suffering muscle cramps and has numbness in both feet. He feels rapidly tired with palpitations when he exerts himself. He has hypertension (treated) and a strong family history of hypothyroidism and cardiovascular disease.

THE FULL BLOOD COUNT

Haemoglobin

Range <130 g/dl in males, <115 g/dl in females (Murphy 2014)

Anaemia, a low haemoglobin, is the most common abnormality we encounter. We see it acutely in haemorrhage with significant compromise or as a function of chronic disease or chronic bleeding. Patients with significant anaemia, particularly with rapid blood loss, may be pale or have cardiovascular dysfunction, low blood pressure or tachycardia (Dingli 2022). Remember, in chronic cases the patient will accommodate to the haemoglobin as it falls, and it is not unusual to see profound anaemia in the absence of clinical signs.

A Stepwise Approach

Haemoglobin (Hb) and Mean Cell Volume (MCV)

If the Hb is low, we initially look at the MCV, a measure of the size of the red blood cells. If the MCV is low (<88), we have small cells – microcytic anaemia – the most common cause of which is iron deficiency (WHO 2022). The bone marrow is deficient in iron creating small cells as it tries to keep pace with requirements. The patient is losing iron, through bleeding (often covert from the bowel), not absorbing iron (coeliac disease or Crohn's disease where the small bowel is diseased) or there is simply not enough iron in the diet. In menstruating women, overt blood loss can be present this way, while children hover on the edge of iron deficiency as they grow. In both scenarios keeping pace with requirement is difficult (Gupta et al. 2016).

If the MCV is raised (>98), the cells are large – macrocytic anaemia. Macrocytic anaemia can be divided into two types; in type 1, megaloblastic red blood cells are large and ovoid in shape due to abnormalities in synthesis secondary to a deficiency of vitamin B12 and/or folate; in type 2, non-megaloblastic red blood cells are typically enlarged and round following direct bone marrow toxicity with, for example, alcohol. In type 2 also, liver disease causes deposition of lipids in red blood cell walls, enlarging the surface area. In this setting B12 and folate are likely to be normal, but the history will inform you (Imashuku et al. 2012).

If the MCV is normal (88–98), the cells are normal sized – normocytic anaemia. Bone marrow function is sensitive to age and chronic disease processes, and cell synthesis is reduced. We commonly see this in chronic kidney disease, chronic heart failure, chronic pulmonary disease and the autoimmune diseases. This often affects the elderly where co-morbidity dictates that we cannot rule out iron or B12 deficiency without checking haematinics (Begum and Latunde-Dada 2019).

Haematinics: Ferritin, B12 and Folate

We check ferritin levels to inform us of circulating iron levels. Most iron is in the red blood cells or liver, hence low serum ferritin indicates significant depletion of stores elsewhere. Vitamin B12 is absorbed in the stomach. Low B12 due to autoimmune destruction of the B12 receptors in the stomach is called pernicious anaemia, the most common cause. Folate is absorbed in the small bowel and is often a feature of Crohn's or coeliac disease whereas small bowel pathology reduces folic acid absorption (Hall 2015).

George's Results

Hb	9.6
MCV	104
WCC	8.3
Plts	210

This is macrocytic anaemia. The most common cause is B12 deficiency due to pernicious anaemia, often found hand in hand with hypothyroidism.

Remember, nothing is absolute and co-pathology is common so, as the MCV is raised, we need to ask about alcohol consumption.

Ferritin	66
B12	110
Folate	5.2

The haematinics confirm the low B12 result. One caveat here is that ferritin is an acute-phase protein, released by the liver when inflammatory processes are at play. This may confound our thinking, but we can address this directly with further testing.

White Cells (Leucocytes)

High numbers of white blood cells (leucocytosis >10 × 10⁹/l) are commonly seen, usually indicating significant infection. Inspection of the subtypes of white cell will help in the assessment (Hall 2015).

Neutrophils are active against bacteria and are raised in significant bacterial infection, and when numbers are low, as in chemotherapy with bone marrow suppression, overwhelming bacterial infection can occur.

Lymphocytes (many types) react to viruses while monocytes assist in bacterial infection. Eosinophils are a marker of allergy and parasite infection.

Blast cells in the circulation are immature cells and may represent a blood cancer, leukaemia. If present, the specialist services will alert you. A raised white cell count (WCC) is also seen in smokers, pregnancy and chronic stress, while a low white cell count can be seen in lymphoma, certain infections (e.g. HIV and sepsis), drug toxicity and bone marrow irradiation.

Platelets (Thrombocytes)

Platelets are the building blocks of blood clots formed as a result of the clotting cascade, a complex series of events driven by clotting factors (produced by the liver), which staunches blood flow.

Raised Platelets (>400)

Raised platelets can predispose to clotting or can give a valuable insight into other disease processes. Platelets can be raised in the early stages of cancer (a paraneoplastic effect) and in other inflammatory conditions. After splenectomy, storage of platelets is lost and the circulating count is raised. Leukaemia and other bone marrow disorders (e.g. primary thrombocythaemia) should be considered (NICE CKS 2021a).

Low Platelets (<150)

Low platelets can raise the risk of haemorrhage. Impaired production in the bone marrow can occur in chemotherapy, Epstein–Barr virus infection, leukaemia, lymphoma, vitamin B12 and folate deficiency. Increased use of platelets will occur because of autoimmune disorders, pregnancy, coagulation disorders, chronic bleeding and following surgery (Hall 2015). Assessment of the bleeding risk is paramount; look at past results and events and take advice if you are unsure.

Inflammatory Markers

The inflammatory response creates the environment for the elements of the immune system to deal with infection or foreign proteins. Once the system is activated, blood vessels dilate to allow fluid, inflammatory proteins and cells into the tissues, creating heat, swelling, redness and pain in the affected area.

C-Reactive Protein

Range <5

In the acute phase of inflammation, the liver releases C-reactive protein (CRP), which activates white blood cells and is released in amounts proportional to the severity of the scenario. It is used to measure the degree of inflammatory response, climbing rapidly in the early stages of illness and falling equally rapidly once treatment is initiated or natural resolution occurs.

Plasma Viscosity

Range <1.72

Another measure of inflammatory response is the plasma viscosity (PV) where release of inflammatory mediators (proteins) in the immune response 'thickens' the blood. It will rise more gradually than CRP and takes time to return to normal. When monitoring chronic inflammatory disease, such as rheumatoid arthritis, it is useful in checking response to medication and disease activity.

George's Results	
Hb	9.6
MCV	104
WCC	8.3
Plts	210
CRP	3
Viscosity	1.67

We see a normal CRP and PV, reassuring us that there is no significant inflammatory process at play.

Renal Function

The kidney is a filter, removing waste products (urea, creatinine, drugs), and is integral to fluid and electrolyte balance. It assists in blood pressure control, secretes erythropoietin to stimulate red blood cell production and activates vitamin D. Estimate of glomerular filtration rate (e-GFR) is now commonplace and gives insight into renal function.

Range

Urea	2.5–7.8 mmol/l (Hall 2015)
Creatinine	♂ 59–104 μmol/l
	♀ 45–84 μmol/l

Creatinine (Cr)

Produced in the liver and excreted by the kidney, this is a measure of kidney function, liver function and muscle mass.

Urea (U)

The breakdown of proteins in the liver creates urea. It is a marker of kidney function and can reflect increased protein levels in the blood, in cases of gastrointestinal bleeding, postoperative states, trauma, infection, malignancy and high-protein diets. It will be reduced in dietary deficiency of protein, malnutrition and liver disease and pregnancy.

Acute Kidney Injury

'The loss of kidney function leading to the retention of urea and other nitrogenous waste products, and dysregulation of extracellular volume electrolytes' (NICE CKS 2021b)

A rise in serum creatinine of at least 50% compared to the patient's normal within the previous seven days, together with a fall in urine output, triggers acute kidney injury (AKI) as a diagnosis. Causes include impaired renal blood flow, sepsis or cardiac failure, renal disease itself, glomerular nephritis or acute interstitial nephritis, and obstruction of urine flow, renal stones, bladder blood clots, bladder tumour or other pelvic malignancy. The likelihood increases over age 65, with coincidental chronic kidney disease or co-morbidities such as diabetes or cardiac failure and nephrotoxic medications: NSAIDS are a major culprit. If urea alone is raised, check fluid status and look for other causes as this may not be a renal issue; we would also look at creatinine to determine renal function (NICE CKS 2021b).

Chronic Kidney Injury

'A reduction in kidney function or structural damage (or both) present for more than three months, with associated health implications' (NICE 2022)

We now monitor and assess renal function chronically, looking to intervene with risk factor modification and management, aiming to minimise vascular risks by tight management of hypertension, diabetes or obesity alongside intrinsic renal disease and obstruction of urine flow, most commonly with prostatic disease.

Electrolytes: Sodium and Potassium

Significant abnormalities in electrolytes can be catastrophic as they are responsible for the normal function of electrical tissue, namely the nervous system and muscle.

- *Sodium* (range 133–146 mmol/l) (Hall 2015). Sodium lives outside cells in the blood plasma, urine or interstitial fluid, so interpretation of sodium results demands a review of fluid status.
- *Low sodium* (hyponatraemia, <133) (NICE CKS 2020, Ball 2013). This is the most common and most complex scenario to assess. Sodium is primarily active in the neurological system, with low levels presenting as confusion, fatigue or seizure. Applying commonality, we can give context to a low sodium, remembering that deficiency is rare and correction of the underlying cause will restore normality.

In oedematous states, fluid moving to the tissues carries sodium with it. The principle of osmosis applies here, where substances will move between compartments to equalise levels. Hence, in heart failure, venous pressure (due to backpressure from a failing heart) forces fluid into tissues, with sodium, hence reducing circulating sodium. Low albumen levels in cirrhosis of the liver also cause fluid to move to the tissues from the bloodstream. The kidneys attempt to normalise sodium levels through water and sodium reabsorption, but this is continually lost into the tissue space until the problem is corrected and balance can be restored. In renal failure and diuretics use, sodium is lost into the urine and not reabsorbed. Diuretics move sodium into the collecting ducts of the kidney to enable the excretion of water, reducing fluid overload in the body. Caution is required here as sodium is used to clear fluid, depleting resources. Once the oedema is cleared, the sodium levels in the blood start to reflect the actual body stores of sodium.

Rarely, high fluid consumption dilutes sodium, but this must be extreme, overwhelming the systems which manage fluid balance. In true deficiency, excess loss in vomit, diarrhoea or sweating occurs. The kidneys are working hard to reabsorb water and sodium, but the issue is true depletion. Assessment of hydration is critical, and replacement of sodium may be required.

Fluid balance is monitored intensively in the kidney and in the central nervous system. The need for water reabsorption drives the pituitary gland to produce antidiuretic hormone (ADH), a normal compensatory mechanism in fluid balance, which drives the kidney to retain water. Excess ADH release leads to retention of too much water and dilutes the sodium in the blood. Syndrome of inappropriate antidiuretic hormone (SIADH) is the most common cause due to a primary brain injury in the elderly, or malignancy and based on a thorough history.

The movement of sodium in the kidney tubule is also under the control of aldosterone, released by the adrenal glands, driven by the pituitary gland, forcing active reabsorption of sodium back into the bloodstream to reset levels and actively maintain blood volume. Absence of aldosterone (Addison disease) can present as addisonian crisis, where failure to resorb sodium, and hence water, leads to an inability to maintain blood pressure with significant infection when the vascular system dilates with the inflammatory response.

- *High sodium* (hypernatraemia, >146) (Hall 2015). This less common scenario reflects either an absence of water in the bloodstream or an excess of sodium in the body. Water loss secondary to excessive loss through the bowel or severe burns is clear. Excess of sodium is more complex with causes including iatrogenic, excess IV saline, hyperaldosteronism driving salt reabsorption from the urine or excess salt ingestion (Ranjan et al. 2020).

- *Potassium* (K+) (range 3.5–5.3 mmol/l) (Hall 2015). Potassium is critical in the function of cardiac muscle, which can react catastrophically to abnormalities with the potential of fatal arrhythmias. Potassium is found in the blood plasma, within the cells of the body and in the fluid around the cells. In contrast to sodium, potassium can move into and out of cells with rapidity, creating real risk in certain clinical scenarios. We test only for blood plasma levels so must assess the context of an abnormal potassium carefully.

- *High potassium* (hyperkalaemia, >5.3 mmol/l). Patients with a potassium above 6 mmol/l need hospital admission as the risk of fatal cardiac arrhythmia is high (Rodan 2017). Causes include renal failure, either acute or chronic, where less potassium is excreted, or overzealous administration of potassium. Extensive cell destruction can precipitate rapid rises in the circulation, for example tumour lysis syndrome during chemotherapy or rhabdomyolysis, extensive muscle damage due to trauma or prolonged lying in the elderly. Potassium is also rapidly moved out of cells in acidosis. In diabetic ketoacidosis (DKA), management is based around normalising blood sugar but potassium is monitored closely due to the rapid shift into cells as insulin is administered.

Pseudo-hyperkalaemia

Elevated potassium may occur during blood taking with prolonged tourniquet time, difficulties in taking blood, use of the wrong anticoagulant, excessive cooling of the specimen and prolonged length of storage. All lead to blood cell damage and subsequent release of intracellular products into the blood sample (Kerr et al. 1985).

Low Potassium – Hypokalaemia (<3.5 mmol/l)

True potassium deficiency occurs if loss is excessive via the kidneys, the GI tract or the skin (severe vomiting and diarrhoea, severe burns) or in malnutrition, failures of total parenteral nutrition or inadequate replacement when on fluids and nil by mouth. In correction of acidosis, potassium moves into cells rapidly. Clearly correction of the issue will help to normalise the result.

George's Results

Sodium	129 (133–146 mmol/l)
Potassium	3.6 (3.5–5.3 mmol/l)
e-GFR	58 (>90)

He has a low sodium and a normal potassium. His e-GFR is low and not ideal for his age.

With his age and co-morbidity (hypertension), this should alert us to look at his blood pressure control and other cardiovascular risk factors.

The sodium is low, but not dramatically so. Here the trend is what we are after and, although we focus on his fatigue, care here is critical for future avoidance of cardiovascular disease.

Electrolytes: Calcium and Magnesium

- *Calcium* (range Ca^{2+} [adjusted] 2.2–2.6 mmol/l) (Hall 2015). Calcium is essential for muscle contraction, nerve conduction, bone structure and cell replication. Calcium binds to albumen in the bloodstream, so results take account of this. The negative feedback loop (Figure 11.1), a frequent concept in hormonal systems, is critical here and with calcium this is managed by the parathyroid glands, sited within the thyroid glands.

- *Low calcium* (hypercalcaemia, range <2.2 mmol/l) (Hall 2015). The parathyroid gland releases parathyroid hormone (PTH), causing bone to release calcium into the bloodstream, and drives the kidney to reabsorb more calcium while conversion of vitamin D into its active form increases GI tract absorption. With poor dietary intake or breakdown of the negative feedback loop, levels drop. If the parathyroid gland is surgically removed (during thyroidectomy), where vitamin D levels are low (poor sun exposure) and in acute pancreatitis (where calcium is neutralised in the circulation), low calcium levels can develop.

- *High calcium* (hypocalcaemia, range >2.6 mmol/l) (Hall 2015). Often a consequence of increased release of calcium from bone due to hyperparathyroidism, excess PTH release or malignancy with bone invasion. Thiazide diuretics increase kidney reabsorption so beware of excess supplementation. Symptoms include bone pain, muscle weakness, kidney stones, constipation and depression, reflecting the impact on muscle and nervous system function. If levels are less than 3.5 and the patient is asymptomatic, monitoring is appropriate while the underlying cause is addressed (NICE CKS 2019).

- *Magnesium* (range Mg^{2+} 0.7–1.0 mmol/l) (Hall 2015). Magnesium is increasingly relevant in practice. The concentration reflects dietary intake and retention through the kidneys and GI tract. Most of it resides in the cells so the relationship between deficiency and plasma level is not strong. This is currently not a common test in primary care, but abnormalities are commonly found in conjunction with other electrolyte disturbances.

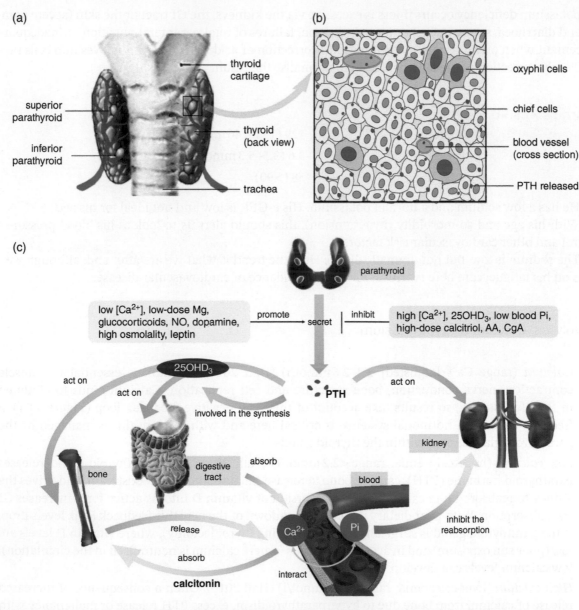

FIGURE 11.1   Calcium and parathyroid feedback loop. a) Cells in the parathyroid, oxyphil cells (bigger but fewer), and chief cells (smaller but more) are compacted. b) The function of parathyroid hormone in the body. Its delivery through blood mainly worked on bones, kidneys, and digestive tract to keep the balance of iron, especially Ca and P concentration. c) Calcium and parathyroid feedback loop. Source: Li et al. (2020)/From John Wiley & Sons/ https://onlinelibrary.wiley.com/doi/full/10.1002/term.3080

Liver Function Tests

The interpretation of liver function tests (LFTs) lends itself to the principle of commonality but remember the resilience of the liver and it ability to regenerate, making tests an unreliable source of reassurance. The liver is active in the creation of waste products, creatinine and urea, synthesis of albumen, clotting factors and inflammatory proteins and storage of fat, glucose and iron (amongst others). It is the primary metaboliser for all substances absorbed from the bowel.

Alanine Aminotransferase (ALT)

Found within hepatocytes, this is an important marker of liver disease. It is an enzyme used by the liver in glucose metabolism and is found only within the liver cells. Elevation is a clear marker of damage to these cells, as in hepatitis. Aspartate aminotransferase (AST) is occasionally seen but it is found in muscle so is less specific.

Alkaline Phosphatase (ALP)

This enzyme is found in the membrane of liver cells in the biliary tree. Hence, biliary pathology (gallstones and cholecystitis commonly) will damage the cells of the biliary tree and release ALP into the bloodstream.

Alkaline phosphatase is also released by bone, placenta, kidney and the intestines. In the absence of other raised LFTs, we need to consider other causes. Both prostate and breast cancer metastasise to bone and hence the ALP we see in the bloodstream may have originated elsewhere.

Bilirubin (Br)

The liver creates bile from the products of red cell destruction arriving from the spleen, storing it in the gall bladder for release when fat digestion is required. Haemolytic anaemia (rapid breakdown of red blood cells) causes a surge in breakdown products, overwhelming the capacity of the liver, and the patient is usually profoundly anaemic.

Patterns of Liver Disease

Liver disease, although insidious, lends itself to commonality and pattern recognition. Table 11.1 defines the common patterns linking to the area of the liver affected. For example, paracetamol overdose will damage liver cells, causing an initial rise in ALT but not ALP or Br. These may follow with severe liver disease. Conversely, bile duct obstruction with a gallstone will cause ALP and Br to rise first, followed later by ALT if the problem persists. Chronic liver disease may not be revealed by blood testing until the liver decompensates, failing rapidly.

George's Results

ALT		66
ALP		45
BR		12
Alb		55

The ALT is slightly elevated with no elevation of ALP or Br. This might indicate low-level hepatic damage and we are pointed, using commonality, to alcohol, non-alcoholic fatty liver disease or medication effects (Hall 2015).

TABLE 11.1   Pattern recognition.

	Prehepatic (Haemolysis)	Acute Hepatocellular Damage (Hepatic)	Chronic Hepatocellular Damage (Hepatic)	Posthepatic (Biliary)
Alanine aminotransferace	Normal	Very raised	Normal or slightly increased	Normal or slight increase
Alkaline phosphatase	Normal	Normal or slight increase	Normal or slightly increased	Very raised
Bilirubin	Raised	Normal or slight increase	Normal or slightly increased	Very raised
	Haemolytic anaemia	Paracetamol overdose	Alcoholic liver disease	Pancreatic carcinoma
	Malaria	Infectious hepatitis, particularly hepatitis A	Non-alcoholic fatty liver disease	Gallstone disease
	Certain medications, anti-tuberculosis drugs	Certain medications	Chronic hepatitis, typically hepatitis B or C	Cholangiocarcinoma

Thyroid Function Tests

Thyroid disease is insidious, presenting subtly with a strong genetic component, frequently autoimmune in origin. The thyroid sets the metabolic rate in the body and is under the control of the hypothalamic pituitary (HPT) axis. Levels of thyroxine (T4) in the body are measured by receptors within the brain; if they are low, the hypothalamus releases thyrotropin releasing hormone (TRH), causing the anterior pituitary to release thyroid stimulating hormone (TSH) which acts on the thyroid gland, increasing production of T4 and T3. Constant balancing is at play as the brain measures the levels of T4 in the blood and acts to increase or decrease the TSH as a response (Figure 11.2).

Hypothyroidism (Underfunctioning)

TSH	>4
Free T4	<9

Patients with excessive tiredness, intolerance of cold, weight gain, muscle pain, dry skin, constipation and low mood may be hypothyroid. This is Hashimoto thyroiditis, in which antibodies destroy the thyroid over years (family history is critical) (NICE CKS 2021d). It is common and managed with thyroxine replacement but think holistically, interpreting the patient's symptoms against the blood test results. This is important when addressing changes to doses according to annual testing.

Hyperthyroidism (Overfunctioning)

TSH	<0.5
Free T4	>24

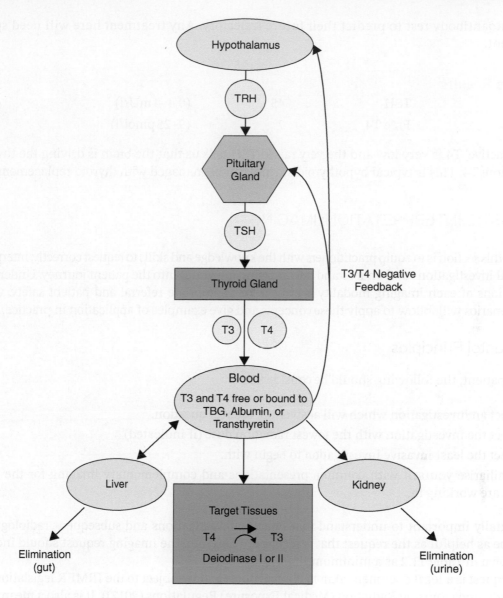

FIGURE 11.2 Thyroid system. *Source*: Baochun Guo et al. (2020).

Graves disease, in which the body produces antibodies which mimic TSH, is the most common cause, leading to overrelease of T4 but bypassing the negative feedback look. Complaints of feeling hot, agitation, diarrhoea, palpitations and anxiety with sleeplessness are usual (NICE CKS 2021c). This group needs specialist management and referral to thyroid services.

Subclinical Hypothyroidism and Hyperthyroidism

TSH	4–10
Free T4	9–25

This group will often have a slightly elevated TSH. They may not be symptomatic but if they are then you may be seeing early disease. Ask about family history and potentially request a thyroid autoantibody test to predict their future trajectory. Any treatment here will need specialist involvement.

> **George's Results**
>
> | | | |
> |---|---|---|
> | TSH | 45 | (0.4–4 mU/l) |
> | Free T4 | 7 | (9–25 pmol/l) |
>
> The 'active' T4 is very low and the very raised TSH tells us that the brain is driving the thyroid to release more T4. This is typical hypothyroidism and can be managed with thyroid replacement.

DIAGNOSTIC INTERPRETATION: IMAGING

The aim of this section is to equip practitioners with the knowledge and skills to request correctly, interpret basic radiological investigations and understand how imaging integrates into the patient journey. Understanding the limitations of each imaging modality is critical for appropriate referral and patient safety. Common clinical scenarios will follow to apply these concepts and give examples of application in practice.

Fundamental Principles

For every patient, the following should be considered.

- Select an investigation which will answer the referral question.
- Select the investigation with the lowest radiation dose (if indicated).
- Select the least invasive investigation to begin with.
- Familiarise yourself with common presentations and complementary imaging for the specialty you are working in.

It is vitally important to understand that imaging investigations and subsequent radiology reports will only be as helpful as the request that is received. Therefore, the imaging request should include the details shown in Table 11.2 as a minimum.

The request is a legal document akin to clinical notes and is subject to the IRMER legislation around ionising radiation (Ionising Radiation (Medical Exposure) Regulations (2017)). It is also a means of communication with the referrer about urgent findings, selecting the most appropriate investigation and choosing how to do the imaging.

TABLE 11.2   Imaging request details.

Patient demographics (name, DOB, address, NHS number)
Clinical presentation/mechanism of injury (including date and time)
Findings on clinical examination (including laboratory results)
The clinical question to be answered.? cause is not one. List your differentials so as to apply logic.
Relevant medical history, e.g. EtOH excess, diabetes, disability, previous trauma, etc.
Body part to be imaged including laterality: left or right
Referrer details (email, professional registration number, job title)

Inaccurate information on the request may lead to:

- delays in imaging
- inappropriate investigations/scan techniques being performed
- false hope with inaccurate expectations of the outcome of the examination
- a breakdown in the logical thought process of patient management
- inaccurate interpretation of the imaging
- misleading clinical information → misdiagnosis → serious clinical consequences → possible legal action.

THE ESSENTIALS OF EACH IMAGING MODALITY ARE CONSIDERED BELOW

Plain Film

The plain film X-ray is a 2D image of a 3D structure and therefore the information gained is limited compared to more complex imaging. It also uses potentially harmful ionising radiation to acquire the image. That said, it requires relatively low amounts of radiation and radiographers are trained to keep the dose as low as reasonably achievable; it is also quick and readily accessible. It is particularly useful in diagnosis of the scenarios shown in Table 11.3.

TABLE 11.3   Plain film imaging studies and their applicable clinical situations.

Investigation	Clinical Scenario
Chest radiograph (CXR)	Placement of lines and tubes Pneumothorax Pleural effusion Lung/lobar collapse Lung mass Consolidation Cardiac failure Foreign body aspiration/penetration Pneumoperitoneum (on erect CXR) Normal and abnormal calcifications Bony thorax abnormalities
Abdominal radiograph (AXR)	Bowel obstruction Toxic megacolon Pneumoperitoneum Foreign body ingestion/penetration Normal and abnormal calcifications
Skeletal radiograph	Fracture – traumatic, pathological, non-accidental Dislocation/subluxation Joint disorders, e.g. arthropathy Joint effusion Lipohaemarthrosis (fat/fluid level within the joint) Soft tissue mass Bone lesions malignant/metastatic/benign/infective Metabolic bone disorders Skeletal dysplasia

A common misconception of the 'black and white' images is that they are easy to interpret and are highly accurate. Interpretation is not straightforward and requires clinical correlation to gain the most accurate diagnosis.

'Normal' can be misleading. Fractures, for example, may be undisplaced or hidden by overlying structures, and sometimes the obvious prevents the viewer from seeing the less obvious; this is known as satisfaction of search (SOS). Here the viewer, having identified an initial abnormality, fails to continue looking for further findings. Technical factors, both equipment and patient presentation, also play a significant role in adequate imaging quality and diagnosis. The prevalence of obesity has more than doubled in England in the last decade and this presents real challenges in image acquisition and interpretation across all imaging modalities (Agha and Agha 2017). There is an unavoidable 'human factor' in radiology reporting, and not all 'misses' mean malpractice. Therefore, attention will be on issues including proof of competence and habits of practice.

The most frequent causes of poor image interpretation are as follows.

- Failure to look at every film. Has every image available been viewed and comparisons made with previous imaging?
- Failure to look at the whole film. Have all abnormalities been picked up?
- Failure to look at the film as a whole. Do the bones display a normal bony architecture or are there generalised features of a metabolic bone disorder?
- Forgetting to look at the soft tissues. Commonly, focusing on the bone and not the adjacent soft tissues, particularly pertinent in imaging of the chest and paediatrics.

A fundamental image used widely in all clinical fields is the chest X-ray. Understanding of how the image is created will help explain key features. The tissues the X-rays hit absorb (attenuate) the beam. Different tissue thicknesses attenuate different amounts of X-rays. More dense tissue results in more X-rays being attenuated, producing a whiter image. If something black is adjacent to something white, then there is greater contrast between the two objects which makes them easier to see.

Now apply this concept to the chest X-ray image in Figure 11.3 which shows normal densities and anatomy.

The importance of assessing image quality for diagnosis is paramount, and the following should be assessed.

- *Rotation*: side lifted from image detector appears lighter. Hila can look distorted.
- *Inspiration*: less than six anterior/eight posterior ribs cause crowding of diaphragm and hila.
- *Penetration*: underexposure can cause false positives, e.g. pulmonary fibrosis or oedema, Overexposure could mimic chronic lung change, e.g. COPD.
- *Angulation*: clavicles should be projected over the lung apices and show no rotation.

After these steps, diagnostic interpretation can be performed. When lung anatomy is shifted or distorted, it is important to decide if it has been pulled to one side or pushed away from the other, or if there is overlying/indwelling disease that is causing obliteration of the normal structural lines.

- Pushed – massive pleural effusion/mass
  - Structures displaced to other side
  - Diaphragm depressed
  - Ribs widened

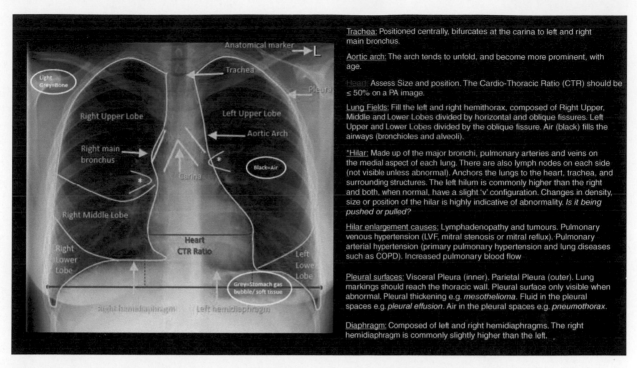

Trachea: Positioned centrally, bifurcates at the carina to left and right main bronchus.

Aortic arch: The arch tends to unfold, and become more prominent, with age.

Heart: Assess Size and position. The Cardio-Thoracic Ratio (CTR) should be ≤ 50% on a PA image.

Lung Fields: Fill the left and right hemithorax, composed of Right Upper, Middle and Lower Lobes divided by horizontal and oblique fissures. Left Upper and Lower Lobes divided by the oblique fissure. Air (black) fills the airways (bronchioles and alveoli).

*Hilar: Made up of the major bronchi, pulmonary arteries and veins on the medial aspect of each lung. There are also lymph nodes on each side (not visible unless abnormal). Anchors the lungs to the heart, trachea, and surrounding structures. The left hilum is commonly higher than the right and both, when normal, have a slight 'v' configuration. Changes in density, size or position of the hilar is highly indicative of abnormality. *Is it being pushed or pulled?*

Hilar enlargement causes: Lymphadenopathy and tumours. Pulmonary venous hypertension (LVF, mitral stenosis or mitral reflux). Pulmonary arterial hypertension (primary pulmonary hypertension and lung diseases such as COPD). Increased pulmonary blood flow

Pleural surfaces: Visceral Pleura (inner). Parietal Pleura (outer). Lung markings should reach the thoracic wall. Pleural surface only visible when abnormal. Pleural thickening e.g. *mesothelioma*. Fluid in the pleural spaces e.g. *pleural effusion*. Air in the pleural spaces e.g. *pneumothorax*.

Diaphragm: Composed of left and right hemidiaphragms. The right hemidiaphragm is commonly slightly higher than the left.

FIGURE 11.3   Chest X-ray densities and normal anatomy. *Source*: Christine Eade (chapter author).

- Pulled – lobular collapse
- Structures displaced to the same side
- Diaphragm pulled up
- Ribs crowded

The example in Figure 11.4 shows a high-quality diagnostic chest X-ray of a 79-year-old male. The left hemithorax shows complete opacification with deviation of the trachea (appearing to be pulled) to the left (yellow arrow), the right hemithorax shows normal lung parenchyma and there is loss of the right heart border as the right medial lung base at the cardiophrenic angle is clearly seen (*). Given the clinical history of 'previous squamous non-small cell lung cancer 12 years ago, treated with left thoracotomy and pneumonectomy, follow-up chest X-ray for surveillance? recurrence', the imaging findings are as expected; thoracotomy noted with surgical resection of the left fifth rib (yellow circle), opacification (white area) of the left hemithorax due to pneumonectomy, deviation of the mediastinal structures to the left and slight overexpansion of the right lung are all normal features of these interventions. Overall appearances are unchanged from the previous chest X-ray of one year previously which was reviewed at the time of reporting. This chest X-ray is entirely normal for this patient.

A final note on consolidation. This is seen as dense (white) areas on the X-ray as fluid fills the alveoli and small airways. Consolidation is a broad term and the underlying cause cannot be differentiated on the plain film. This requires clinical correlation (it does not always imply infection).

- *Pneumonia* – airways full of pus/fluid, caused by bacteria, viruses or fungi.
- *Cancer* – airways full of cells.
- *Pulmonary haemorrhage* – airways full of blood.
- *Pulmonary oedema* – airways full of fluid.

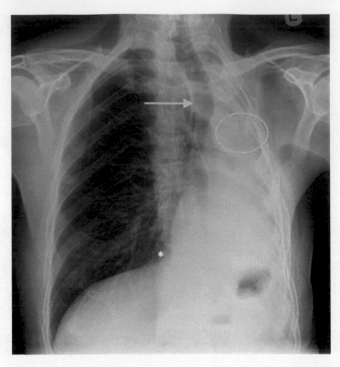

FIGURE 11.4 A 79-year-old male with history of squamous non-small cell lung cancer treated with left thoracotomy and pneumonectomy.

Figure 11.5 shows a chest X-ray of a 34-year-old female non-smoker who presented with two weeks of new cough, increased temperature and raised CRP of 40 mg/l, clinical question;? Infection. The chest X-ray appearances are consistent with infective consolidation with dense opacification in the right upper lobe 'settled' on the horizontal fissure.

Ultrasound

Ultrasound is a non-invasive diagnostic tool used to complement other imaging modalities. It uses the basic principle of a handheld transducer (and is therefore hugely operator dependent) that both emits and detects sonographic waves. When the waves hit substances (fluid/soft tissue/bone), they reflect back to the transducer to create electrical signals which generate a 2D real-time image on the ultrasound scanning machine for visualisation. Ultrasound does not use ionising radiation and is a safe imaging modality when used by trained practitioners, for the assessment of, but not limited to, acute kidney injury, jaundice, cholecystitis, postmenopausal bleeding, some musculoskeletal disorders and ovarian pathology. For the purposes of advanced practice, we will focus here on lung ultrasound, focused assessment with sonography for trauma (FAST) and cardiac echo scans.

Lung Ultrasound

Lung ultrasound (LUS) is role specific and an established point-of-care tool for the evaluation of patients in the emergency department. During the SARS-CoV-2 pandemic, LUS was used as a diagnostic tool for patients with COVID-19. Findings in LUS such as bilateral B-lines, pleural irregularity and/or subpleural consolidations lead to an increased suspicion of COVID-19. Pleural effusions are rare (Moynihan et al. 2021). LUS can only be undertaken by practitioners who have had extensive experience in undertaking scans and interpretation.

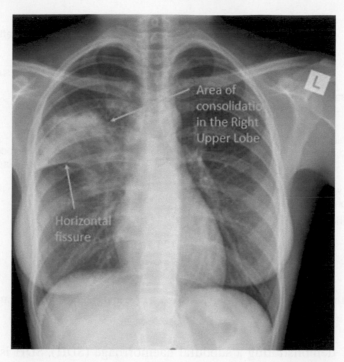

FIGURE 11.5 Chest X-ray of a 34-year-old female showing consolidation in the right upper lobe.

FAST Scan

FAST scans are a point-of-care ultrasound (POCUS) examination performed at presentation of major trauma patients. The study is used as a 'rule in' tool rather than a means of exclusion as large amounts of intraperitoneal free fluid (approx. 500 ml) need to be seen to make an accurate diagnosis. It is helpful in time-critical patients where immediate management may include surgical intervention/referral to theatre. In most trauma situations, when the patient is stable for transfer, a CT scan is preferrable for a more detailed, accurate diagnosis. That said, if the operator is sufficiently competent, consolidation, pleural effusion and pneumothoraces can be accurately diagnosed.

Echo

Focused echo sonography is used by some cardiology and intensive care specialists in the emergency department to assess for pericardial effusion and during resuscitation to assess cardiac motion.

Computed Tomography

A computed tomography (CT) scan is a form of cross-sectional image of the body using high doses of radiation. CT multi-trauma, or whole-body CT, is an increasingly used investigation in patients with multiple injuries sustained after significant trauma. Clinical assessment and mechanism of injury may underestimate injury severity by 30% (Linder et al. 2016). The primary purpose of the scan is the rapid evaluation of life-threatening injury and secondly to accurately assess known and diagnose unknown pathologies.

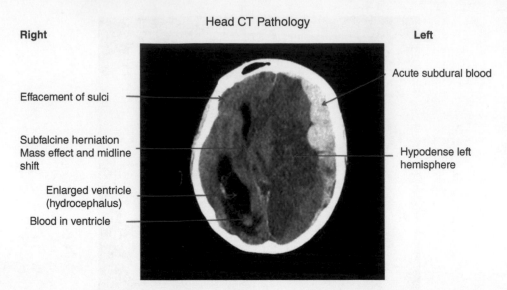

Head CT Pathology

Right

Left

Effacement of sulci

Acute subdural blood

Subfalcine herniation
Mass effect and midline
shift

Hypodense left
hemisphere

Enlarged ventricle
(hydrocephalus)

Blood in ventricle

FIGURE 11.6 Axial slice through the head showing left-sided acute subdural haemorrhage and surrounding mass effects (red arrows).

Figure 11.6 is a CT demonstrating a subdural haemorrhage (SDH). SDH is a collection of blood accumulating in the subdural space, the *potential* space between the dura and arachnoid mater of the meninges around the brain. SDH can happen in any age group. in this case, a 43-year-old male was involved in a motorcycle accident in which his bike 'T-boned' a car, throwing the victim several metres from the collision. CT scans are the gold standard for this type of diagnosis.

To conclude, CT imaging is a high radiation dose modality that offers complex scans. CT is the gold standard in trauma scenarios. Interpretation is difficult, requires lengthy training, and in particular, full body scan interpretation can only be undertaken by highly competent radiologists. Accurate, relevant clinical history is vital for accurate interpretation and diagnosis.

Imaging Summary

In summary, imaging investigations impact patient care in the following ways.

- **Cons**
  - Cost (high tariff for some modalities, e.g. CT/MRI)
  - Radiation dose (CT)
  - Time
  - Incidental findings may lead to unnecessary follow-up/clinical uncertainty
- **Pros**
  - Aids clinical diagnosis
  - Patient triage (discharge, observation, surgery, medical)
  - Fast
  - Accurate
  - Minimally invasive

Take Home Points
- Advanced level practitioners must develop and utilise a systematic approach to ordering and interpreting laboratory tests. They must use their underpinning knowledge and integrate this into their decision-making processes.
- Advanced level practitioners must have the ability to underpin all clinical tests and work with other healthcare professionals when working outside their scope of practice.
- Advanced level practitioners must be accurate in their interpretation of lab results in the context of the disease process by recognising patterns of disease through testing to inform patient management.

REFERENCES

Agha, M. and Agha, R. (2017). The rising prevalence of obesity: part a: impact on public health. *International Journal of Surgical Oncology* 2 (7): 1–6.

Ball, S.G. (2013). How I approach hyponatraemia. *Clinical Medicine* 13 (3): 291–295.

Baochun Guo, D.L., Liang, Q., Liu, Z. et al. (2020). Tissue-engineered parathyroid gland and its regulatory secretion of parathyroid hormone. *Journal of Tissue Engineering and Regenerative Medicine* 14 (10): 1363–1377.

Begum, S. and Latunde-Dada, G.O. (2019). Anemia of inflammation with an emphasis on chronic kidney disease. *Nutrients* 11 (10): 2424.

Dingli, D. (2022) Anemia. https://www.mayoclinic.org/diseases-conditions/anemia/symptoms-causes/syc-20351360

Gupta, P.M., Perrine, C.G., Mei, Z., and Scanlon, K.S. (2016). Iron, anemia, and iron deficiency anemia among young children in the United States. *Nutrients* 8 (6): 330.

Hall, J. (2015). *Guyton and Hall Textbook of Medical Physiology*, 13e. London: Elsevier.

Health Education England (2017). Multi-professional Framework for Advanced Clinical Practice in England. www.hee.nhs.uk/sites/default/files/documents/multi-professionalframeworkforadvancedclinicalpracticeinengland.pdf

Imashuku, S., Kudo, N., and Kaneda, S. (2012). Spontaneous resolution of macrocytic anemia: old disease revisited. *Journal of Blood Medicine* 3: 45–47.

Ionising Radiation (Medical Exposure) Regulations (IR(ME)R) (2017). www.legislation.gov.uk/uksi/2017/1322/made

Kerr, D.J., McAlpine, L.G., and Dagg, J.H. (1985). Pseudohyperkalaemia. *British Medical Journal (Clinical Research Ed.)* 291 (6499): 890–891.

Li, D., Guo, B., Liang, Q. et al. (2020). Tissue-engineered parathyroid gland and its regulatory secretion of parathyroid hormone. *Journal of Tissue Engineering and Regenerative Medicine* 14: 1363–1377.

Linder, F., Mani, K., Juhlin, C., and Eklöf, H. (2016). Routine whole-body CT of high energy trauma patients leads to excessive radiation exposure. *Scandinavian Journal of Trauma, Resuscitation and Emergency Medicine* 24: article no. 7.

Moynihan, R., Sanders, S., Michaleff, Z. et al. (2021). Impact of COVID-19 pandemic on utilisation of healthcare services: a systematic review. *BMJ Open* 11 (3): e045343.

Murphy, W.G. (2014). The sex difference in haemoglobin levels in adults – mechanisms, causes, and consequences. *Blood Reviews* 28 (2): 41–47.

NICE CKS (2019). `https://cks.nice.org.uk/topics/hypercalcaemia`

NICE CKS (2020). `https://cks.nice.org.uk/topics/hyponatraemia`

NICE CKS (2021a). `https://cks.nice.org.uk/topics/platelets-abnormal-counts-cancer/background-information/causes-of-thrombocytosis/`

NICE CKS (2021b). `https://cks.nice.org.uk/topics/acute-kidney-injury/diagnosis/responding-to-aki-warning-stage-test-results`

NICE CKS (2021c). `https://cks.nice.org.uk/topics/hyperthyroidism/diagnosis`

NICE CKS (2021d). `https://cks.nice.org.uk/topics/hypothyroidism/diagnosis/diagnosis`

NICE CKS (2022). `https://cks.nice.org.uk/topics/chronic-kidney-disease/diagnosis/diagnosis`

Ranjan, R., Lo, S.C., Ly, S. et al. (2020). Progression to severe hypernatremia in hospitalized general medicine inpatients: an observational study of hospital-acquired hypernatremia. *Medicina* 56 (7): 358.

Rodan, A.R. (2017). Potassium: friend or foe? *Pediatric Nephrology* 32 (7): 1109–1121.

World Health Organization (WHO) (2022). Anemia. `www.who.int/health-topics/anaemia#tab=tab_1`

FURTHER READING

Clarke, C. and Dux, A. (2015). *Abdominal X-Rays for Medical Students*. Oxford: Wiley-Blackwell.

Gee, C., Young, A., Rodrigues, M. et al. (2020). *The Unofficial Guide to Radiology: 100 Practice Orthopaedic X Rays with Full Colour Annotations and Full X Ray Reports*. London: Zeshan Qureshi.

Hamilton, P. (2022). *Blood Tests Made Easy*. Philadelphia: Elsevier.

SELF-ASSESSMENT QUESTIONS

1. As a trainee ACP, what are your learning needs in relation to diagnostic interpretation?
2. How will you identify your diagnostic interpretation needs for supervision and what documents and guidance will support this?
3. How will you evaluate and assess your diagnostic interpretation skills to prove your competency and capability in practice?
4. How can you ensure that you continue to develop your ability to refine your diagnostic interpretation practice?

GLOSSARY

Acute kidney injury (AKI)   The causes of acute kidney injury can be divided into pre-renal (for example, hypovolaemia, decreased cardiac output), intrinsic renal (for example, nephrotoxic drugs, interstitial nephritis) and postrenal (for example, renal stones, bladder outflow obstruction from prostate enlargement).

Anaemia   Anaemia is a condition in which the body does not have enough healthy red blood cells. Red blood cells provide oxygen to body tissues. Different types of anaemia include anaemia due to vitamin B12 deficiency, anaemia due to folate (folic acid) deficiency, anaemia due to iron deficiency, anaemia of chronic disease, haemolytic anaemia, idiopathic aplastic anaemia, megaloblastic anaemia, pernicious anaemia, sickle cell anaemia and thalassaemia. Iron deficiency anaemia is the most common type of anaemia.

Biochemistry   Biochemistry is the branch of science that explores the chemical processes within and related to living organisms. It is a laboratory-based science that brings together biology and chemistry. By using chemical knowledge and techniques, biochemists can understand and solve biological problems.

CT scan   A computed tomography (CT) scan combines a series of X-ray images taken from different angles around the body and uses computer processing to create cross-sectional images (slices) of the bones, blood vessels and soft tissues inside the body. CT scan images provide more detailed information than plain X-rays do.

Haemorrhage   Haemorrhage is an acute loss of blood from a damaged blood vessel. The bleeding can be minor, such as when the superficial vessels in the skin are damaged, leading to petechiae and ecchymosis, or major (catastrophic), requiring immediate action and correction

Neurology   Neurology is the science of diagnosis, treatment and management of conditions affecting the brain and spinal cord, and disorders of the nerves and muscles that activate movement and transmit sensations from around the body to the brain.

Plasma   Plasma is one of the four fundamental states of matter. It contains a significant portion of charged particles – ions and/or electrons.

CHAPTER 12

Public Health: Prevention, Promotion and Empowerment

Joanna Lavery and Sharon Riverol

Aim

The aim of this chapter is to explore public health, prevention, promotion and empowerment in the context of advanced clinical practice. This will support the reader to utilise aspects of local and national frameworks and policy to consider their advanced practice role.

LEARNING OUTCOMES

After reading this chapter the reader will:

1. understand the overarching public health approach that underpins advanced practice within the community setting
2. identify the key health policies and strategies relating to the care of individuals with long-term conditions
3. recognise the role of the advanced practitioner in providing patient education and empowerment to support or improve patient health
4. understand how the HEE Multi-professional Framework (MPF) supports the advanced practitioner to deliver patient-centred, holistic care.

INTRODUCTION

The impact of chronic diseases on the health of the nation was recognised in the NHS plans for reform, aiming to place people at the 'heart of public services', leading to the publication of the National Service Framework for Long Term Conditions quality standards (DOH 2000, 2004, 2005a, 2005b). The focus on

The Advanced Practitioner: A Framework for Practice, First Edition. Edited by Ian Peate,
Sadie Diamond-Fox, and Barry Hill.
© 2024 John Wiley & Sons Ltd. Published 2024 by John Wiley & Sons Ltd.

evidence-based guidance sought to improve medical care and treatment for individuals, families and communities with chronic long-term conditions. During this time, the DOH (2002) publication 'Liberating the Talents' added a new dimension to the response in managing populations with complex healthcare needs. The strategy offered leadership opportunities to nurses and allied health professionals to shape the delivery and organisation of local health services. Advanced clinical practice featured as a key component, to innovate, encourage decision making at a higher level, break down barriers and challenge traditional ways of working (Howkins and Thornton 2003). More recent key government papers such as 'Five Year Forward View', 'The Long-term Plan' and 'Advancing Our Health: Prevention in the 2020s' focus on person-centred care, integrated care models and the enablement of patients to self-manage conditions (NHS England 2014a, 2014b; DOH 2019, NHS 2019).

The World Health Organization (WHO 2022) highlighted that 74% of all international deaths were a direct result of chronic illness and must be prioritised by healthcare services. In England, 15 million people are living with a long-term condition and generate 50% of GP appointments, utilise 70% of bed days and absorb 70% of the acute and primary care budgets due to treatment costs (Coulter et al. 2013). The cost of ill health to individuals and informal carers in managing conditions from a health and social care perspective requires consideration and is often overlooked and understudied (Stafford et al. 2021). Also, understanding quality of life in chronic disease is also important to inform decision making in practice and of prognostic importance to help predict treatment success (Haraldstad et al. 2019).

Current statistics demonstrate that while the health of the world's population is progressively improving, a caveat for this lies with each country's relationship with health and sociodemographic indices (Lancet 2020). In 2000, life expectancy from birth was 67.2 years, which increased to 73.5 in 2019 (Lancet 2020). In the UK, from 2001 to 2018 the leading causes of death remained consistent, with the top causes in 2018 demonstrated in the table below (Office for National Statistics 2020).

Leading Causes of Death in 2018	Number of Deaths
Ischaemic heart diseases (IHD)	40 214
Dementia and Alzheimer	26 579
Malignant neoplasm of trachea, bronchus and lung	18 587
Chronic lower respiratory diseases	17 988
Cerebrovascular diseases	15 437
Influenza and pneumonia	14 708

Data from the Office for National Statistics (ONS 2021) refer to avoidable mortality in England, where deaths are defined as either preventable or treatable, with 22.5% UK deaths in 2019 being considered avoidable. The main diseases which cause early death in the under-75s are cancers, diseases of the circulatory system, respiratory disease, liver disease and self-harm in the form of drug and alcohol abuse.

The burden of ill health is further compounded when considering serious mental illness (SMI). Data from 2016 to 2018 suggested that individuals with SMI in England are 4.5 times more likely to die prematurely and there is a 1.4–2 increased risk of developing physical co-morbidities such as cardiovascular disease, which can further reduce life expectancy (Department of Health and Social Care 2022; Firth et al. 2019). Mental health disorders made up 20% of the global disease burden prior to COVID-19 and the literature highlights the complexities of tackling such conditions which are transglobal and not isolated to one demographic (Campion et al. 2020).

Consequently, parliamentary drivers and advances in technology are reinforcing the vital role of the advanced clinical practitioner (ACP) within community and public health services. The diverse skill set of an ACP is crucial to cope with the demands of an ever progressive healthcare system and ageing population. ACPs are able to implement exacting standards of care encompassing the four pillars of advanced practice, against the current backdrop of workforce shortages within primary and community care (HEE 2017; Edwards and Palmer 2019).

Multi-Professional Framework for Advanced Clinical Practice (HEE 2017)

This chapter relates to the following areas of the MPFfACP:

Clinical practice
1.1, 1.2, 1.3, 1.4, 1.5, 1.6, 1.7, 1.8, 1.9, 1.10

Leadership and management
2.1, 2.2, 2.6, 2.9, 2.11

Education
3.1, 3.2, 3.4, 3.6, 3.7, 3.8

Research
4.3, 4.4, 4.6, 4.7

Accreditation Considerations

This chapter is applicable to the following specialist curricula:

- Royal College of General Practitioners. VTE guidance; Efficient Multimorbidity Management (rcgp.org.uk)
- Royal College of Physicians. Measurement of lying and standing blood pressure: a brief guide for clinical staff; Stroke rehabilitation in adults – NICE guideline; London Fall Safe resources – original (rcp.ac.uk/)
- Royal Pharmaceutical Society. Professional standards; prescribing-specials.pdf; Polypharmacy (rpharms.com)
- Chartered Society of Physiotherapy. Physiotherapy works falls – a community approach (csp.org.uk)
- Royal College of Nursing. Professional standards; prescribing-specials.pdf (rcn.org.uk)

Case Study 1

Field of practice – Community matron
    PC – Swollen, red leg
    HPC – 3/7 patient reports her lower leg feeling heavy, swollen with worsening erythema and agitation secondary to pain. No invasive laboratory investigations had taken place prior to examination.

The 80-year-old female patient had a significant past medical history of pulmonary embolism postoperatively (2017), rheumatoid arthritis, obesity, stage 3 chronic kidney disease, recurrent cellulitis of the lower limbs, type 2 diabetes, insulin dependent, 4/52 diagnosis of COVID-19. Surgical history pertains to right knee replacement (2017) and hysterectomy over 30 years ago for fibroids.

At the time of presentation, there were functional deficits in the following instrumental activities of daily living (IADLs) – handling finances, cooking, shopping and exercise tolerance of <50 yards requiring a mobility aid. She lives with her husband who has Parkinson disease; he continues to be fully independent and known to a local neurological centre specialist nurse, with no other regular healthcare input. Their daughter is her main carer and lives across the road with their grandson, who goes shopping for them.

The patient was a retired factory worker, an ex-smoker with a 30-pack-year history, drinking two glasses of wine a night. No illegal drug use, although her grandson smokes marijuana and often asks for money. Family history recalls her mother having dementia in her 80s, and unknown cause of death of her father.

GREEN FLAG

The case history identified a grandson smoking illegal drugs and asking for money in unspecified amounts. County lines as an emerging phenomenon must be considered, with evidence suggesting that frontline practitioners are overworked and underresourced, causing difficulties in identifying vulnerable young people and their families (Windle et al. 2020).

Public Health England (2020) identified that vulnerable populations who self-isolated were disproportionately at risk during COVID-19. ACPs must work together with individuals and organisations to safeguard children and adults to promote a life free from abuse or neglect (Anka et al. 2020). ACP awareness of practice guidance will help to direct practitioners and inform the safeguarding process. Six principles of protection – protection, proportionality, empowerment, prevention, partnership and accountability – underpin safeguarding adults in practice, closely correlating to the Mental Capacity Act 2005 and the Human Rights Act 1998.

Review of symptoms noted, with pertinent negatives.

Cardio – No reports of chest pain, palpitations or evidence of syncope.
Neuro – No witnessed seizures or loss of consciousness. No reports of trauma to her head or leg.
Resp – No acute or chronic breathlessness or wheeze, no sputum production or haemoptysis. Exercise tolerance remains unchanged.
Gastro – Weight steady, good appetite, bowel habits unchanged and no complaints of indigestion.
GUM – Patient has known nocturia and urgency for several years and wears incontinence pads to bed.
MH – She reveals low mood partly due to shielding and not being fully mobile to enjoy physical activity.

ORANGE FLAG

There is recognition that social distancing as a consequence of COVID-19 has adversely affected the mental and physical health of older people, resulting in feelings of social disconnectedness, perceived loneliness and symptoms of anxiety and depression (Santini et al. 2020). ACPs therefore need to consider physical, psychological and non-medical strategies for this population, such as social prescribing to enable self-management of conditions whilst helping to address the wider determinants of health (Sepúlveda-Loyola et al. 2020; Drinkwater et al. 2019).

Current medications

Butrans patch 5 mcg 7/7, recently increased
Butrans 10 mcg 7/7
Paracetamol 1 g QDS/PRN
Alfacacidol 500 ng OD
Sitagliptin 100 mg OD
Novo mix 30 morning 10 units and teatime 12 units s/c
Atorvastatin 80 mg nocte
No over-the-counter medications
Allergies – can't take penicillin since a child, was ill with it and had a rash

CLINICAL EXAMINATION

Directives for the use of the National Early Warning Score 2 (NEWS2) are in place for acute services and ambulance trusts but not enforceable in primary care (NHS England 2018; NICE 2017a). Subsequently, this may result in the unreliable identification of people at risk of acute deterioration and a lack of structured guidance for healthcare professionals (NCEPOD 2015). It has been suggested that NEWS 2 scoring can play an integral role in prioritising acute community referrals during the emergency process and prevent adverse patient outcomes (Inada-Kim et al. 2020).

NICE (2017) lists high-risk groups for developing sepsis, such as vulnerable elderly with long-term conditions, the very young, pregnant women and neonates, all of whom may have contact with an ACP. The assessment of vital signs as incorporated into the NEWS2 system is recommended to identify sepsis early on and avoid poor outcomes, given that 37 000 deaths in the UK are attributed to sepsis each year (Pope 2020). Recommendations are that individuals suspected to have sepsis in a community setting must have a complete set of observations to support prognostication (NICE 2017a,b). The introduction of an adapted community NEWS system not only supports best practice but demonstrates benefits for staff and patients alike (Pope 2020) (Table 12.1).

NEWS 2 = 1

- BP 165/77 mmHg
- Pulse 89 bpm
- RR 19
- Temperature 38.1
- Oxygen saturations 96% R/A
- CBG 6, alert and orientated

TABLE 12.1 Example of an adapted NEWS tool.

Element	Score						
	3	2	1	0	1	2	3
Respiratory rate	≤ 8		9–11	12–20		21–24	≥25
SpO$_2$	≤91	92–93	94–95	≥96%			
Oxygen		Yes		No			
Systolic blood pressure	≤90	91–100	101–110	111–219			≥220
Pulse	≤40		41–50	51–90	91–110	110–130	≥131
ACVPU				A			C, V, P, U
Temperature, °C	≤35.0		35.1–36.0	36.1–38.0	38.1–39.0	≥39.1	

Score ≥ 3: discuss with duty nurse, senior colleague; score ≥ 6: immediate discussion with advancer clinical practitioner or a doctor. Concern about patient or difficulty obtaining a single parameter requires escalation regardless of score. Complete a sepsis screen on all patients with a NEWS ≥with signs of infection.
AVPU, Alert, Confusion, Voice, Pain, Unresponsive; SPO$_2$, peripheral capillary oxygen saturation; NEWS, National Early Warning Score.

Resp – Chest clear – no wheeze or crackles audible, percussion note resonant.
Cardio – HS 1 + 11 + 0 – no murmurs, pulse regular, JVP <2 cm on 45° assessment, unilateral peripheral oedema left leg, to knee level.
Abdominal – Soft, non-tender, no organomegaly/masses, bowel sounds present, percussion note tympanic.
Neuro – PEARL, GCS 15/15, no focal neurology/deficit, wears glasses, poor vision without.

RED FLAG

The differential diagnosis for this patient must consider and exclude any life-threatening conditions. Differentials could include a DVT, gout, ruptured Baker's cyst, superficial thrombophlebitis and erysipelas. ACPs must consider Virchow's triad (republished in 1998) and the three factors of endothelial injury, blood stasis and blood hypercoagulability, which contribute to the risk of thrombus. Non-reversible risk factors for further thrombus include earlier pulmonary emboli, reduced mobility, obesity and COVID-19 (Prins et al. 2018, 2020; Lavery 2021; Hotoleanu 2020). Venous thromboembolism (VTE) is a leading cause of death and disability in the UK and worldwide, affecting 1 in every 1000 of the UK population (NHS Litigation Authority 2015). Therefore, lower limb examination is essential to correctly treat and manage the patient in the community setting and to prevent unnecessary hospital admissions, as advocated by NICE (2020a–d).

Lower limb examination in both limbs to determine any differences.

- Assessment of legs for oedema by pressing the skin firmly for five seconds to identify whether it is pitting and unilateral.

- Lower limb assessment of femoral, popliteal, dorsalis pedis and posterior tibial pulses were palpated, with capillary refill time under two seconds (Bickley and Szilagyi 2017).
- Assess the skin colour and elevation of the patient's leg in a supine position to ascertain colour changes, warmth and note Buerger's sign which demonstrates pallor on elevation, dependent rubor and indicates limb ischaemia (Insall et al. 1989).
- Caution is needed for patients with darker skin colour as some of the critical cellulitic signs may prove ambiguous and it is important that associated symptoms are considered to aid diagnosis (Thakrar and Sultan 2021).

Perform Wells score assessment to assess risk of a deep vein thrombosis (DVT) (Table 12.2) (Wells et al. 1997, 2003).

Leg assessment

Wells score = 0

Erythema, redness and pain to mid-calf region, measurement 10 cm from tibial tuberosity, <2 cm in symptomatic leg. Colour, sensation, movement and pedal pulses intact. Unilateral leg oedema. Clinical impression of cellulitis therefore DVT unlikely.

Clinical Investigation – Point-of Care (POC) D-dimer Testing

Blood clots which develop in the deep venous system can progress and travel through the heart towards the pulmonary vasculature, resulting in a pulmonary embolism (Barco et al. 2020). The signs and symptoms of a VTE have a low positive predictive value (PPV) which can make clinical diagnosis difficult (Jones and Round 2021). A blood test can be taken for a D-dimer which is a by-product

TABLE 12.2   Wells score assessment.

Clinical Feature	Points
Active cancer (on treatment, treated in the last 6 mo or palliative)	1
Paralysis, paresis or plaster immobilisation of the lower limb	1
Bedridden for 3 d or more, or major surgery in the past 12 wk requiring general or regional anaesthesia	1
Localised tenderness along the distribution of the deep venous system	1
Calf swelling 3 cm larger than the symptomatic side	1
Pitting oedema confined to the symptomatic leg	1
Collateral superficial veins (non-varicose)	1
Previous DVT	1
Alternative diagnosis is at least as likely as DVT	−2

Clinical Probability Simplified Score	Points
DVT likely	2 points or more
DVT unlikely	1 point or less

Source: Adapted from Wells et al. (2003).

of blood coagulation released once there is degradation of a thrombus in the blood (Bounds and Kok 2021).

POC D-dimer testing is performed in primary care first contact and ambulatory centres, often referred to as qualitative POC testing (Lucassen et al. 2015). Studies have proven qualitative POC D-dimer testing to be safe and effective in excluding VTEs in a primary care environment (Reynen and Severn 2017; Buller et al. 2009).

POC D-dimer testing has historically had a sizeable number of false-positive outcomes which can result in patients being needlessly referred to secondary care settings for further investigation (Lucassen et al. 2015). A current evidence-based addition of the age-adjusted D-dimer cut-off level to rule out a low suspicion PE exists in the form of the pulmonary embolism rule-out criteria (PERC) whereby the clinician can exclude a PE if no risk criteria exist and estimate a likelihood of PE to be less than 15% from clinical impression, with other workable differential diagnoses (NICE 2020a, b; Kline et al. 2004, 2008). However, these stratifications are not widely used in primary care having derived from their use in emergency departments and ACPs advocating investigations should only initiate this after an individual clinical assessment to inform decision making (Righini et al. 2014; Schouten et al. 2013; Jones and Round 2021; NICE 2020a–d).

Diagnosis – Class 1 Cellulitis

Cellulitis is defined as an acute infection of the dermis and subcutaneous tissue, frequently occurring after localised skin trauma (Bailey and Kroshinsky 2011; Sullivan and de Barra 2018) (Table 12.3).

Management for this patient as per NICE guidance (2021a,b) includes:

- demarcation of the erythema on the affected limb (using a permanent marker pen) to evaluate its spread on follow-up assessment
- paracetamol and ibuprofen to manage pain
- patient to keep a CBG diary for review on next visit
- encourage fluid intake, leg elevation whenever possible
- Red Flag advice on who to contact on deterioration of condition
- elevate leg to prevent further swelling and oedema
- documentation to medical team via the correct electronic system
- review of bloods, FBC, U&E, CRP, LFT, clotting if resources support this to inform follow-up clinical assessment.

Pharmacology

NICE guidance (2021a,b) for adults with class 1 uncomplicated cellulitis of the limb (no uncontrolled comorbidities or systemic toxicity)

TABLE 12.3   Classification of cellulitis.

Class I	There are no signs of systemic toxicity, and the person is well other than the cellulitis
Class II	The person is systemically unwell but does not have any unstable co-morbidities
Class III	The patient has significant systemic features such as acute confusion, tachycardia, tachypnoea, hypotension or unstable co-morbidities which may interfere with a response to treatment, or a limb-threatening infection with vascular compromise
Class IV	The person has sepsis syndrome or a severe life-threatening infection such as necrotising fasciitis

Source: Eron (2000).

Prescribe flucloxacillin 500–1000 mg four times daily for 5–7 days. If this is unsuitable, or the person has a penicillin allergy, prescribe:

- clarithromycin 500 mg twice daily for 5–7 days
- doxycycline 200 mg on the first day then 100 mg once daily, for a total of 5–7 days
- erythromycin (in pregnancy) 500 mg four times daily for 5–7 days.

Follow-up Plan

Follow up at 24–48 hours post treatment to review progress and/or inflammatory markers to exclude progressive severe infection. If the patient's condition is not improving, the matron may need to consider referring the patient via an ambulatory emergency care unit for assessment for intravenous antibiotics or admission. Recurring cellulitis is identified as more than two episodes in a year for the same site and guidance necessitates a routine secondary care referral for advice on prophylactic antibiotic therapy (NICE 2021b). Further interventions may require a case management approach. Qualitative studies illustrate that case management provides care that is continuous, person centred and emotionally supportive; however, ongoing communication of information is required from ACPs for this model of care to be efficacious (Joo and Liu 2018). Interprofessional collaborations with the GP, diabetes specialist services and AHPs for re-enablement, social services or referrals to the safeguarding team may be appropriate. A medication reconciliation to assess contraindications, adverse clinical outcomes of polypharmacy and promote awareness of diabetic complications is best practice (Huang et al. 2019; Wastesson et al. 2018).

Case Study 2

Field of practice – General practice, advanced nurse practitioner.

PC and HPC – A 50-year-old male with a 12-year history of diabetes, attendance for diabetic reviews has been sporadic at best. Last recorded diabetic blood tests over 12 months ago, HbA1c was raised and the condition was classed as uncontrolled as per NICE (2022b). Known hypertension, last blood pressure checks 18 months ago but within acceptable parameters as per NICE (2019b), last estimated glomerular filtration rate (eGFR) placed patient as chronic kidney disease stage 2 (NICE 2021a,b), last urine test completed more than 12 months ago. Body Mass. Index 55 – clinically obese. The patient has received numerous invitations to attend the practice for a diabetic review and for health assessments/checks to be carried out, but no appointments were made.

Presenting complaint was an uncomfortable left ear with reduced hearing, wife had noted television was on louder than normal. On presentation, the only issue expressed by the patient was a dull ache in the left ear and reduced hearing; on examination, the left ear was blocked with wax, the tympanic membrane was not visible and the right ear was clear and normal on examination. The patient used a telephone headset that sat in the left ear, probably contributing to wax build-up. Ear care advice given and advised of treatments available such as irrigation. As per Making Every Contact Count which is set out in the NICE (2019a,b) Long-Term Plan diabetic care was then discussed. It was noted that the patient's non-verbal and verbal communication changed considerably.

Vogel et al. (2018) discuss the importance of effective communication, verbal and non-verbal, and patient satisfaction with the care they receive is often linked to the healthcare professional's communication skills. The patient was given the opportunity to express any concerns he had; it was at this moment he advised that due to previous experiences, he did not wish to have his diabetes monitored. The patient had felt he had been judged unkindly by the healthcare professionals monitoring his condition, and that although he knew he could do better with his lifestyle, he was overwhelmed by his diabetes, the possible consequences of the disease and the changes which had to be made to improve the condition.

GREEN FLAG

With increasing rates of chronic disease, there has been a focus on self-management of conditions, with many trusts providing NHS patient expert programmes following on from the pilot study which started in 2002. This has improved patient outcomes and, in some cases, delayed the onset of disease (DOH 2013). Franklin et al. (2018) discuss the issues of promoting self-management of long-term conditions when the current medical model used in healthcare assumes the patient as a passive member of the team. ACPs must engage with individuals to understand the distinction between managing a condition versus managing a condition well (Morgan et al. 2016). The four pillars of advanced practice will support the advanced practitioner in providing patient-centred care (HEE 2017). Drescher et al. (2019) promote the ACP as the link between the multidisciplinary team but also as a key factor in patient education and support for patients being able to manage their own medical condition.

The patient was offered one main contact for diabetes care, which was agreed, and he consented for a diabetic review to be completed.

Review of symptoms noted, with pertinent negatives.

Cardio – No issues noted.
Neuro – No issues noted.
Resp – Stated he has become increasing breathless on minimal exercise; chest sounds clear and breath sounds heard in all areas equal air entry. Admits he feels his weight is an issue, he has never smoked and has no history of asthma, chest X-ray ordered and review with results.
Gastro – No weight loss, some indigestion not regular.
GUM – Increased nocturia probably due to uncontrolled diabetes, urine sample requested.

Current medications (amount taken in 24 hours):

Ramipril 5 mg
Amlodipine 5 mg
Indapamide 2.5 mg
Metformin 2 g
Gliclazide 160 mg

Dapagliflozin 10 mg
Atorvastatin 20 mg
Over the counter:
    Aspirin 75 mg – taking as concerned about weight and blood clots after reading an article online
    Occasional paracetamol
Allergies: none known.

CLINICAL EXAMINATION

When completing a clinical examination in a diabetic patient, the advanced practitioner must be aware of the NICE guidelines for the diabetic patient which when managing a long-term condition will differ from those without diabetes (NICE 2022b).

NEWS2 score 0 – although NEWS2 is not used within primary care
Temperature: 36.8
Pulse: 87 bpm regular
Respiration rate: 18
Oxygen saturations: 97% on room air
Blood pressure: 168/94 – NICE guidelines would advise a diabetic patient has a blood pressure taken a minimum of once a year.
Alert and orientated to time and place.
Patient states skin intact, minimal swelling to ankles and feet.
Cardiac examination S1 + S2 + 0, pulse regular, normal JVP, no abnormalities on visual inspection of chest and abdomen.

CLINICAL INVESTIGATIONS

A diabetic review as per NICE guidance (2022b) includes a blood test, BMI and foot check; the patient agreed to attend for these checks. He attended for HbA1c, U&E, LFT, lipids, FBC. He was also reviewed by a healthcare assistant for BMI, blood pressure and foot check. The supervision of staff within the MDT whose investigations and assessments contribute to the ongoing management is of great importance. ACPs must demonstrate role modelling and make effective use of the full range of skills and experiences that members of the team can bring, as identified by the NHS People Plan (Bailey 2020). This can maximise efficiency and quality of care, whilst creating mutual respect between colleagues. It is the ACP's role to interpret investigations and explain them to the patient to ensure a patient-centred approach and support the improvement, slowing disease progression, and in maintenance of a long-term conditions. It is vital that the ACP considers the patient's level of health literacy. There are reports of a rise in health literacy across all population studies, and it is recognised as a determining factor in health which poses a challenges for practitioners (Nutbeam and Lloyd 2020).

RED FLAG

A diabetic foot check is important to exclude peripheral artery disease (PAD). PAD is a progressive condition referred to as a complete or partial occlusion and/or stenosis of the peripheral vessels in upper and lower limbs, occurring due to universal atherosclerosis in the coronary and cerebral arteries (Soyoye et al. 2021; Shu and Santulli 2018). Patients with diabetes are known to have a 20–30% higher incidence of PAD than the general population with peripheral neuropathy signalling the latter stages of the disease process (Vrsalovic et al. 2017).

Therefore, community ACPs require diligence and awareness to recognise PAD early and ensure secondary prevention of cardiovascular disease is instigated. Following NICE (2016, 2020a–d) guidance can safeguard patients from major cardiovascular events as PAD can contribute to amputations in diabetics (Fowkes et al. 2017).

Results

HbA1c: 87 mmol/mol
UE: within acceptable levels
LFT: gamma-GT raised but normal for patient
FBC: within acceptable levels
Lipids: controlled with medication
Foot check: abnormal referral to podiatry completed
BMI: 58
Blood pressure: 148/80, NEWS2 = 0 but BP remains raised

Management

Over the next 12 months this patient was managed by regular reviews. His hypertension was monitored, and ramipril was increased as per NICE guidance for hypertension (NICE 2019b). Diabetic medication was optimised, and drugs changed with the patient using a partnership approach to care. During sessions, realistic changes the patient could make to his lifestyle to improve his health were discussed. He started a one meal a day approach, making small achievable targets; this was observed as part of the success in bringing the HbA1c down.

Pharmacology

This patient required an increase in antihypertensive medication – angiotensin converting enzyme (ACE) rather than calcium channel blocker (CCB), a kidney protective element and less likely to cause ankle swelling than CCB. A meta-analysis by Zhang et al. (2020) concluded that the use of ACE lowers the risk of kidney and cardiac events. The NHS (2020a–d) Specialist Pharmacy Service advises that if a patient cannot tolerate CCB due to ankle swelling, the best course of action is to change to ACE, for control of blood pressure and reduction of ankle swelling (NHS 2020).

Review of diabetic medication – Patient on triple therapy including Gliclazide which is associated with weight gain and not controlled on triple therapy, as per NICE (2022b).

On discussion, compliance with medications could be improved. Patient is currently taking metformin – discussion regarding side-effects such as diarrhoea and vomiting. The patient is not experiencing any of these and is taking 2 g daily.

Gliclazide – concerns regarding weight and the use of a sulfonylurea medication known to cause weight gain and hypoglycaemia; patient is not checking blood sugars but not reporting any symptoms of low blood sugars. Currently taking 80 mg twice a day with meals; he admits not always remembering to take with the evening meal.

Dapagliflozin – 10 mg once a day.

The patient does not wish to inject himself and wishes to continue with oral medications. As per NICE (2022a,b), the medication must be discussed in conjunction with the patient and the treatment plan agreed.

The patient agreed to continue with metformin and dapagliflozin. However, once he had been advised of the potential for weight gain with gliclazide (NICE 2022b; BNF 2022), he wanted to change. Over a period of two months, he was taken off the gliclazide and commenced on linagliptin at his request; this medication is also less likely to cause hypoglycaemia (BNF 2022).

This procedure not only helped the patient to feel part of the decision-making process but also reduced his risk of complications from hypoglycaemia and the likelihood of medication-associated weight gain. Settineri et al. (2019) found that even just listening to what the patient has to say can help improve the relationship the patient will have with the ACP and the educational opportunities so the patient will have the opportunity to self-manage their long-term condition.

ORANGE FLAG

Himmelstein and Puhl (2021) found that diabetic patients reported they were subjected to weight stigma and blamed for their condition. This also leads to self-judgement and low self-esteem. Flint et al. (2018) discussed the role of the media in supporting the stigma that comes with being overweight and the impact on patients' mental health. For example, headlines within the newspapers linking obesity with laziness can cause patients with long-term conditions such as diabetes to feel that they are responsible for their condition and have a lower social standing.

It is important to consider the patient as an individual and understand the unique way each person's experience or condition impacts upon their quality of life (NICE 2012). The evaluation of their experience can help to improve quality of care, foster partnership working and enhance the patient–clinician therapeutic relationship.

The HEE Multi-Professional Framework (2017) outlines the importance of working with patients and their families/carers alongside other members of the multidisciplinary team. This is to ensure holistic care and at the heart of this is communication and including the patient within the care plans Van Dusseldorp et al. (2019) discussed how the care given by the ACP empowers patients and states that the patient satisfaction rates remain high for the ACP.

Case Study 3

PC – Fall

HPC – The fall took place three days previous after a loss of balance on standing quickly from a sitting position in the evening. The patient became light-headed and acutely dizzy and described having an awareness she was about to fall. She declined to attend the local hospital so was assessed at home. She was referred via her GP for assessment by the ACP who tended to the patient in her own home.

The 72-year-old female patient had a past medical history of hypertension (2012), CKD progressed to stage 3 (2015), asthma and osteoporosis. Surgical history of cholecystectomy in her 40s.

She was a retired teacher and widowed over 20 years ago. She had never smoked, seldom drank alcohol. She lived alone in a bungalow, and was usually independently mobile. The patient's daughter and family lived next door and provided daily support with social care. There were no functional deficits in the IADLs.

Review of symptoms noted, with pertinent negatives.

Cardio – No reports to suggest a cardiac event, palpitations or syncope.

Neuro – No features to suggest seizures such as tongue biting, incontinence or loss of consciousness. No head trauma observed.

Resp – Nil acute ET unchanged.

Gastro – Weight steady, good appetite, bowel habits unchanged and no complaints of indigestion.

GUM – No urinary dysfunction,

MH – Mood steady.

Medications

Ramipril 7.5 mg OD
Amlodipine 10 mg OD
Bendroflumethiazide 2.5 mg OD
Atenolol 25 mg OD
Citalopram 10 mg nocte
Alendronic acid 70 mg once a week
Co-codamol 15/500 mg PRN
Clenil Modulite 200 mcg BD
Salbutamol MDI 100 mcg QDS

CLINICAL EXAMINATION

NEWS2 – 0 But Blood Pressure Found to Be Hypotensive

Lying and standing BP – the patient had been lying for around 15 minutes; on arrival blood pressure 98/50 mmHg, standing blood pressure 91/52 mmHg, no postural drop noted but both readings were hypotensive. All other nursing observations are within acceptable limits.

Neuro assessment

Alert and orientated
PEARL, GCS 15/15, no focal neurology/deficit
No papilloedema
Wears glasses and poor vision without
Difficult to assess balance as mobility poor
Neuro Rx completed for falls/fall history
Ear assessment – tympanic membranes seen, no abnormalities, the patient reports hearing normal

RED FLAG

Echoing previous case studies, a differential diagnosis must exclude life-threatening or life-limiting conditions. Differential diagnoses in this case could include cerebellar stroke, labyrinthitis, benign paroxysmal positional vertigo (BPPV), postural hypotension under the terminology of orthostatic dysregulation, medication side-effects, migrainous vertigo or vestibular neuritis (Sarikaya and Steinlin 2018). Cerebellar strokes account for 2% of all ischaemic strokes and this patient group is thought to be at higher risk for persistent disability and mortality (Macdonell et al. 1987; Sarikaya and Steinlin 2018). Furthermore, Macdonell et al. (1987) estimate the risk of a successive infarct of the brainstem post cerebellar stroke to be 13%. The National Institutes of Health Stroke Scale is used in clinical examination to calculate the risk of a stroke but can often underestimate patients with a cerebellar stroke (Brott et al. 1989; Nickel et al. 2018). Consequently, posterior circulation strokes are missed more than anterior, even by acute services (Arch et al. 2016). Therefore, ACPs require extensive skills to inform decision making when assessing presentations such as those in the case study with what would be deemed as a non-life-threatening symptom. Case-based discussions may provide a beneficial strategy for ACPs to share complex cases and atypical presentations, particularly for those predominantly working in isolation.

Abbreviated Mental Test Score (AMTS) – The AMTS was introduced to assess elderly patients rapidly for possible signs of dementia. It is best practice as an accompaniment to neurological examination in the elderly (Hodkinson 1972). The questions in Table 12.4 are put to the patient. Each question correctly answered scores one point.

Diagnosis – Iatrogenic drug interaction. Iatrogenic diseases are a result of prophylactic, diagnostic and therapeutic interventions, meaning that they are brought about by the medical treatment of an individual (Shoukath et al. 2018).

TABLE 12.4   Abbreviated Mental Test Score questions.

1. What is your age?
2. What is the time to the nearest hour?
3. Give the patient an address, and ask him or her to repeat it at the end of the test, e.g. 42 West Street
4. What is the year?
5. What is the name of the hospital or number of the residence where the patient is situated?
6. Can the patient recognise two persons (the doctor, nurse, home help, etc.)?
7. What is your date of birth (day and month sufficient)?
8. In what year did World War 1 begin?
9. Name the present monarch/prime minister/president.
10. Count backwards from 20 down to 1.

A score of 6 or less suggests delirium or dementia, although further tests are necessary to confirm the diagnosis.

CLINICAL INVESTIGATION

The measurement of lying and standing blood pressure (BP) is important to exclude orthostatic hypertension (OH), also known as postural hypotension, which is common in older people, during acute illness and can increase the risk of falls (O'Riordan et al. 2017). BP measurements are taken in a supine position and standing position. A manual sphygmomanometer is preferred, and the patient is required to lie down for five minutes, BP is measured prior to standing, again after standing in the first minute, and again after the patient has been standing for three minutes (RCP 2017).

Orthostatic hypertension is defined as a drop in systolic BP of ≥ 20 mmHg (or 30 mmHg in hypertensive patients) and/or ≥ 10 mmHg diastolic blood pressure of at least 10 mmHg within three minutes of standing (Gilani et al. 2021). It is worth noting that OH is recognised as an investigation which is poorly reproducible and thought to underestimate the correct prevalence of the condition (Cremer et al. 2019). The dissemination of evidence-based care and accurate procedural skill for junior staff is of the utmost importance, as it will help them develop their skills and underpin the validity of patient assessments.

MANAGEMENT

A multifactorial risk assessment for this individual would be required (Figure 12.1) (NICE 2019a).

- Completion of a Falls Risk Assessment Tool is warranted to establish the cause of the fall.
- Referral to a specialist falls service is advised to provide a more in-depth assessment in strength and balance training, home hazard assessment and intervention, vision assessment and medications review.

There are countless medications management and prescribing considerations for the ACP in community settings. When dealing with an elderly population, polypharmacy has been associated with multiple unintended therapeutic outcomes and increased incidents of serious drug-to-drug interactions and use of inappropriate medication (Al-Musawe et al. 2020). ACPs who follow up patients after discharge need to be aware of any changes to medications because medication-related harm (MRH) is more common in older adults after hospital discharge, and accounts for substantial uptake of healthcare resources (Parekh et al. 2018).

Pharmacology

The NHSBSA estimates (2021) that the cost of medication to the NHS for 2020–21 was £17.1 billion, which was an increase of 4.56% on the previous year, with 55% of the total expenditure being win primary care. Le Fanu (2018) highlights the mass medicalisation in current medicine and the related polypharmacy-induced iatrogenesis which exists in even routine practices. This is something ACPs need to consider when assessing patients with multimorbidity and polypharmacy and in the case study, a medicines reconciliation was initiated. STOPP (Screening Tool of Older Persons' Prescriptions) and START (Screening Tool to Alert to Right Treatment) are useful criteria to guide prescribers (NHS England 2014a). These tools can facilitate medication reviews in older people or those with multiple co-morbidities in most clinical settings, to prevent adverse drug reactions and inappropriate prescribing (O'Mahony 2019; NHS England, 2014b).

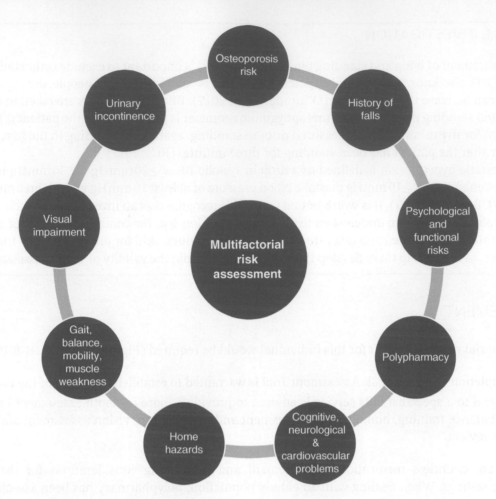

FIGURE 12.1   A multifactorial risk assessment.

The list of medications for this patient was extensive due to hypertensive disease, with three antihypertensive medications prescribed for this alone. Atenolol was added following an episode of palpitations which resulted in a hospital admission (more than eight years previously), and the antidepressant citalopram was added following the death of her husband 20 years previously. Calcium tablets daily and once-weekly alendronic acid for osteoporosis for more than seven years. Furthermore, she has a prescription for low-dose co-codamol for pain as and when required and inhaled therapy of Clenil (ICS) inhalers two puffs BD and salbutamol (SABA) to be taken as and when required for asthma.

On review of medications within the patient's home, it was clear that some medications were being overordered, with several packets unopened and out of date. Medication errors are a wider public health issue and adverse events can occur because of out-of-date medications, posing a substantial risk for all prescribers (Rodziewicz et al. 2018). Therefore, ACPs need to understand the indications and contraindications for medications to make decisions on discontinuation. Involving patients in a provider-initiated medication discontinuation process is beneficial because patients often prefer to take fewer medications but do not always share their beliefs with healthcare providers (Linsky et al. 2015)

REFLECTIONS

Admission Avoidance

The pressure on acute services is often widely publicised in the media and there can be a dependence on community ACPs to prevent hospital admissions as an integral part of their role. Patients and families are often reluctant to attend acute and emergency departments for further assessments when advocated. This can pose an additional burden to decision making, management plans and follow-up care provided to patients who decline acute admissions. ACPs, like any registered professional, are required to be aware of their individual scope of practice and professional conduct in association with their governing body. Nevertheless, the level of responsibility and risk associated with the role must be emphasised, with the pillars of advanced practice fundamental to their actions and choices (HEE 2017).

The case studies explored provide examples of the complexities of the role and the demands of caring for people within the social context and home environment. Community ACPs often have limited resources and investigations to guide their diagnoses, therefore it is important to engage in collaborative practice and shared decision making wherever possible to ensure optimal patient outcomes.

Advanced Care Practitioner and Patient Empowerment

The relationship between the patient and the ACP can be a fruitful partnership, resulting in improved outcomes for long-term conditions and reduced hospital admissions (Mileski 2020). However, in case study 2 it was evident that previous poor experience from health services had contributed to a reluctance to engage with services, resulting in the patient having diabetes which was unmonitored and uncontrolled. The ACP–patient relationship needs to be cultivated and based on honesty, trust and teamwork. The HEE Framework for Advanced Practice (2018) can support the development of the skills required to facilitate these relationships, with beneficial outcomes for the patient. There are societal pressures on patient populations to self-manage and the health system is under duress to improve health outcomes; patients may feel overwhelmed and develop low self-esteem. It is important that the ACP produces a management plan in partnership with the patient that is both attainable and in their best interests, prioritising their wishes, whilst providing patient education to empower them to make positive changes. If the relationship between the patient and healthcare systems breaks down then the whole process would need to start again, and patients may feel distrust or anxiety about accessing medical help.

Take Home Points
- ACPs in the community face the challenge of managing acute episodes of care in individuals with multiple co-morbidities in complex environments.
- Decision making requires consideration of the severity of the presenting complaint, disease process and the ability to competently manage this outside a secondary care environment.
- Community ACPs 'make every contact count'. The promotion of a partnership approach to care is vital to support individuals with the self-management of complex conditions.
- Admission avoidance is key to the role of the community matron and ACP; however, this must be in line with current guidance, positive health outcomes and in the best interests of the patient.

REFERENCES

Al-Musawe, L., Torre, C., Guerreiro, J.P. et al. (2020). Polypharmacy, potentially serious clinically relevant drug-drug interactions, and inappropriate medicines in elderly people with type 2 diabetes and their impact on quality of life. *Pharmacology Research & Perspectives* 8 (4): e00621.

Anka, A., Thacker, H., and Penhale, B. (2020). Safeguarding adults practice and remote working in the COVID-19 era: challenges and opportunities. *Journal of Adult Protection* 6: 415–427.

Arch, A.E., Weisman, D.C., Coca, S. et al. (2016). Missed ischemic stroke diagnosis in the emergency department by emergency medicine and neurology services. *Stroke* 47 (3): 668–673.

Bailey, S. (2020). The NHS people plan. *BMJ* 370: m3398.

Bailey, E. and Kroshinsky, D. (2011). Cellulitis: diagnosis and management. *Dermatologic Therapy* 24 (2): 229–239.

Barco, S., Mahmoudpour, S.H., Valerio, L. et al. (2020). Trends in mortality related to pulmonary embolism in the European Region, 2000–15: analysis of vital registration data from the WHO Mortality Database. *Lancet Respiratory Medicine* 8 (3): 277–287.

Bickley, L. and Szilagyi, P. (2017). *Bates' Guide to Physical Examination and History Taking*, 12e. Philadelphia: Wolters Kluwer.

Bounds, E.J. and Kok, S.J. (2021). *D Dimer*. Treasure Island: Stat Pearls Publishing.

British National Formulary (2022) Type two diabetes. https://bnf.nice.org.uk/treatment-summary/type-2-diabetes.html

Brott, T., Adams, H.P. Jr., Olinger, C.P. et al. (1989). Measurements of acute cerebral infarction: a clinical examination scale. *Stroke* 20 (7): 864–870.

Buller, H.R., Ten Cate-Hoek, A.J., Hoes, A.W. et al. (2009). Safely ruling out deep venous thrombosis in primary care. *Annals of Internal Medicine* 150: 229–235.

Campion, J., Javed, A., Sartorius, N., and Marmot, M. (2020). Addressing the public mental health challenge of COVID-19. *Lancet Psychiatry* 7 (8): 657–659.

Coulter, A., Roberts, S., and Dixon, A. (2013). *Delivering better services for people with long-term conditions. Building the house of care*, 1–28. London: The King's Fund.

Cremer, A., Rousseau, A.L., Boulestreau, R. et al. (2019). Screening for orthostatic hypotension using home blood pressure measurements. *Journal of Hypertension* 37 (5): 923–927.

Department of Health (2000). The NHS Plan: A Plan for Investment, A Plan for Reform. Department of Health, London.

Department of Health (2002). Liberating the Talents: Helping Primary Care Trusts and Nurses to Deliver the NHS Plan. Department of Health, London.

Department of Health (2004). The NHS Improvement Plan: Putting People at the Heart of Public Services. Department of Health, London.

Department of Health (2005a). The National Service Framework for Long-Term Conditions. http://assets.publishing.service.gov.uk/government/uploads/system/uploads/attachment_data/file/198114/National_Service_Framework_for_Long_Term_Conditions.pdf

Department of Health (2005b). Supporting People with Long Term Conditions: Liberating the Talents of Nurses Who Care for People with Long Term Conditions. Department of Health, London.

Department of Health (2013). The Expert Patients Programme. www.gov.uk/government/case-studies/the-expert-patients-programme

Department of Health and Social Care (2019). Advancing Our Health: Prevention in the 2020s – Consultation Document. Executive summary. Department of Health and Social Care: London.

Department of Health and Social Care (2022). Premature mortality in adults with severe mental illness. Department of Health and Social Care: London.

Drescher, H., Lissoos, T., Hajisafari, E., and Evans, E.R. (2019). Treat-to-target approach in inflammatory bowel disease: the role of advanced practice providers. *Journal for Nurse Practitioners* V15 (9): 676–682.

Drinkwater, C., Wildman, J., and Moffatt, S. (2019). Social prescribing. *BMJ* 364: 1285.

van Dusseldorp, L., Groot, M., Adriaansen, M. et al. (2019). What does the nurse practitioner mean to you? A patient-oriented qualitative study in oncological/palliative care. *Journal of Clinical Nursing* 28 (3–4): 589–602.

Edwards, N. and Palmer, B. (2019). A preliminary workforce plan for the NHS. *BMJ* 365: 4144.

Eron, L.J. (2000). Infections of skin and soft tissue: outcomes of a classification scheme. In: *Clinical Infectious Diseases*. Chicago: University of Chicago Press.

Firth, J., Siddiqi, N., Koyanagi, A. et al. (2019). The Lancet Psychiatry Commission: a blueprint for protecting physical health in people with mental illness. *Lancet Psychiatry* 6: 675–712.

Flint, S.W., Nobles, J., Gately, P., and Sahota, P. (2018). Weight stigma and discrimination: a call to the media. *Lancet Diabetes and Endocrinology* 6 (3): 169–170.

Fowkes, F.G.R., Aboyans, V., Fowkes, F.J. et al. (2017). Peripheral artery disease: epidemiology and global perspectives. *Nature Reviews Cardiology* 14 (3): 156–170.

Franklin, M., Lewis, S., Willis, K. et al. (2018). Patients' and healthcare professionals' perceptions of self-management support interactions: systematic review and qualitative synthesis. *Chronic Illness* 14 (2): 79–103.

Gilani, A., Juraschek, S.P., Belanger, M.J. et al. (2021). Postural hypotension. *BMJ* 373: n922.

Haraldstad, K., Wahl, A., Andenæs, R. et al. (2019). A systematic review of quality-of-life research in medicine and health sciences. *Quality of Life Research* 28 (10): 2641–2650.

Health Education England (2017). Multi-professional framework for advanced clinical practice in England. www.hee.nhs.uk/sites/default/files/documents/multi-professionalframeworkforadvancedclinicalpracticeinengland.pdf

Himmelstein, M.S. and Puhl, R.M. (2021). At multiple fronts: diabetes stigma and weight stigma in adults with type 2 diabetes. *Diabetic Medicine* 38 (1): e14387.

Hodkinson, H.M. (1972). Evaluation of a mental test score for assessment of mental impairment in the elderly. *Age and Ageing* 1 (4): 233–238.

Hotoleanu, C. (2020). Association between obesity and venous thromboembolism. *Medicine and Pharmacy Reports* 93 (2): 162.

Howkins, E. and Thornton, C. (2003). Liberating the talents: whose talents and for what purpose? *Journal of Nursing Management* 11 (4): 219–220.

Huang, Z., Lum, E., Jimenez, G. et al. (2019). Medication management support in diabetes: a systematic assessment of diabetes self-management apps. *BMC Medicine* 17 (1): 1–12.

Inada-Kim, M., Knight, T., Sullivan, M. et al. (2020). The prognostic value of national early warning scores (NEWS) during transfer of care from community settings to hospital: a retrospective service evaluation. *BJGP Open* 4 (2): bjgpopen20X101071.

Insall, R.L., Davies, R.J., and Prout, W.G. (1989). Significance of Buerger's test in the assessment of lower limb ischaemia. *Journal of the Royal Society of Medicine* 82 (12): 729–731.

Jones, N.R. and Round, T. (2021). Venous thromboembolism management and the new NICE guidance: what the busy GP needs to know. *British Journal of General Practice* 71 (709): 379–380.

Joo, J.Y. and Liu, M.F. (2018). Experiences of case management with chronic illnesses: a qualitative systematic review. *International Nursing Review* 65 (1): 102–113.

Kline, J.A., Mitchell, A.M., Kabrhel, C. et al. (2004). Clinical criteria to prevent unnecessary diagnostic testing in emergency department patients with suspected pulmonary embolism. *Journal of Thrombosis and Haemostasis* 2 (8): 1247–1255.

Kline, J.A., Courtney, D.M., Kabrhel, C. et al. (2008). Prospective multicentre evaluation of the pulmonary embolism rule-out criteria. *Journal of Thrombosis and Haemostasis* 6 (5): 772–780.

Lancet (2020). Global health: time for radical change? *Lancet* 396 (10258): 1129–1306.

Lavery, J. (2021). Clinical assessment of the leg for a suspected deep vein thrombosis. *Nursing Times* 117 (5): 18–21.

Le Fanu, J. (2018). Mass medicalisation is an iatrogenic catastrophe. *BMJ* 361: k2794.

Linsky, A., Simon, S.R., and Bokhour, B. (2015). Patient perceptions of proactive medication discontinuation. *Patient Education and Counseling* 98 (2): 220–225.

Lucassen, W.A., Erkens, P.M., Geersing, G.J. et al. (2015). Qualitative point-of-care D-dimer testing compared with quantitative D-dimer testing in excluding pulmonary embolism in primary care. *Journal of Thrombosis and Haemostasis* 13 (6): 1004–1009.

Macdonell, R.A., Kalnins, R.M., and Donnan, G.A. (1987). Cerebellar infarction: natural history, prognosis, and pathology. *Stroke* 18 (5): 849–855.

Mileski, M., Pannu, U., Payne, B. et al. (2020). The impact of nurse practitioners on hospitalizations and discharges from long-term nursing facilities: a systematic review. *Healthcare* 8 (2): 114.

Morgan, H.M., Entwistle, V.A., Cribb, A. et al. (2016). We need to talk about purpose: a critical interpretive synthesis of health and social care professionals' approaches to self-management support for people with long-term conditions. *Health Expectations* 20: 243–259.

National Confidential Enquiry into Patient Outcome and Death (2015). Just Say Sepsis! www.ncepod.org.uk/2015sepsis.html

National Health Service. (2019). The NHS Long Term Plan. www.longtermplan.nhs.uk/publication/nhs-long-term-plan

National Health Service (2020). Specialist Pharmacy Service. How should ankle oedema caused by calcium channel blockers be treated? www.sps.nhs.uk/articles/how-should-ankle-oedema-caused-by-calcium-channel-blockers-be-treated

NHS England (2014a). Five Year Forward View. www.england.nhs.uk/wp-content/uploads/2014/10/5yfv-web.pdf

NHS England (2014b). Toolkit for general practice for supporting older people living with frailty. www.england.nhs.uk/publication/toolkit-for-general-practice-in-supporting-older-people-living-with-frailty/#:~:text=Toolkit%20for%20general%20practice%20in%20supporting%20older%20people%20living%20with%20frailty,-Document%20first%20published&text=This%20document%20provides%20GPs%2C%20practice,older%20people%20living%20with%20frailty

NHS England (2018). NHS Improvement. Patient Safety Alert: Resources to support the safe adoption of the revised National Early Warning Score (NEWS2). https://improvement.nhs.uk/documents/2508/Patient_Safety_Alert_-_adoption_of_NEWS2.pdf

NHS Litigation Authority (2015). Thrombosis risk. https://thrombosisuk.org/downloads/Venous_Thromboembolism_Leaflet-NHS-COST_2016.pdf

NICE (2012). Patient experiences in adult NHS services: improving the experience of care for people using adult NHS services. CG138. www.nice.org.uk/guidance/cg138

NICE (2016). Cardiovascular disease: risk assessment and reduction, including lipid modification. CG181. www.nice.org.uk/guidance/cg181

NICE (2017a). Sepsis: recognition, diagnosis and early management. www.nice.org.uk/guidance/ng51

NICE (2017b). Falls in older people. QS86. www.nice.org.uk/guidance/qs86

NICE (2019a). Falls in older people: assessing risk and prevention. CG161. www.nice.org.uk/guidance/cg161

NICE (2019b). Hypertension in adults: diagnosis and management. www.nice.org.uk/guidance/ng136

NICE (2020a). Venous thromboembolic diseases: diagnosis, management, and thrombophilia testing. NG158. www.nice.org.uk/guidance/ng158

NICE (2020b). Venous thromboembolic diseases: diagnosis, management, and thrombophilia testing. NICE guideline (NG158) Published:26 March 2020. Overview | Venous thromboembolic diseases: diagnosis, management and thrombophilia testing | Guidance | NICE Last accessed 21/04/22.

NICE (2020c). Venous Thromboembolic Diseases: Diagnosis, Management and Thrombophilia Testing.

NICE (2020d). Peripheral artery disease: diagnosis and management. Clinical guideline (CG147) Recommendations | Peripheral arterial disease: diagnosis and management | Guidance | NICE Last accessed 19/05/22.

NICE (2021a). Chronic kidney disease: assessment and management. www.nice.org.uk/guidance/ng203

NICE (2021b). Cellulitis – acute. https://cks.nice.org.uk/topics/cellulitis-acute/

NICE (2022a). British National Formulary. https://bnf.nice.org.uk

NICE (2022b). Type 2 diabetes in adults: management. CG 28. www.nice.org.uk/guidance/ng28

Nickel, A., Cheng, B., Pinnschmidt, H. et al. (2018). Clinical outcome of isolated cerebellar stroke – a prospective observational study. *Frontiers in Neurology* 9: 580.

Nutbeam, D. and Lloyd, J.E. (2020). Understanding and responding to health literacy as a social determinant of health. *Annual Review of Public Health* 42: 159–173.

Office for National Statistics (2020) Leading causes of death, UK: 2001 to 2018. www.ons.gov.uk/peoplepopulationandcommunity/healthandsocialcare/causesofdeath/articles/leadingcausesofdeathuk/2001to2018#uk-leading-causes-of-death-for-all-ages

Office for National Statistics (2021). Avoidable Mortality in the UK: 2019. www.ons.gov.uk/peoplepopulationandcommunity/healthandsocialcare/causesofdeath/bulletins/avoidablemortalityinenglandandwales/2019#:~:text=proportioned%20between%20both.-,In%202019%2C%2022.5%25%20of%20all%20deaths%20in%20the%20UK%20were,time%20series%20began%20in%202001.

O'Mahony. D (2019). STOPP/START Criteria for Potentially Inappropriate Medications/potential Prescribing Omissions in Older People: Origin and Progress. *Expert Review of Clinical Pharmacology* 13: 15–22.

O'Riordan, S., Vasilakis, N., Hussain, L. et al. (2017). Measurement of lying and standing blood pressure in hospital. *Nursing Older People* 29: 20–26.

Parekh, N., Ali, K., Stevenson, J.M. et al. for the PRIME Study Group(2018). Incidence and cost of medication harm in older adults following hospital discharge: a multicentre prospective study in the UK. *British Journal of Clinical Pharmacology* 84 (8): 1789–1797.

Pope, D.T. (2020). Improving community recognition of sepsis using early warning scores. *Nursing Times* 116 (1): 20–22.

Prins, M.H., Lensing, A.W., Prandoni, P. et al. (2018). Risk of recurrent venous thromboembolism according to baseline risk factor profiles. *Blood Advances* 2 (7): 788–796.

Prins, M.H., Lensing, A.W., Prandoni, P. et al. for Public Health England(2020). *Disparities in the Risk and Outcomes of COVID-19*. London: Public Health England.

Public Health England (2020) Disparities in the risk and outcomes of COVID-19. https://assets.publishing.service.gov.uk/government/uploads/system/uploads/attachment_data/file/908434/Disparities_in_the_risk_and_outcomes_of_COVID_August_2020_update.pdf

Reynen, E. and Severn, M. (2017). Point-of-care D-dimer testing: a review of diagnostic accuracy, clinical utility, and safety. www.ncbi.nlm.nih.gov/books/NBK526296/

Righini, M., van Es, J., Den Exter, P.L. et al. (2014). Age-adjusted D-dimer cutoff levels to rule out pulmonary embolism: the ADJUST-PE study. *JAMA* 311: 1117–1124.

Rodziewicz, T.L., Houseman, B., and Hipskind, J.E. (2018). *Medical Error Reduction and Prevention*. Treasure Island: StatPearls.

Royal College of Physicians (2017). Lying and standing BP timeline. www.rcplondon.ac.uk/projects/outputs/measurement-lying-and-standing-blood-pressure-brief-guide-clinical-staff http://www.rcplondon.ac.uk/guidelines-policy/fallsafe-resources-original

Santini, Z., Jose, P., Cornwall, E. et al. (2020). Social disconnectedness, perceived isolation, and symptoms of depression and anxiety among older Americans (NSHAP): a longitudinal mediation analysis. *Lancet Public Health* 2020 (5): e62–e70.

Sarikaya, H. and Steinlin, M. (2018). Cerebellar stroke in adults and children. *Handbook of Clinical Neurology* 155: 301–312.

Schouten, H.J., Geersing, G.J., Koek, H.L. et al. (2013). Diagnostic accuracy of conventional or age adjusted D-dimer cut-off values in older patients with suspected venous thromboembolism: systematic review and meta-analysis. *BMJ* 346: f2492.

Sepúlveda-Loyola, W., Rodríguez-Sánchez, I., Pérez-Rodríguez, P. et al. (2020). Impact of social isolation due to COVID-19 on health in older people: mental and physical effects and recommendations. *Journal of Nutrition, Health and Aging* 25: 1–10.

Settineri, S., Frisone, F., Merlo, E.M. et al. (2019). Compliance, adherence, concordance, empowerment, and self-management: five words to manifest a relational maladjustment in diabetes. *Journal of Multidisciplinary Healthcare* 12: 299.

Shoukath, U., Khatoon, F., Mahveen, S., and Uddin, M.N. (2018). Iatrogenic disease. *Asian Journal of Pharmaceutical Research* 8 (2): 113–116.

Shu, J. and Santulli, G. (2018). Update on peripheral artery disease: epidemiology and evidence-based facts. *Atherosclerosis* 275: 379–381.

Soyoye, D.O., Abiodun, O.O., Ikem, R.T. et al. (2021). Diabetes and peripheral artery disease: a review. *World Journal of Diabetes* 12 (6): 827.

Stafford, M., Deeny, S.R., Dreyer, K., and Shand, J. (2021). Multiple long-term conditions within households and use of health and social care: a retrospective cohort study. *BJGP Open* 5 (2): 2020:0134.

Sullivan, T. and de Barra, E. (2018). Diagnosis and management of cellulitis. *Clinical Medicine* 18 (2): 160.

Thakrar, D.B. and Sultan, M.J. (2021). Cellulitis: diagnosis and differentiation. *Journal of Wound Care* 30 (12): 958–965.

Virchow, R. (1998). *Thrombosis and Emboli (1846–1856)*. Cambridge: Science History Publications.

Vogel, D., Meyer, M., and Harendza, S. (2018). Verbal and non-verbal communication skills including empathy during history taking of undergraduate medical students. *BMC Medical Education* 18 (1): 157.

Vrsalovic, M., Vucur, K., Vrsalovic Presecki, A. et al. (2017). Impact of diabetes on mortality in peripheral artery disease: a meta-analysis. *Clinical Cardiology* 40 (5): 287–291.

Wastesson, J.W., Morin, L., Tan, E.C., and Johnell, K. (2018). An update on the clinical consequences of polypharmacy in older adults: a narrative review. *Expert Opinion on Drug Safety* 17 (12): 1185–1196.

Wells, P.S., Anderson, D., Bormanis, J. et al. (1997). Value of assessment of pre-test probability of deep-vein thrombosis in clinical management. *Lancet* 350 (9094): 1795–1798.

Wells, P.S., Anderson, D., Rodger, M. et al. (2003). Evaluation of D-dimer in the diagnosis of suspected deep-vein thrombosis. *New England Journal of Medicine* 349 (13): 1227–1235.

Windle, J., Moyle, L., and Coomber, R. (2020). 'Vulnerable' kids going country: children and young People's involvement in county lines drug dealing. *Youth Justice* 20 (1–2): 64–78.

World Health Organization (2022). Noncommunicable diseases. www.who.int/news-room/fact-sheets/detail/noncommunicable-diseases

Zhang, Y., He, D., Zhang, W. et al. (2020). ACE inhibitor benefit to kidney and cardiovascular outcomes for patients with non-dialysis chronic kidney disease stages 3–5: a network meta-analysis of randomised clinical trials. *Drugs* 80 (8): 797–811.

FURTHER READING

British Association of Dermatologists bad.org.uk

National Institute for Health and Care Research (2021). Multiple long-term conditions (multimorbidity): making sense of the evidence. https://evidence.nihr.ac.uk/collection/making-sense-of-the-evidence-multiple-long-term-conditions-multimorbidity/.

NHS England (2014) Toolkit for general practice for supporting older people living with frailty. www.england.nhs.uk/publication/toolkit-for-general-practice-in-supporting-older-people-living-with-frailty/#:~:text=Toolkit%20for%20general%20practice%20in%20supporting%20older%20people%20living%20with%20frailty,-Document%20first%20published&text=This%20document%20provides%20GPs%2C%20practice,older%20people%20living%20with%20frailty

NICE (n.d.) https://cks.nice.org.uk/topics/

NICE (2016). Multimorbidity: clinical assessment and management. www.nice.org.uk/guidance/ng56

The Lymphoedema Support Network https://www.lymphoedema.org/

SELF-ASSESSMENT QUESTIONS

1. Consider the use of clinical decision-making tools within the case studies to support and promote the safety of the patient in the community environment.

2. As this patient's healthcare professional, how would you proceed? Take time to write a plan of action to encourage engagement with health services and realistic goals from which to construct a therapeutic relationship.

3. Reflect on the process of the drugs reconciliation as a method to empower the patient.

4. Consider how interprofessional working could enhance the patient's journey within the given scenarios.

GLOSSARY

Advanced clinical practitioner   Advanced clinical practitioners (ACPs) are healthcare professionals, educated to Master's level or equivalent, with the skills and knowledge to allow them to expand their scope of practice to better meet the needs of the people they care for.

Abbreviated Mental Test Score   This quick screening test was first introduced in 1972. Developed by geriatricians, this is probably the best known test in general hospital usage. The Abbreviated Mental Test Score lacks validation in primary care and screening populations; most validity data refer to correlation to the Mini Mental State Examination (MMSE).

Angiotensin converting enzyme   Angiotensin-converting enzyme (ACE) inhibitors are medications that help relax the veins and arteries to lower blood pressure. ACE inhibitors prevent an enzyme in the body from producing angiotensin II, a substance that constricts blood vessels. This narrowing can cause high blood pressure and forces the heart to work harder. Angiotensin II also releases hormones that raise blood pressure.

Benign paroxysmal positional vertigo   BPPV occurs when pieces of calcium carbonate material break off from a part of your inner ear and move to another part of the inner ear. When you move your head a certain way, the crystals move inside the canal and stimulate the nerve endings, causing you to become dizzy.

Estimated glomerular filtration rate   The estimated glomerular filtration rate (eGFR) is a test that measures your level of kidney function and determines your stage of kidney disease. Your healthcare team can calculate it from the results of your blood creatinine test, your age, body size and gender.

Falls Risk Assessment Tool   This is a quick and easy tool to assess an individual's falls risk. It can be used for all individuals you think may be at risk of falling and gives guidance on specific areas surrounding the individual's falls risk.

National Institutes of Health Stroke Scale   The National Institutes of Health Stroke Scale (NIHSS) is the most widely used deficit rating scale in modern neurology; over 500 000 healthcare professionals have been certified to administer it using a web-based platform. Every clinical trial in vascular neurology – prevention, acute treatment, recovery – requires a severity assessment, and the NIHSS became the gold standard for stroke severity rating after the first successful trial in acute stroke therapy, the National Institute of Neurological Disorders and Stroke recombinant tissue-type plasminogen activator for Acute Stroke Trial.

Pulmonary embolism rule-out criteria   The Pulmonary Embolism Rule-out Criteria (PERC) is an eight-item block of clinical criteria that can identify patients who can safely be discharged from the ED without further investigation for PE.

STOPP & START   STOPP (Screening Tool of Older Persons' Prescriptions) and START (Screening Tool to Alert to Right Treatment) are criteria used by clinicians to review potentially inappropriate medications in older adults and have been endorsed as best practice by some organisations.

CHAPTER 13

Managing Complexity

Jaclyn Proctor and Sadie Diamond-Fox

Aim

The aim of this chapter is to develop a greater appreciation around the role of complexity and its application to practice and beyond, drawing on theory to grow understanding around the healthcare phenomenon of complexity. Our journey through complexity will apply a specific lens that examines the following aspects: medical complexity, situational complexity and systems complexity.

LEARNING OUTCOMES

After reading this chapter the reader will have a comprehensive knowledge of:

1. Medical complexity theory
2. Situational complexity theory
3. Systems complexity theory
4. Application of the above theories to advanced practice within the health and social care settings.

INTRODUCTIONS

Complexity is not a new term; in fact, we hear it used in healthcare practice daily, but what do we mean by this? Complexity is certainly a concept that requires deeper exploration into this emerging field to enhance our understanding.

> For every complex problem there is a solution that is clear, simple . . . and wrong.
>
> H. L. Mencken (American writer, 1880–1956)

In 2013 Cohn et al. provided a definition that has been frequently cited in numerous papers: 'Complexity is described as a dynamic and constantly emerging set of processes and objectives that not only interact with each other but come to be defined by those interactions'. Moving from a generic definition to a focused one around NHS and social care, complexity is 'a complex adaptive system where there are high levels of connectivity, interdependence, unpredictability, competing, and changing demands, as well as a need to work with emergence' (NHS England Digital Transformation n.d.). Braithwaite (2018) stated that no other system, not banking, manufacturing, military or even education, is as complex as healthcare, representing the size of the challenge for practitioners, managers and executive teams. Exploring this further, Braithwaite (2018) adds that no comparison can be made with any other sector or industry that has the same span and scope, experiencing constantly changing landscapes that are intricate and often subject to multiple moving parts such as funding models.

It is necessary to consider our own thoughts when referring to complexity. Are we merely alluding to the patient's clinical condition? Or are we applying this terminology to a local healthcare system utilised by both patients and practitioners where system application or navigation may be complex (Manning 2017)? Or are we merely focusing on the complexity of the wider national health service and social care system in its entirety?

It is well acknowledged by all healthcare teams at every level that healthcare has become undeniably more complex (Plsek and Greenhalgh 2001). Despite this acknowledgement, to some extent, there remains a lack of shared or conscious agreement around the meaning and what it describes (Meleis 2007). Valderas et al. (2009) refer to complexity as being understood in several ways which makes an overarching definition challenging, particularly in relation to healthcare.

At the clinical practice level, we may be more familiar with the term complexity being applied to patient care/clinical service when in fact, as supported by the earlier statements, complexity is often multifaceted and the impacts are multi-layered, ultimately involving the wider healthcare system, which we perhaps are all more aware of since the COVID-19 pandemic.

Multi-professional Framework for Advanced Clinical Practice (MPFfACP) (HEE 2017)

This chapter maps to the following areas of the MPFfACP:

1.2   Demonstrate a critical understanding of their broadened level of responsibility and autonomy and the limits of own competence and professional scope of practice, including when working with complexity, risk, uncertainty, and incomplete information

1.4   Work in partnership with individuals, families and carers, using a range of assessment methods as appropriate (e.g. of history-taking; holistic assessment; identifying risk factors; mental health assessments; requesting, undertaking and/or interpreting diagnostic tests; and conducting health needs assessments).

1.6   Use expertise and decision-making skills to inform clinical reasoning approaches when dealing with differentiated and undifferentiated individual presentations and complex situations, synthesising information from multiple sources to make appropriate, evidence-based judgements and/or diagnoses.

1.8   Exercise professional judgement to manage risk appropriately, especially where there may be complex and unpredictable events and supporting teams to do likewise to ensure safety of individuals, families, and carers

2.9   Continually develop practice in response to changing population health need, engaging in horizon scanning for future developments (e.g. impacts of genomics, new treatments and changing social challenges)

Accreditation Considerations – Advanced Critical Care Practitioners (ACCP)

This chapter maps to the following areas of the Faculty of Intensive Care Medicine Curriculum (FICM) for ACCP training:

4.3   Diagnosis and disease management within the scope of critical care.

Accreditation Considerations – ACPs in Emergency Care (ACP-EC)

This chapter maps to the following areas of the Royal College of Emergency Medicine (RCEM) curriculum for training ACP-EC:

SLO 1   Care for physiologically stable adult patients presenting to acute care across the full range of complexity

SLO 4   Care for acutely injured adult patients across the full range of complexity

(RCEM 2022).

Accreditation Considerations – ACPs in Acute Medicine

This chapter maps to the following areas of the Health Education England (HEE) Acute Medicine curriculum for training:

3.1.2   Manages the assessment, diagnosis, and plans future management of patients in an outpatient clinic, ambulatory, or community setting, including the management of long-term conditions, in the context of complexity and uncertainty.

Manages a multi-professional team, including the planning and management of discharge planning in complex, dynamic situations. Manages end-of-life care and applies palliative care skills in the context of complexity and uncertainty.

3.2   Demonstrates capability in dealing with complexity and uncertainty.

MEDICAL COMPLEXITY

This area may feel the most comfortable for many reading this section of the book. With advances in health science alongside the application of health promotion and health protection, life expectancy has increased. However, these developments have also led to patients living with multimorbidity, one research publication (Nicolaus et al. 2022) postulating that two-thirds of older (65 years and older) people are affected by multimorbidity. Patients who present with co-morbidities may also have a decreased quality of life which in turn may lead to an increase in psychological distress. We are aware that the above can influence the patient's length of hospital stay if they are admitted acutely and if a surgical procedure is required, there may be increased complications postoperatively, ultimately resulting in increased costs of delivering health care. We must not forget that clinicians are dealing with this level of complexity every day. However, it does not detract from the diagnostic uncertainty when these co-morbidities interact in unpredictable ways.

Complexity often extends beyond the realms of diagnosis: for example, there are a variety of management strategies and multiple treatment options including chemical measures (for example, medications) alongside mechanical support (physiotherapy, occupational therapy). Clinicians are often simultaneously navigating appropriate treatment plans for patients whilst holding difficult discussions and initiating social care supportive interventions to prepare the patient for home. This often involves a multiagency approach, with financial funding decisions adding to the complex nature of medical care and indeed the ability of patients and their families to navigate the system.

We can consider clinical complexity in a different way with a more real-life scenario; let us take antibiotics as an example here and consider the interactions. It is well known that antibiotic resistance is an issue for patients and the wider healthcare community. If we take this a step further and consider what is occurring at a biochemical level, then we know that micro-organisms are in a process of continual adaption just like our complex systems. The consequence for patients of the process of adaption is that the condition may be more complex to treat due to antimicrobial resistance (Plsek and Greenhalgh 2001), leading to a prolonged hospital stay or a longer duration of community treatment.

It is, however, important to acknowledge that the complex nature of healthcare brings with it clinical risk. Statistically around 10% of adverse events occur in healthcare and it is imperative that these cases are carefully explored to generate understanding of how these events occurred. Viewing these events through an investigative lens enables clinical/managerial teams to review procedures and establish processes that avoid recurrence. However, it is rare to hear about the remaining 90% where clinical teams are delivering care to patients with no harm being experienced (Braithwaite 2018).

Stafford et al. (2007) acknowledge that patient complexity is more than just co-morbidity. They suggested that additional contributing factors include socio-economic, behavioural, environmental and cultural.

Measuring Complexity in a Healthcare Context

The World Health Organization (WHO) utilises a 'Family of International Classifications' (FIC) which are key for effective knowledge representation and data transfer between organisations (Table 13.1).

The FIC includes three reference classifications which serve as a global standard for health data, clinical documentation and statistical aggregation (WHO 2022a).

- International Statistical Classification of Diseases and Related Health Problems (ICD) (Figure 13.1) (WHO 2022b) – allows systematic recording, analysis, interpretation and comparison of mortality and morbidity data. ICD-11 is the most current iteration at the time of publishing this chapter and is effective from January 2022.
- International Classification of Functioning, Disability and Health (ICF) – describes functional health status and social impact via a bio-psycho-social model/framework (Figure 13.2) (WHO 2022c). It acknowledges the significance of personal and environmental factors in clinical

TABLE 13.1   International organisations' usage of FIC (WHO 2022a).

Organisations	Usage of FIC
Government	Allocation of resources
Researchers/academics	International collaboration
Healthcare professionals and providers	Documentation of patient presentations/case and utilised in algorithms for decision support
Hospitals	To count the frequency of presentations
Laboratories	To exchange investigative data
Insurance companies	For billing purposes
International organisations	To assess trends in public health

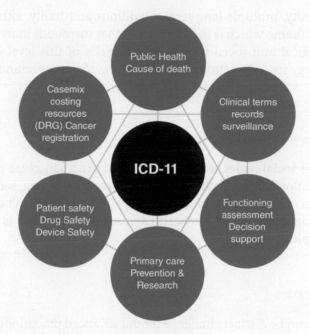

FIGURE 13.1   International Statistical Classification of Diseases and Related Health Problems (ICD) (WHO 2022b).

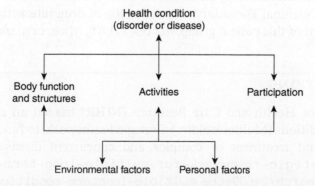

FIGURE 13.2   A pictorial representation of the elements included in the International Classification of Functioning, Disability and Health (ICF) by Kuipers et al. (2011). *Source*: Adapted from WHO (2022b).

complexity and can be used to inform understanding of healthcare complexity at individual and systems levels.

- International Classification of Health Interventions (ICHI) – a common tool for reporting and analysing health interventions for clinical and statistical purposes (WHO 2022d).

Fields of Practice – Paediatrics

The International Classification of Functioning, Disability and Health (ICF) now includes the International Classification of Functioning, Disability and Health for Children and Youth (ICF-CY).

RED FLAGS – PATHOLOGICAL CONSIDERATIONS

Co-morbidity, multimorbidity, multiple long-term conditions and frailty, although interchangeable terms, all share a common theme which is the complexity that surrounds individuals presenting with multiple health, psychological and social issues. The presence of this level of clinical complexity, regardless of the terminology used, has strong links to decreased life expectancy.

ORANGE FLAGS – PSYCHOLOGICAL CONSIDERATIONS AND GREEN FLAGS – SOCIAL CONSIDERATIONS

Physical, psychological and social issues are intertwined and can all increase perceived clinical complexity. Unidentified psychological (e.g. anxiety, depression) and social (e.g. social and/or economical marginalisation) issues can create barriers to improving patient outcomes. The NHS Long Term Plan (2019) emphasises a multiagency approach to health and social care, which is particularly important in the case of clinical complexity.

Pharmacological Principles

Managing multimorbidity can be distinct challenge for the advanced practitioner. Those with prescribing rights have an added layer of complexity when considering managing multimorbidity as patients will often be receiving pharmacotherapy in multiple forms which increases the risk of drug–drug interactions. The British National Formulary interactive list of drug interactions is a useful tool for ensuring safe management of this patient group: https://bnf.nice.org.uk/interactions

CLINICAL INVESTIGATIONS

The National Institute for Health and Care Research (NIHR) has set an ambitious goal via the Multiple Long-term Conditions (Multimorbidity) Strategic Framework, to fund high-quality research into the investigation and treatment of complex and concurrent diseases: www.nihr.ac.uk/documents/nihr-strategic-framework-for-multiple-long-term-conditions-multimorbidity-mltc-m-research/24639#the-multiple-longterm-conditions-multimorbidity-strategic-framework

SITUATIONAL COMPLEXITY

Although much of the published literature focuses on co-morbid and multimorbid conditions, it is important to broaden understanding here, which leads into the discussion around situation complexity. When introducing situational complexity, it quickly becomes apparent that research within this area is vast, but searching this specific term does not produce a vast array of articles. It could simply be that the terminology is used interchangeably, ironically making this complex.

The focus within situational complexity is around two aspects. First, environmental factors, which include the impact of a patient's physical and social environment and the influence this has on how the patient lives. Second, personal factors such as lifestyle, life events, upbringing, gender, race; this is not an exhaustive list but these may have an influence/impact on a patient's health conditions and health status. This is perhaps more succinctly summarised in a Government paper released in 2018 where the authors state 'Good or bad health is not simply the result of individual behaviours, genetics, and medical care. A substantial part of the difference in health outcomes is down to the social, economic, and environmental factors that shape people's lives'.

Fields of Practice – Mental Health

When considering the environment and its impact on health, this leads naturally to focusing on housing which is frequently cited as a key social determinant of a patient's health. As a result, there is the potential to develop numerous negative effects on both health and well-being due to poor housing circumstances (Rolfe et al. 2020). In 2018 the World Health Organization associated poor housing with the potential development of a wide array of health conditions, such as respiratory disease, cardiovascular diseases, mental health and infectious diseases, to name only a few. Prior to this WHO publication, in 2017 the Health Foundation published the stark statistic that one in five dwellings in England does not meet decent standards.

The number of emergency department visits in the UK for respiratory conditions accounts for 6 million inpatient beds and more than 700 000 hospital admissions in the UK each year (NICE, https://indepth.nice.org.uk/respiratory-reducing-emergency-pressure/index.html). Recognition of the contribution that poor housing conditions can make to an individual's health and well-being is only part of the issue; understanding how to address these complexities to improve individuals' health is another.

Data from NHS Digital (2020–2021) demonstrated that the rate of attendance to emergency departments from the most deprived areas accounted for 2.2 million visits, while it was 1.1 million from the least deprived areas, a statistic that no one should have to be reading in the twenty-first century but that is sadly becoming all too familiar.

Lifestyle impact on health has been well documented and each year there are campaigns to support reducing alcohol intake (Dry January), stop smoking (Stoptober) and prostate cancer awareness (Movember), to name only a few. In addition to this, we have specific events for charities supporting research into health conditions such as Alzheimer disease. All these interventions are aimed at increasing awareness around conditions and supporting individuals to modify lifestyle choices.

In 2014–2016, the variance in life expectancy between the most and least deprived areas within England was 9.3 years in males and 7.3 years in females (Gov.uk 2018). There are many reasons behind this in terms of the development of health conditions such as cancer and cardiovascular disease. Higher rates of mental health problems, smoking and alcohol consumption have been observed. Access to healthcare is not always simple, not all patients attend screening appointments and not all patients have access to transport.

The challenges and complexities around how to balance the inequalities in life expectancy are only one part of a multifaceted picture and the question often posed is around how to change this. In the latter part of this chapter, we will be discussing the NHS Long Term Plan (2019) and will undoubtedly note many efforts that are being made to address much of the above.

SYSTEMS COMPLEXITY

Over the last decade, within healthcare there has been significant growth in digital working, e-observations, electronic patient records, electronic patient prescribing, robot machines in pharmacy departments and interest in artificial intelligence and its potential opportunities for healthcare. This connects the vision from the NHS Long Term Plan (2019) where one of the most ambitious improvements surrounded the transformation of technological advances for the future NHS. The above examples demonstrate that healthcare is developing through the exploration of opportunities that the digital world may offer.

Although these system developments lead to more effective ways of working, this inherently leads to more complexity within the system. For example, not all healthcare providers utilise the same digital platform – some systems 'speak' to each other whilst others do not. In addition to this, not all patients have digital access and as we develop digital momentum, it is important not to exclude patients for whom this approach is not readily available.

However, the possibilities are endless – many will have experienced the ability to book online vaccinations during COVID and have access to online evidence of the vaccination being completed. This is probably one of the most intricate systems that we have all experienced to date on a national level. However, it is necessary to provide a word of warning here, around the issue of maintaining patient confidentiality as we move to a more digitalised provision of healthcare and how this can be assured. In 2019, NICE published guidance around best practice standards for new technologies commissioned by the NHS.

More recently, we have seen the new integrated care boards (ICBs) launched in July 2022. This partnership between healthcare providers and commissioners enables a more collaborative approach to planning health and care systems/services to meet the needs of the local population (Charles 2021). The ICBs throughout England are geographically based and to date 42 are operational with the expectation that this will continue to develop over time. The ICB development was a key part of the NHS Long Term Plan 2019 (Charles 2021). There is no doubt that this implementation of ICBs will initially bring challenges whilst healthcare practitioners and the ICB teams themselves become more familiar with their roles and responsibilities. Advancements in healthcare will always be complex, but the moving landscape and the need for the health and social care system to adapt to meet the needs of a growing population require innovative thinking and the formation of ICBs reflects this.

On another level, we must consider the interplay between patient, health conditions and healthcare system complexity; these are influential components that when combined add to the challenges faced by the NHS at both local and national level.

NHS LONG TERM PLAN (2019)

Having analysed complexity using three distinctive components, we now direct the discussion to reflect on the NHS Long Term Plan and the influence of this White Paper. Many will be familiar to some extent with this paper and the plans that have been set out. This document builds upon the NHS five year forward view which focused on the need to integrate care to meet the needs of a changing population. This is perhaps the most comprehensive plan covering a range of issues (Charles et al. 2019).

- Improving services – clinical priorities: cancer, cardiovascular disease, maternity, neonatal, mental health, stroke, diabetes and respiratory care, with a focus on the health of children and young people.
- Primary care and community services – general practices will join to form primary care networks; these groups of neighbouring practices will cover around 30–50 000 people, with a focus on digital consultations online or via the phone (something which increased during COVID). Increased capacity within the crisis support services and an enhancement in social prescribing.
- Mental health and learning disabilities – the plan commits to improving mental health services for adults, children and young people, with a strong focus on improving care and support for people with learning disabilities and autism.
- Acute service, urgent and emergency care – significant measures aimed at reducing accident and emergency attendances. Commitment to establishing urgent treatment centres. The development of same-day emergency care facilities (SDEC) located within secondary care accident and emergency departments.
- Wider acute services – introducing digital technology into outpatient services; again we have seen this established during COVID and to a large extent it remains in place.
- Finance and productivity.
- Digital – as previously discussed.
- Leadership and support for staff – the developments here lead on from the national strategic framework.
- Developing people and improving care. This also incorporates BAME representation across the senior leadership team.
- Role of patient and carers.
- Tackling inequalities in health – again as we have previously explored.
- Workforce – which also leads us to introduce advanced clinical practice here which featured within the long-term plan, stating that ACPs are an important part of meeting the current and future workforce demands (Diamond-Fox and Stone 2021).

Fields of Practice – Learning Disability and Autism (LD&A)

The NHS Long Term Plan aims to reduce health inequalities of individuals with LD&A via several initiatives.

- Offering annual health checks.
- Prescribing initiatives via:
  - STOMP: Stopping The Over-Medication of children and young People with a learning disability, autism or both
  - STAMP: Supporting Treatment and Appropriate Medication in Paediatrics.
- LeDeR: Learning from deaths reviews.

When the plan was released in 2019, no one knew that we had a pandemic looming and thus some of the key features of the plan were evoked earlier and quicker than expected. Perhaps not to the degree of what the plan envisioned, however digital consultations maintained contact between healthcare providers and the public during the height of the pandemic. We are now witnessing elements of the plan move to reality, as emergency departments and same-day emergency care units are being built as we write this chapter. There is, of course, some way to go but changes are being made and that was the purpose of this comprehensive plan. The complexity arises when trying to implement these modifications which often involve multiagency approaches, with leadership teams across health, social care and the funding sector.

ADVANCED CLINICAL PRACTICE

Advanced clinical practice, much like complexity, is not necessarily a new concept, although the terminology applied to the roles has evolved over time (Leary and MacLaine 2019). Discussion to date has circulated around these roles not being a replacement for medical models, but rather a role that complements the current NHS workforce (Diamond-Fox and Stone 2021). This workforce is continually growing and developing each year due to investment from Health Education England and engagement from higher educational institutes, clinical supervisors and organisations; the wider benefits of advanced practice for patients, families and NHS services are there for all to see.

The promotion of these roles within the NHS Long Term Plan (2019) placed this group of highly skilled professionals within one of the most progressive documents driving forward the NHS to meet future demands. The multiprofessional nature of these positions means that they lend themselves to experienced clinicians who seek to grow and extend their professional knowledge with the four pillars of advanced practice. In 2017 Health Education England released the Multi-professional Framework for Advanced Practice, and for the first time clinicians were able to provide a definition to their role.

Whilst the above forms a nice way to introduce this section, we must not overlook the complexity of advanced practice. First, terminology, an area that was widely discussed in Hooks and Walker's (2020) exploration of the advanced clinical practitioner role. At the present time, there exists only the initial registration that the practitioner holds as a verification of professional qualification to practise, but this does not capture the advanced level of practice. The hope is that this will change over time; however, how this qualification will be added and the timeline for its implementation are currently unknown. Therefore, it currently falls to individual organisations to ensure that job descriptions are specific and the role is supervised within clinical practice during training and into qualification.

Advanced clinical practice requires the practitioner to consider complexity on multiple levels, including assessment of a patient's clinical history, interpretation of diagnostic tests and prescribing decisions, but is not restricted to these example activities. The Multi-professional framework for Advanced Clinical Practice (HEE 2017) refers to the term 'complex' throughout the four pillars of practice and their applied capabilities. When we analyse this more closely, the reference is often managing complexity in terms of patient care or in relation to leading a team and this widely represents daily practice for an ACP.

If we now apply all this information to the following patient scenario, then we can begin to appreciate complexity in the reality of clinical care.

Case Study

A patient has presented to your department with an exacerbation of chronic obstructive pulmonary disease (COPD). They also have diabetes and have been prescribed steroids for this exacerbation, thus causing a temporary destabilisation of their diabetic control resulting in the patient potentially requiring an alteration in their diabetic regimen. Due to the stress, the patient's blood pressure could be higher. Whilst clinically this may not be complex, for the patient there is a disturbance to their usual regimen and the involvement from an additional clinical team (diabetes) in their care. During the assessment process, the patient has a chest X-ray (CXR), which is flagged for suspected cancer and the radiology department has suggested a computed tomography (CT) scan and a referral to respiratory care.

As the ACP managing the patient's care, you now need to inform the patient why the CT scan has been requested. These conversations are highly stressful for the patient due to the unexpected nature of the finding and for the clinician delivering this information. The patient now has the involvement of another team in their care, the lung multidisciplinary team, where the CT scan will be reviewed and care planned accordingly. The patient has an anxious wait for the report in an unfamiliar often isolating environment. Not only are they no longer self-managing their diabetes, they are also faced with the distressing wait around the CT scan; the patient's control of these variables is limited.

The CT scan confirms lung cancer and following explanation of the results, the lung cancer nurse specialist attends to support the patient and answer any questions. As a result of the above, the patient may experience physiological and psychological effects, both of which have been directly affected by the clinical condition and unexpected diagnosis in an environment that is unfamiliar. The patient is now navigating a new, unknown system of care that can feel complex.

Presenting Complaint: 77 year old, identifies as female. Presented to primary care provider with shortness of breath (SOB).

History of Presenting Complaint: recent infective exacerbation of COPD. Completed course of antibiotics and steroids, but SOB persists. Nil recent pulmonary rehab.

Past Medical History: COPD, hypertension, atrial fibrillation, type 2 diabetes, high cholesterol, depression and osteoporosis.

Drug History: amlodipine 5 mg OD, atorvastatin 10 mg OD, alendronic acid 70 mg + cholecalciferol 5600 UI (weekly), metformin BD, perindopril 5 mg, salbutamol inhaler PRN and salbutamol 500 mg + fluticasone furoate 50 mg inhaler BD. Recent vaccinations of influenza, SARS-CoV-2, and pneumococcus.

Family History: nil of note.

Social History: carer for husband.

On exam

General survey: nil signs of respiratory distress. Denies pain. BP 148/95 mmHg. HR 72 bpm (irregularly irregular). Chest auscultation NAD (nil wheeze or crackles). Heart sounds: I + II + 0. Nil peripheral oedema. Abdo soft, non-tender.

Body mass index (BMI): 24.8 kg/m^2.

Recent investigations

Spirometry; post bronchodilator FEV_1/FVC 58.

- Chest X-ray: NAD.
- Nil eosinophils on recent full blood count.
- HbA1c 60 mmol/ml.

Impression/Problems

Multiple long-term conditions/multimorbidity (MLTC-M).

- Poorly controlled COPD.
  - Post bronchodilator FEV_1/FVC <0.7 indicates persistent airflow obstruction despite combined long-acting muscarinic and beta-2 receptor agonists.
  - Unsuitable for inhaled corticosteroids due to osteoporosis and diabetes.
  - Nil recent pulmonary rehab engagement since last exacerbation.
- Poorly controlled hypertension – BP >140/90 mmHg.
- Poorly controlled type 2 diabetes – HbA1c >48 mmol/ml

Before we conclude this chapter, it is important to take a moment to consider management theory which seems pertinent to the discussion. There are two terms that come to mind here: tame and wicked problems (Keith Grint) and for those familiar with these terms you will notice the tangible link immediately. However, for many this will be an entirely new concept and warrants a breakdown explanation. For example, a tame problem is something that can be easily defined, and the solution may be equally as visible. A wicked problem is more complex, and it may be difficult to define the nature of the problem in detail. Figures 13.3 and 13.4 demonstrate this well; you will notice that the three themes become more intertwined and as they do so, the wickedness in terms of complexity increases and becomes more challenging.

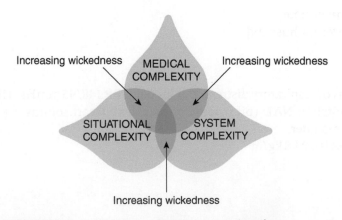

FIGURE 13.3 Dimension of healthcare and 'wickedness' Kuipers et al. (2011).

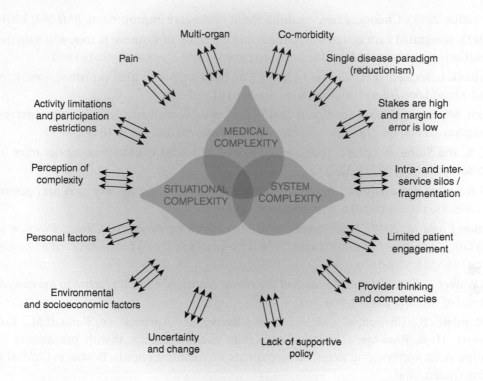

Multi-organ

Co-morbidity

Pain

Single disease paradigm
(reductionism)

Activity limitations
and participation
restrictions

Stakes are high
and margin for
error is low

MEDICAL
COMPLEXITY

Perception of
complexity

SITUATIONAL
COMPLEXITY

SYSTEM
COMPLEXITY

Intra- and inter-
service silos /
fragmentation

Personal factors

Limited patient
engagement

Environmental
and socioeconomic factors

Provider thinking
and competencies

Uncertainty
and change

Lack of supportive
policy

FIGURE 13.4 Factors associated with healthcare complexity and 'wickedness' Kuipers et al. (2011).

CONCLUSION

There is still much to learn from exploring complexity and this chapter by no means covers the subject area in its entirety but we hope it will increase your awareness of the ever-changing landscape of complexity within health and social care.

Take Home Points

- To practise effectively and within your professional registration, you must possess the correct knowledge, skills and professional behaviours to undertake your role with proficiency whilst working with complex patient groups.

- Advanced practitioners must be able to demonstrate a critical understanding of their knowledge surrounding the management of complex patients. They must acknowledge the limits of their own competence and professional scope of practice, including when working with complexity, risk, uncertainty and incomplete information.

- Advanced practitioners must be aware of the legalities and ethical complexities associated with their practice when leading the care of complex patient groups and work with other healthcare professionals to offer an integrated package of care.

REFERENCES

Braithwaite, J. (2018, 2018). Changing how we think about healthcare improvement. *BMJ* 361: k2014.

Charles, A (2021). Integrated care systems explained: making sense of systems, places, and neighbourhoods. `www.kingsfund.org.uk/publications/integrated-care-systems-explained`

Charles A, Ewbank L, McKenna H, Wenzel L (2019). The NHS long-term plan explained. `www.kingsfund.org.uk/publications/nhs-long-term-plan-explained`

Cohn, S., Clinch, M., Bunn, C., and Stronge, P. (2013). Entangled complexity: why complex interventions are just not complicated enough. *Journal of Health Services Research and Policy* 18 (1): 40–43.

Diamond-Fox, S. and Stone, S. (2021). The development of advanced clinical practitioner roles in the UK. *British Journal of Nursing* 30 (1): 32–33.

Gov.uk (2018). Research and analysis, Chapter 6: wider determinants of health. `www.gov.uk/governement/publications/health-profile-for-england-2018`

Health Education England (2017). Multi-professional Framework for Advanced Clinical Practice. `www.hee.nhs.uk/sites/default/files/documents/multi-professionalframeworkforadvancedclinicalpracticeinengland.pdf`

Hooks, C. and Walker, S. (2020). An exploration of the role of advanced clinical practice in the east of England. *British Journal of Nursing* 29 (15): 864–869.

Kuipers, P., Kendall, E., Ehrlich, C., McIntyre, M., Barber, L., Amsters, D., Kendall,M., Kuipers, K., Muenchberger, H. & Brownie, S (2011). Complexity and healthcare: Health practitioner workforce, services, roles, skills and training to respond topatients with complex needs. Brisbane: Clinical Education and Training Queensland.

Leary, A. and MacLaine, K. (2019). The evolution of advanced nursing practice: past, present, and future. *Nursing Times* 115 (10): 18–19.

Manning, E. (2017). The complex patient: a concept clarification. *Nursing and Health Sciences* 19 (1): 13–21.

Meleis, I. (2007). *Theoretical Nursing: Development and Progress*. New York: Lippincott, Williams and Wilkins.

NHS (2019). The Long-Term Plan. `www.longtermplan.nhs.uk`

NHS Digital (2021). Hospital Accident and Emergency Activity 2020–21. `https://digital.nhs.uk/data-and-information/publications/statistical/hospital-accident--emergency-activity/2020-21`

NHS England Digital Transformation (n.d.). `www.england.nhs.uk/digitaltechnology`

Nicolaus, S., Crelier, B., Donze, J.D., and Aubert, C.E. (2022). Definition of patient complexity in adults: a narrative review. *Journal of Multimorbidity and Comorbidity* 12: 26335565221081288.

Plsek, P.E. and Greenhalgh, T. (2001). Complexity science – the challenge of complexity in health care. *BMJ* 323 (7313): 625–628.

Rolfe, S., Garnham, L., Godwin, J. et al. (2020). Housing as a social determinant of health and wellbeing: developing an empirically-informed realist theoretical framework. *BMC Public Health* 20: 1138.

Royal College of Emergency Medicine (2022). Emergency Medicine. `https://rcem.ac.uk/`

Safford, M.M., Allison, J.J., and Kiefe, C.I. (2007). Patient complexity: more than comorbidity. The vector model of complexity. *Journal of General Internal Medicine.* 22 (Suppl 3): 382–390.

Valdera, J.M., Starfield, B., Sibbald, B. et al. (2009). Defining comorbidity: implications for understanding health and health services. *Annals of Family Medicine* 7 (4): 357–363.

World Health Organization (2018). Housing impacts health: new WHO guidelines in housing and health. `www.who.int/news/item/26-11-2018`

World Health Organization (2022a). Classifications and Terminologies – WHO Family of International Classifications (FIC). `www.who.int/standards/classifications`

World Health Organization (2022b). International Statistical Classification of Diseases and Related Health Problems (ICD). www.who.int/standards/classifications/classification-of-diseases

World Health Organization (2022c). International Classification of Functioning, Disability and Health (ICF). www.who.int/standards/classifications/international-classification-of-functioning-disability-and-health

World Health Organization (2022d). International Classification of Health Interventions (ICHI). www.who.int/standards/classifications/international-classification-of-health-interventions

FURTHER READING

Health Education England (2017). Multi-professional framework for advanced clinical practice in England. www.hee.nhs.uk/sites/default/files/documents/multi-professionalframeworkforadvancedclinicalpracticeinengland.pdf

Health Education England (2020). Core Capabilities Framework for Advanced Clinical Practice (Nurses) Working in General Practice/Primary Care in England. www.hee.nhs.uk/sites/default/files/documents/ACP%20Primary%20Care%20Nurse%20Fwk%202020.pdf

SELF-ASSESSMENT QUESTIONS

1. As an advanced practitioner, consider the intricacies of your patient groups and why you believe them to be complex.
2. How do you determine that you are competent with the correct knowledge, skills and behaviours to assess and treat an individual with complex needs?
3. As an advanced practitioner, who are the health and social care professional groups you work with most frequently and how do these groups affect your practice?
4. What is complex care and what do you believe to be the differences in leading such care as an advanced level practitioner? Can you justify your role and your uniqueness?

GLOSSARY

Alzheimer's disease   A progressive neurological disorder that causes the brain to shrink (atrophy) and brain cells to die.

Autism   A lifelong developmental disability which affects how people communicate and interact with the world.

Bronchodilator   Medication used to dilate the lungs' airways.

Co-morbidity   More than one illness or disease occurring in one person at the same time.

Complexity   A state or quality of being intricate or complicated.

Frailty   A syndrome arising from the ageing process in which multiple body systems gradually lose their in-built reserves.

Long-term condition   A health condition (physical or psychological) that requires ongoing management for a year or longer and affects a person's life.

Multimorbidity   More than two illnesses or diseases occurring in the same person at the same time.

NHS Long Term Plan   A 10-year plan which includes measures to prevent 150 000 heart attacks, strokes and dementia cases, and provide better access to mental health services for adults and children.

Spirometry   A test that measures lung function, specifically the amount (volume) and/or speed (flow) of air that can be inhaled and exhaled.

CHAPTER 14

Frailty: Principles of Rehabilitation and Reablement, Palliative Care and Organ Donation

Esther Clift and Stevie Park

Aim

The aim of this chapter is to enable advanced practitioners to develop an understanding of frailty as a long-term condition, the principles of rehabilitation and reablement, palliative care and organ donation pathways.

LEARNING OUTCOMES

After reading this chapter the reader will:

1. Understand the process of flow through reablement or rehabilitation pathways.
2. Identify frailty syndromes, understand the process of comprehensive geriatric assessment, and offer appropriate interventions for people living with frailty.
3. Understand the principles of palliative and end-of-life care and organ donation pathways.
4. Understand the possible discharge pathways and the imperative of appropriate communication.

INTRODUCTION

All four pillars of advanced practice (clinical, leadership and management, education and research) are relevant when considering the complex boundaries between the different care settings described in this chapter. The four pillars are each needed in a practitioner working with older people, and with those

The Advanced Practitioner: A Framework for Practice, First Edition. Edited by Ian Peate,
Sadie Diamond-Fox, and Barry Hill.
© 2024 John Wiley & Sons Ltd. Published 2024 by John Wiley & Sons Ltd.

approaching the end of their days, where highly attuned communication skills meet clear diagnostics and a thorough understanding of expected trajectories. When working in a rehabilitation context, a combination of advanced skills and capabilities can make the difference between a good recovery experience and a poor one. This chapter will describe some of the complexity which an advanced practitioner needs to understand to be effective, and the capabilities necessary to become a highly performing team member.

Accreditation Considerations

- The British Geriatrics Society Diploma in Geriatric Medicine – for expertise in frailty.
- Palliative care, rehab credential . . . yet to be published – HEE Centre for Advanced Practice.
- HEE Advanced Clinical Practice in Older People Curriculum Framework: `https:// healtheducationengland.sharepoint.com/sites/APWC/Shared%20Documents/ Forms/AllItems.aspx?id=%2Fsites%2FAPWC%2FShared%20Documents%2FCredential s%2FCredentials%20Endorsement%20Documents%2FAdvanced%20clinical%20prac-tice%20older%20people%20curriculum%20framework%20%20%2Epdf&parent=%2Fsi tes%2FAPWC%2FShared%20Documents%2FCredentials%2FCredentials%20Endorse-ment%20Documents&p=true&ga=1`
- NHSBT – NHS Blood and Transplant.

DISCHARGE PLANNING

Discharge planning is described as 'an interdisciplinary approach to continuity of care' (Lin et al. 2012). The discharge process is described as subjective, complex, risky and challenging, and requires significant experience (Rees and Chapman, 2022). Advanced practitioners in a hospital setting need to know what the discharge options are for their patients, and actively engage in facilitating a 'home first' approach to onward care, while fully engaging patients and their families in the discharge process. This is a legal requirement.

The discharge process needs to be systematic and well documented. Every discharge should ensure that the patient is at the centre by regularly asking their wishes. A good understanding of the Mental Capacity Act (2005) and the process to safeguard people who may lack capacity around decision making is fundamental to all advanced practitioners undertaking discharge planning. Advanced practitioners will need to be able to assess mental capacity and how to make decisions in a person's best interest, using independent mental capacity advocates where required. These are highly skilled communication and assessment processes, which require careful documentation and communication with others who may be involved in care provision, such as social care providers and family members. Understanding the legal process of Lasting Power of Attorney for Health, Wellbeing and Finances is critical to ensuring good outcomes for patients.

NHS England has defined four specific pathways for discharge, depending on the intensity of the care needs once discharged. Pathway 0 is a straightforward return to home with no additional requirements. Pathway 1 may require an intervention from community nursing, therapy or domiciliary social care, or an early supported discharge using a virtual ward or hospital at home model, but a return to home. Pathway 2 requires a bed-based intermediate care option and rehabilitation; and Pathway 3 is a transfer into a care home, when care needs can no longer be met at home. This is most often due to deterioration in function at night which is unsafe and unsustainable (Figure 14.1).

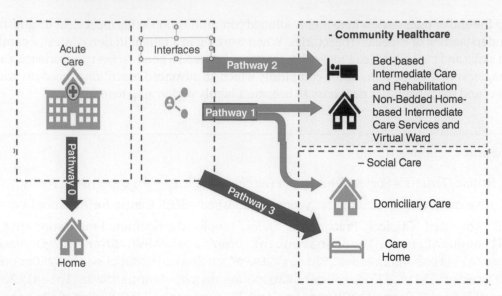

FIGURE 14.1   Discharge pathways.

Engaging with third sector providers and community care navigators may be part of the discharge process to ensure that older people are not left isolated or lonely on discharge from a hospital. The Better Care Fund has enabled integrated pathways to develop in local communities which wrap around individuals to ensure they can stay well at home and avoid unnecessary admissions to hospital. Advanced practitioners in the community will need to have relationships with their community navigators to ensure that the best possible services are offered to people in their own homes – and that they can access support. Any discharge from service marks a measurable change and therefore a well-documented discharge summary to support the transfer of care, and a summary of care given in a hospital setting, is a vital information-sharing exercise. Advanced practitioners in any setting may be expected to complete discharge summaries, including person-centred goals and clinical information, as well as expected onward care needs for other colleagues to follow up, such as further review of renal function after an acute kidney injury in hospital.

INTERMEDIATE CARE

Intermediate Care offers short interventions to aid recovery and regain independence (NICE 2017). Intermediate care includes rehabilitation, reablement, crisis response, home-based and bed-based support, which may be in a hospital or care home. By its very nature, intermediate care is multiprofessional, with integration between health and social care services and systems. Practitioners may be occupational therapists, physiotherapists, speech and language therapists, doctors and nurses as well as care home staff.

NICE describes four stages of intermediate care. (1) Before it starts, advanced practitioners may make clinical decisions, regarding the need for onward referral into intermediate care services. (2) At the start, where advanced practitioners are likely to be managing complex person-centred goal setting with individuals and their families, to establish the expected outcomes of intermediate care interventions. (3) The third stage of intermediate care is while receiving the service, where advanced practitioners may be responsible for delivering or supervising the delivery of clinical and social interventions and care.

(4) Finally, at the end of the intervention, an advanced practitioner may be responsible for discharging the person from one service and ensuring that a smooth transfer takes place into another service, such as ensuring ongoing care needs are met, if required.

Intermediate care is complex due to sitting between health and social care which may be in a variety of phases of integration.

Rehabilitation

Rehabilitation takes many forms but its goal is to help people recover from illness or regain/maintain function-maximising quality of life and independence, despite underlying disease both chronic and acute (O'Hanlon and Smith 2021). Advanced practitioners in rehabilitation may have a background in any specialty (therapies or nursing). The focus is on ensuring holistic care and person-centred, highly specialised interventions, using a multidisciplinary team. Some specialties are further developed such as stroke rehabilitation which may follow a person who has had a stroke through several rehabilitation settings, from hospital-based acute care through bed-based rehabilitation to home or care home.

An advanced practitioner will have a thorough understanding of the underlying illness which caused the functional decline which requires rehabilitation, such as stroke, frailty or falls-related fractures, and be able to offer appropriate evidence-based interventions in any setting, using highly developed diagnostic skills, clinical reasoning and treatment planning. Treatment interventions will be prescribed by highly skilled clinicians who may be advanced practitioners or clinical specialists. The interventions may be delivered by support workers under the oversight of highly specialised therapists.

Unfortunately, commissioned services often do not facilitate evidence-based rehabilitation pathways. Interventions are often curtailed before full potential is achieved, such as falls pathways where evidence indicates that a 12-week intervention is most efficacious in preventing future falls, but most systems offer a six-week therapy intervention at most (Sherrington et al. 2008). Advanced practitioners will be able to present evidence to support investment in developing pathways to enable robust rehabilitation to prevent future deterioration and deconditioning and reduce the burden of care from both health and social care budgets.

Not surprisingly, rehabilitation is not always the responsibility of formal health provision, and advanced practitioners will need to work within the mixed economy of private provision for highly specialised rehabilitation, for sports injuries and third sector providers for local provision. They will need to have a good understanding of the evidence base for their area of rehabilitation to support development of appropriate third sector provision and signpost support staff (such as care navigators, social prescribers and other practitioners) to select appropriate interventions for people to continue their rehabilitation journey and maintain their functional capacity.

Rehabilitation includes specialist areas, such as speech and language, podiatry, weight management, sensory rehabilitation, cognition (including dementia), vestibular rehabilitation and continence, to name but a few. An advanced practitioner will have a basic understanding but know where specialist help can be sought if these are included as the patient's particular areas of concern or goals for rehabilitation. This will include specialist equipment provision to enable independence, as well as physical therapeutic interventions such as specific exercise or more general physical activity. There are clear guidelines on the expected dose of activity for adults published by Public Health England.

All systems have a finite provision for rehabilitation, and often there are arbitrary boundaries placed on provision. This has often historically been described as not having 'rehabilitation potential'. Rehabilitation potential is a process, which involves complex clinical judgement and prognostication on the projected benefits of undertaking a targeted programme of rehabilitation. The assessment of rehabilitation potential should consider physical and psychological factors identified during multidisciplinary assessments along with the patient's needs and wants and the availability of family support. It involves developing an understanding of who will participate with rehabilitation, in and outside the therapy setting, who can support this and who is likely to benefit (Cowley et al. 2021). This description includes the invaluable role which families and carers play in the process of rehabilitation. Family provides the ongoing context and experience of a person, which is invaluable in setting realistic goals and expectations for the rehabilitation process. An advanced practitioner will develop highly skilled communication strategies to ensure that their interventions sit within a continuum of an appropriate pathway of care.

Reablement

Reablement is the assessment and interventions provided to people in their home (or care home) aiming to help them recover skills and confidence and maximise their independence. For most people interventions last up to six weeks. Reablement is delivered by a multidisciplinary team but most commonly by social care practitioners and occupational therapists.

Pathways

Intermediate care is focused on integrated working, with a single point of access and a single assessment process, with shared understanding of aims for benchmarking and reporting. Some people, often older people living with frailty, may be referred in a step-down pathway, where they have had a hospital stay, and others in a step-up pathway, when they have had a functional decline but not a bed-based stay.

Comprehensive geriatric assessments (CGA) form a core offering within the intermediate care environment. An advanced clinical practitioner may undertake this or contribute to the CGA. Every encounter during a reablement intervention should be an opportunity for health education, using techniques such as Making Every Contact Count (MECC). A key focus for reablement is delivering person-centred goals, which take account of preferences ('what matters to me') and are culturally sensitive. Facilitation skills to enable engagement with self-management are key for good outcomes. Coaching skills and understanding patient activation levels will enable better outcomes for individuals (Hibbard and Gilburt 2014).

Technology

Reablement teams often use technology to prompt self-care, such as an alarm to alert someone to take their medication or monitoring changes in activity, such as pressure sensors to alert to a risk of falling over. This technology enables people to live longer and more independently at home. This is a rapidly growing area, and advanced practitioners should be aware of new developments and participate in trials to develop this work further.

Home-based Care

Home-based care offers several care services and benefits to the service user and the healthcare provider (Figure 14.2).

Urgent and emergency care (UEC) has traditionally taken place within the boundaries of hospital care, usually with access via an emergency department. Recent challenges to hospital provision as the

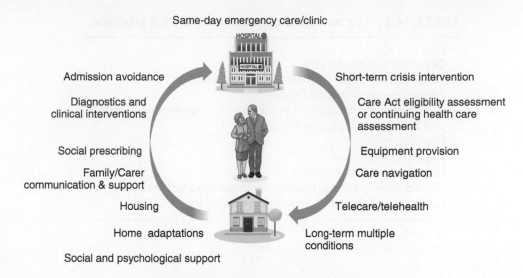

Same-day emergency care/clinic

Admission avoidance

Diagnostics and clinical interventions

Social prescribing

Family/Carer communication & support

Housing

Home adaptations

Social and psychological support

Short-term crisis intervention

Care Act eligibility assessment or continuing health care assessment

Equipment provision

Care navigation

Telecare/telehealth

Long-term multiple conditions

Ongoing rehabilitation and self-management

FIGURE 14.2   Home-based care.

best place for care, and the additional pressures of the COVID-19 pandemic, have hastened advances to deliver highly specialised care closer to home. This includes diagnostics and interventions which would have traditionally been delivered within a hospital setting.

Virtual Wards

A virtual ward is defined as a safe and efficient alternative to NHS bedded care that is enabled by technology. Virtual wards, including frailty and acute respiratory infections (ARI) virtual wards, support patients who would otherwise be in hospital to receive the acute care, monitoring and treatment they need in their own home or place of residence. This includes allowing the patient to be cared for at home or to go home sooner (NHSE 2022). The workforce delivering virtual wards should include highly skilled advanced practitioners who are capable of undertaking diagnostics and interventions to manage acute illness at home. The governance of each service is the responsibility of the advanced practitioners within the service and the individual providers within the integrated care system.

Urgent Community Response

Two-hour urgent community response (UCR) teams in England provide assessment, treatment and support to people over the age of 18 in their own home or usual place of residence who are experiencing a health or social care crisis and are at risk of hospital admission within 2–24 hours. Assessment and care should start within two hours of the referral being received, where clinically appropriate, with short-term interventions typically lasting under 48 hours. Teams are expected to work in an interdisciplinary way, and often consist of advanced clinical practitioners, physiotherapists, paramedics, occupational therapists, nurses, support staff and social workers. Further support may come from other relevant professionals including GPs and geriatricians, all of whom will require the digital capability to ensure safe assessment and monitoring of virtual care. The nine conditions included in UCR provision can be seen in Table 14.1.

TABLE 14.1   The nine conditions included in UCR provision.

– Falls
– Decompensation of frailty
– Reduced function/deconditioning/reduced mobility
– Palliative/end-of-life crisis support
– Urgent equipment provision to support a person experiencing a
  crisis/at risk of hospital admission
– Confusion/delirium
– Urgent catheter care
– Urgent support for diabetes
– Unpaid carer breakdown which, if not resolved, will result in a
  healthcare crisis for the person they care for (NHSE 2022)

PALLIATIVE OR END-OF-LIFE CARE

End-of-life care is defined by NHS England as care that is provided in the 'last year of life' although for some conditions, end-of-life care may be provided for months or years. Palliative care describes care for people living with a terminal illness. This builds on the work of Dame Cicely Saunders, the founder of the modern hospice movement, whose aspiration for good end-of-life care was motivated by the fact that how people die remains in the memory of those who live on.

The focus of palliative care is holistic care.

- Managing any symptoms.
- Offering emotional, spiritual and psychological support.
- Offering practical support, including planning or securing equipment.
- Giving you a good quality of life.

Advanced practitioners are likely to be involved in both delivering specialist palliative care and symptom control, and determining when patients are moving into a palliative trajectory or approaching the end of their lives. These are emotive and highly challenging decisions and conversations to have, and often require the input of the whole MDT, but this may not always be possible. These decisions involve the highest level of clinical decision making, using person-centred care skills, thorough understanding of the disease process and life course for the individual and highly skilled communication to ensure that the expectations and outcomes of any interventions are understood and agreed with each person.

A clinician needs to have a high degree of medical understanding of the terminal illness leading to palliation and be able to express the pros and cons of further medical interventions with the patient, their family and significant others. The probabilities of outcomes of interventions as well as the side-effects need to be well understood and articulated in a way that is understood by the person, before a decision to move to palliation is made. NICE (2019) recognises the following for palliative care treatment: advanced, progressive, incurable conditions; general frailty and co-existing conditions that mean the person is at increased risk of dying within the next 12 months; existing conditions if the person is at risk of dying from a sudden acute crisis in their condition; life-threatening acute conditions caused by sudden catastrophic events.

Gold Standard Framework

The Gold Standard Framework is a practical, systematic, evidence-based end-of-life care service improvement programme, identifying the right people, promoting the right care, in the right place, at the right time, every time.

The aspiration for end-of-life care is for each person to have a good death. Although every individual may have a different idea about what would, for them, constitute a 'good death', the Department of Health (2008) suggested the following factors.

- Being treated as an individual, with dignity and respect.
- Being without pain and other symptoms.
- Being in familiar surroundings.
- Being in the company of close family and/or friends.

Care Plans

Preparing and forward planning are important when considering future health needs. This may involve writing a treatment escalation plan, an advanced care plan or an anticipatory care plan. Advanced practitioners are well placed to facilitate this process as part of an MDT, with positive open conversations with patients and significant others.

The key components of a care plan are as follows.

1. *Initiation* – propose the conversation and identify who needs to be part of the discussion; gather pertinent background information about who the person is and their underlying presentation, clinical and functional.
2. *Exploration* – present a draft document and identify specific wishes and preferences and discuss what clinical options may be available.
3. *Documentation* – clarify understanding and record preferences, including ceilings of care; consider organ donation and agree review interval.
4. *Sharing* – ensure that the document is shared with all who might need the information, and that the person has their own copy.

There are broadly four levels of treatment escalation which can be shared with a person.

1. *Palliation* – symptom control in the preferred place of care.
2. *Home-based care* with possible oral or intramuscular intervention, or basic intravenous interventions if available locally.
3. *Ward-based care* with no high-dependency care escalations.
4. *Intensive interventions* – including intubation and ventilation.

It is helpful to define some specific possible clinical scenarios for a person to help them understand what might happen in a particular situation, such as lower respiratory tract infection, urinary tract infection, stroke, fall or COVID-19.

Do Not Attempt Cardiopulmonary Resuscitation (DNACPR)

Most NHS Trusts assume that all people are for cardiopulmonary resuscitation (CPR) unless a valid DNACPR decision has been made and documented, or an advanced decision to refuse treatment (ADRT) prohibits CPR. DNACPR decisions are based on legal guidance. Survival rates for CPR for adults are 5–20% depending on the circumstances. In most hospitals, the average survival to discharge rate is 15–20%. Out-of-hospital resuscitation has a survival rate of between 5–10%.

Undertaking the discussion and completing the documentation for DNACPR requires advanced clinical understanding of the person's disease process and trajectories as well as a good understanding of the Mental Capacity Act (2005). This capability is not profession specific, although most forms require an NMC or GMC registration number; HCPC registered professions are also able to complete them with the required capability.

Decisions are categorised as 1A, where CPR is deemed unlikely to be successful and would not be in the person's best interest. This would include terminal diagnoses including frailty and end-stage dementia. The reasons for the unsuccessful CPR need to be clearly articulated on the form. 1 B decisions may be made if CPR may be successful but would lead to a length and quality of life which may not be of overall benefit to the person. The discussion and agreement around this decision need to be clearly documented, and if a person does not have capacity themselves, then family must be included in the conversation. If there are no family available, then an independent mental capacity advocate (IMCA) may be sought. If a Lasting Power of Attorney is in place, they must be included in the discussions. A 1 C decision is when a DNACPR is in accord with the recorded, sustained wishes of the person who is mentally competent.

Pain and Symptom Control

Recognition and management of the last days of life in any care setting are important for the patient and their family as this will influence the family's bereavement and the way they will cope with the loss of their loved one. Frequent symptoms in the last hours of life are pain, restlessness, agitation and terminal respiratory secretions ('death rattle'). Adequate recognition and treatment of these symptoms are vital (BGS Silver Book 2021). During the last days of life, the focus is on relief of symptoms. Pain and shortness of breath can be mostly controlled by continuous opioids delivered intravenously or subcutaneously. In opioid-naive patients, morphine should be started at low doses (10–20 mg intravenously over 24 hours after a bolus of 2 mg in patients with severe pain). For previous opioid users, adequate doses and opioid should be chosen depending on the opioid already used.

Death rattle is caused by respiratory secretions which can no longer be cleared independently. This noisy breathing may be more distressing for the family than for the patient. Giving families information about the origin of the death rattle is the first step. There is some controversy in the literature about the evidence for the use of anticholinergic drugs at the end of life. Anticholinergic medication such as hyoscine hydrobromide (0.5 mg/4 h SC, IM) or glycopyrronium (200–400 µg given every 4–6 hours SC, IM) may be considered if the aim is to diminish the production of respiratory secretions. These drugs can be added to a syringe driver or as a patch to the skin. For patients with terminal restlessness, the use of psychotropic medications, such as midazolam, can be considered and if there are also hallucinations, the use of haloperidol or clotiapine. These can also be delivered subcutaneously. Enteral or parenteral food or fluids have no proven benefit for symptoms of dehydration or prolongation of life and can possibly harm the dying patient. The pros and cons of their use should be discussed with the next of kin.

Advanced practitioners need to be able to recognise end of life and manage the appropriate care. For most people who are dying, this approach will enable management of the symptoms causing discomfort. In complex cases, urgent advice from palliative care teams could be considered.

Verifying Death

Notification of death to a coroner falls under the statutory regulations and can be found in the 2019 legal framework. Anyone verifying death needs to understand the process for notifying the coroner.

Many Trusts will have a training process to enable clinicians other than medical colleagues to undertake the process of verifying a death. This can support families in the event of an expected death as no new personnel need to be involved in the final stage of verification that the end has come. The process has several steps, all of which need to be completed.

1. Confirm the identity of the patient.
2. Inspect for obvious signs of life such as movement and respiratory effort.
3. Assess the patient's response to verbal stimuli (e.g. *'Hello, Mrs Smith, can you hear me?'*).
4. Assess the patient's response to pain using a trapezius squeeze.
5. Assess the patient's pupillary reflexes using a pen torch; after death, the pupils become fixed and dilated.
6. Palpate the carotid artery for a pulse: after death, this will be absent.
7. Perform auscultation to identify any heart or respiratory sounds.
   - Listen for heart sounds for at least **two** minutes.
   - Listen for respiratory sounds for at least **three** minutes.
8. The recommended amount of time to listen for heart and respiratory sounds can vary, but it is generally accepted that a minimum of five minutes of auscultation is required to establish that irreversible cardiorespiratory arrest has occurred.
9. Confirm with family members that the person has died.

Organ Donation

Advanced practitioners (APs) play an important role in helping to support donation. It is important that they are aware of the process as they often play a role in optimising and caring for the donor and supporting the patient's family. Potential donors can save and improve up to eight other people's lives. Organs that can be donated include the heart, lungs, kidneys, liver, pancreas and intestine.

There are two ways in which a person can go on to donate: through donation after cardiac death (DCD) or donation after brainstem death (DBD). During DCD, withdrawal of life-sustaining treatment will take place, usually in theatre, and the wait for patient to reach asystole will begin. When the patient is confirmed dead, they can then be taken into theatre where the operation will begin. For this to happen, the patient must die within a three-hour window. If they do not die, they will usually be taken back to the critical care unit. During DBD, diagnosis of death will be sought through brainstem testing where each of the cranial nerves is assessed via several tests.

Diagnosing Death by Neurological Criteria (Brainstem Death Testing)

When managing a potential organ donor, the aim is to maintain physiological stability as well as possible. Diagnosing death by neurological criteria is completed once a set of tests have been carried out to assess the cranial nerves in the brainstem. This is defined as the irreversible loss of capacity for consciousness, combined with irreversible loss of the capacity to breathe – and therefore irreversible cessation of the integrative function of the brainstem. Preconditions include identifying a cause for the patient's loss of consciousness, excluding reversible and non-neurological causes, and ensuring the patient's physiological stability during testing.

Brainstem function is tested by two senior GMC-registered doctors, one of which must be a consultant; neither can be part of the transplant team. The completion time for the first set of tests denotes the time of death to be registered.

Role of the SN-OD and Referral Process

Once the medical team has determined that further treatment would be futile and the decision has been made to withdraw life-sustaining treatment, the patient can be referred via the National Referral Centre. They will briefly screen the patient and allocate a specialist nurse for organ donation (SN-OD) to the patient. The SN-OD attends the hospital where the patient is located and screens the patient further to see if they are appropriate to donate organs and which organ is acceptable to use. The SN-OD is crucial when discussing the option of donation with the patient or their family. Studies have shown an increase in family consent when a SN-OD leads the donation discussion. Not only do they help with communication between the family and the hospital staff, they support the nursing and medical team and provide expert information on how to manage and optimise a patient going for donation.

Tissue Donation

Where solid organ donation is not suitable, tissue donation may still be considered. Corneas and heart valves are consistently in high demand, with skin, bone, cartilage and tendons all offering transformational life change. As retrieval may be undertaken up to 48 hours after death, the assessment process can be performed after the patient has died by specialist nurses in tissue donation following a referral to the National Referral Centre. The patient does not need to have died in the critical care setting to be considered as a tissue donor.

CLINICAL FRAILTY

Healthy ageing is defined as a process of developing and maintaining the functional ability that enables well-being in older age – with functional ability. Population ageing is accelerating across the globe. The trajectory indicates an increase from 461 million people over 65 in 2004 to an estimated 2 billion by 2050 (Kinsella and Philips 2005). Defining 'later life' is complex, as chronology alone is not an acceptable marker. The clinical condition of frailty is an expression of population ageing (Clegg et al. 2013). Frailty is defined as 'a state of increased vulnerability to poor resolution of homeostasis after a stressor event, which increases the risk of adverse outcomes, including falls, delirium, and disability' (Clegg et al. 2013, p.752).

Diagnosis Tools for Diagnosis and CGA

Determining degrees of frailty can help to determine appropriate interventions (Cameron et al. 2013). Frailty is not synonymous with disability or co-morbidity, although there is some overlap (Syddall et al. 2003). There are a number of markers characterising frailty used by clinicians and researchers. They include a calculation of the accumulation of particular deficits (cumulative deficit model) (Rockwood et al. 2005) (Table 14.2); the seven-point PRISMA clinical frailty score (Table 14.3) (Rockwood et al. 2005);

TABLE 14.2   Rockwood clinical frailty scale.

Clinical Frailty Scale[a]

 1. **Very Fit** – People who are robust, active, energetic and motivated. These people commonly exercise regularly. They are among the fittest for their age.

 2. **Well** – People who have **no active disease symptoms,** but are less fit than category 1. Often, they exercise or are very **active occasionally,** e.g. seasonally.

 3. **Managing Well** – People whose **medical problems are well controlled**, but are **not regularly active** beyond routine walking,

 4. **Vulnerable** – While **not dependent** on others for daily help, often **symptoms limit activities**. A common complaint is being "slowed up", and/or being tired during the day.

 5. **Mildly Frail** – These people often have **more evident slowing**, and need help in **high order IADLS** (finances, transportation, heavy housework, medications). Typically, mild frailty progressively impairs shopping and walking outside alone, meal preparation and housework.

 6. **Moderately Frail** – People need help with **all outside activities** and with **keeping house**. Inside, they often have problems with stairs and need **help with bathing** and might need minimal assistance (cuing standby) with dressing.

 7. **Severely Frail** – **Completely dependent for personal care**, from whatever cause (physical or cognitive). Even so, they seem stable and not at high risk of dying (within - 6 months).

 8. **Very Severely Frail** – Completely dependent. approaching the end of life. Typically, they could not recover even from a minor illness.

 9. **Terminally Ill** – Approaching the end of life. This category applies to people with **a life expectancy <6 months**, who are **not otherwise evidently frail**.

Scoring frailty in people with dementia
The degree of frailty corresponds to the degree of dementia. Common symptoms in mild dementia include forgetting the details of a recent event, though still remembering the event itself repeating the same question/story and social withdrawal. In moderate dementia, recent memory is very impaired, even though they seemingly can remember their past life events well. They can do personal care with prompting In severe dementia, they cannot do personal care without help.

[a] 1. Canadian Study on Health & Aging Revised 2008.
  2. K. Rockwood et al. (2005)A global clinical measure of fitness and frailty in elderly people CMAJ, 173: 489–495, 2007–2009.

TABLE 14.3   PRISMA clinical frailty score.

1. Are you older than **85 years**?
2. Are you **male**?
3. In general, do you have any health problems that require you to **limit you activities**?
4. Do you need someone to **help you on a regular basis**?
5. In general, do you have any health problems that **require you to stay at home**?
6. In case of need, can you **count on someone** close to you?
7. Do you regularly **use a stick, walker or wheelchair** to get about?

evidence of problems in at least two areas of physical, nutritive, sensory and cognitive domains (Strawbridge et al. 1998), dependency or requirements for care from others (Rockwood et al. 2005); grip strength (Syddall et al. 2003); and Timed Up and Go Test (Lyndon and Stevens 2014).

The criteria outlined by Fried et al. (2001) have been most widely accepted and used as an objective marker for frailty (phenotype model). Here, frailty is defined as being present if there is evidence for at least three of the following: weight loss, weakness, exhaustion, slowness and low activity. This can be determined using a five-question questionnaire such as a Modified Cardiovascular Health Study tool (Malmstrom et al. 2014). Older people living with frailty are more likely to be admitted to hospital for an unplanned stay and require care home placement (Oliver et al. 2014). Presence of frailty is also indicative of a higher incidence of falls, disability and mortality (Fried et al. 2001). The accompanying physical and mental impairment often restrict the ability to complete Activities of Daily Living (McPhee et al. 2016). There is a bidirectional link between frailty and psychological well-being (Gale et al. 2014). Any assessment of frailty should be undertaken when the person is well and in their usual environment. If this is not possible then their functional ability two weeks prior to the assessment should be considered, to allow for any acute and reversible decompensation.

Determining frailty status, like any other long-term condition, allows clinicians to plan for specific interventions which may be most appropriate for that person. It should not be used as a service rationalisation tool without specific further clinical assessment. For example, most people living with severe frailty would not be physically able to survive long surgical procedures, but there may be some exceptions, and the frailty score should comprise only one factor for risk benefit analyses. Any person diagnosed with frailty should undergo a CGA, which is a detailed process for identifying a person's health, social and environmental needs. The CGA leads to holistic care planning to enable priorities for life to be set (British Geriatrics Society 2014) (Figure 14.3).

There is mounting evidence for undertaking CGA while in hospital (Turner and Clegg 2014), which reduces the possibility of admission to nursing homes, and there is growing evidence that providing CGA within home and community settings, and nursing homes, could lower hospital admissions and support people to live at home for longer (Lansbury et al. 2017). The CGA comprises a holistic assessment including medical assessment, medication review, goal setting and advanced care planning. The assessment should include components from all relevant members of the MDT. The CGA leads to an individualised care and support plan which may include an anticipatory care plan as well as advanced care planning for escalations in anticipation of deterioration. The priority of the assessment is to rationalise and optimise clinical conditions and manage expectations for the future.

Frailty is likely to increase with ageing, but there are several interventions which can reduce the impact.

Exercise

There is significant evidence that undertaking regular exercise can reduce and decelerate the development of frailty (Merchant et al. 2021). Systematic reviews demonstrate that regular exercise improves functional independence (Merchant et al. 2021). Advanced practitioners should be familiar with recommended guidelines for activity for older people (see Table 14.2) and be confident in prescribing activity for older people.

Nutrition

Sarcopenia, or loss of muscle mass, is a significant factor in frailty, and people with severe frailty often exhibit significant sarcopenia. Oral intake is multifactorial and appetite as well as access to food and oral health can affect nutritional intake.

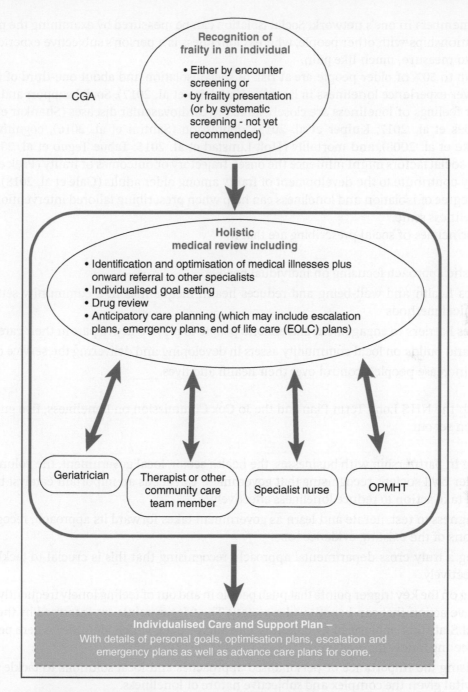

**Recognition of
frailty in an individual**

• Either by encounter
  screening or
• by frailty presentation
  (or by systematic
  screening - not yet
  recommended)

CGA

**Holistic
medical review including**

• Identification and optimisation of medical illnesses plus
  onward referral to other specialists
• Individualised goal setting
• Drug review
• Anticipatory care planning (which may include escalation
  plans, emergency plans, end of life care (EOLC) plans)

Geriatrician

Therapist or other
community care
team member

Specialist nurse

OPMHT

Individualised Care and Support Plan –
With details of personal goals, optimisation plans, escalation and
emergency plans as well as advance care plans for some.

FIGURE 14.3   Fit for Frailty. *Source*: Adapted from Turner and Clegg (2014).

Social Isolation and Loneliness

There is growing evidence relating to social isolation and health. Social isolation is a complex phenomenon that can be characterised by five key attributes: decreased number of social contacts, decreased feeling of belonging, reduced or lack of fulfilling relationships, decreased engagement with others and reduced quality of the members in one's network. Social isolation can be measured by examining the presence or absence of relationships with other people, whereas loneliness is a person's subjective experience and is more difficult to measure, much like pain.

Globally, up to 50% of older people are at risk of social isolation and about one-third of those aged 60 years and over experience loneliness in later life (Landeiro et al. 2017). Social support and social disengagement or feelings of loneliness are closely linked to cardiovascular diseases (Shankar et al. 2011), dementia (Dröes et al. 2017; Kuiper et al. 2015), depression (Santini et al. 2016), cognitive decline, disability (Janke et al. 2008), and mortality (Holt-Lunstad et al. 2015; Tabue Teguo et al. 2016). Taken together, these social factors might influence the onset, trajectory or outcomes of frailty (Peek et al. 2012). Loneliness may contribute to the development of frailty among older adults (Gale et al. 2018). Measures to determine degree of isolation and loneliness can help when prescribing tailored interventions, such as the UCLA loneliness scale.

The core principles of social prescribing are that it:

- is a holistic approach focusing on individual need
- promotes health and well-being and reduces health inequalities in a community setting, using non-clinical methods
- addresses barriers to engagement and enables people to play an active part in their care
- utilises and builds on local community assets in developing and delivering the service or activity
- aims to increase people's control over their health and lives.

In line with the NHS Long Term Plan and the Jo Cox Commission on Loneliness, five guiding principles have been set out.

- Working in partnership with businesses, the health sector, local government, the voluntary sector and wider civil society, recognising that government can act as an important catalyst but that we must all take action to reduce loneliness effectively.
- A willingness to test, iterate and learn as government takes forward its approach, recognising the limitations of the existing evidence base.
- Ensuring a truly cross-departmental approach, recognising that this is crucial to tackling loneliness effectively.
- Focusing on the key trigger points that push people in and out of feeling lonely frequently, alongside preventive action that can benefit wider society. The trigger points are informed by the Office for National Statistics' analysis of Community Life Survey data, which identifies where people are at risk of feeling lonely more often.
- Recognising the importance of personalised approaches and local solutions to tackle loneliness. This is vital given the complex and subjective nature of loneliness.

Advanced practitioners working with people with frailty need to work across systems, using population data and with a good understanding of person-centred care to prescribe appropriate interventions for loneliness.

Case Study

Mrs Jones, who has a Clinical Frailty Score of 7, fell in her kitchen. She lives alone. A neighbour helped her up, and she asked not to go to hospital but needed a review. The Urgent Community Response team attended; there was no long bone fracture, no catastrophic bleed or head injury. A full examination was performed and blood screen taken, leading to a NEWS 2 score of 3 with BP 110/70 and RR 20. No new infection but significant microcytic anaemia, with low ferritin but folate replete, Na 130 and AKI of 1 with eGFR 30. Next day Mrs Jones was painful to mobilise so she was taken to a same-day clinic for pelvic X-ray which showed fractured pubic ramus. Care was started three times a day for personal care and to meet hydration and nutrition needs, with a hot meal delivery at lunch time. Started fumarate 210 mg daily. Provided pressure-relieving and mobility equipment. Repeat blood in three days showed Na 135 and eGFR 45. Ongoing rehabilitation for six weeks to meet goal of preparing own meals again. DNACPR completed for irreversible frailty, and anticipatory care plan with specific goals and treatment escalations was completed.

CONCLUSION

Advanced practice in rehabilitation, discharge planning and end-of-life care is complex and highly skilled, requiring all the diagnostic skills described in other chapters in this book. The role of the advanced practitioner is imperative to smooth pathways and facilitation the best patient outcomes.

Take Home Points
- Better health outcomes are achieved for older people when holistic care is provided, considering 'what matters to me' and addressing social factors such as loneliness, as well as activity levels.
- Highly skilled communication combined with in-depth clinical knowledge is required to support end-of-life care and possible organ donation.
- Pathways into rehabilitation are complex, but an advanced practitioner needs to fully understand 'what matters to me' for each person in their care in order to ensure they have access to appropriate recovery and intermediate care options.

REFERENCES

British Geriatrics Society (2014) "The BGS Toolkit for Comprehensive Geriatric Assessment in Primary Care Setting" CGA in Primary Care Settings.pdf (bgs.org.uk) Last accessed June 2023.

British Geriatrics Society (2021). Silver Book. www.bgs.org.uk/resources/silver-book-ii-geriatric-syndromes

Cameron, I., Fairhall, N., Langron, C. et al. (2013). A multifactorial interdisciplinary intervention reduces frailty in older people: randomized trail. *BioMed Central* 11: 65.

Clegg, A., Young, J., Iliffe, S. et al. (2013). Frailty in elderly people. *Lancet* 38: 752–762.

Cowley, A., Goldberg, S., Gordon, K.M., and Logan, P. (2021). Exploring rehabilitation potential in older people living with frailty: a qualitative focus group study. *BMC Geriatrics* 21 (1): 1–11.

from them (Lang 2019). Unconscious bias functions below the level of consciousness and is evolutionary in nature, arising from a time when speed was more important than accuracy, leading to information processing shortcuts. It is associated with, amongst other things, stereotypes, social influence and emotional and moral motivation. It requires work and self-awareness to identify it in yourself, and in others, as it can also be institutional and societal.

There are numerous identified unconscious biases and we recommend you become more familiar with them, as this will allow you to identify the bias(es) that you or your colleagues/service may be most prone to. One example of unconscious bias is ascertainment bias, whereby we see what we expect to see, like a self-fulfilling prophecy. This can be linked to diagnostic overshadowing, and confirmation bias, whereby we look for information that confirms what we suspect/think and disregard information that does not fit the picture.

MENTAL HEALTH AND ETHNICITY

MIND (2021) has identified several noteworthy facts in relation to mental health and ethnicity. Black men are more likely to have experienced a psychotic disorder in the last year than white men. Additionally, black people are four times more likely to be detained under the Mental Health Act than white people; older south Asian women are an at-risk group for suicide; refugees and asylum seekers are more likely to experience mental health problems than the general population, including higher rates of depression, anxiety and posttraumatic stress disorder (PTSD). People of Indian, Pakistani and African-Caribbean origin show higher levels of mental well-being than other ethnic groups. Suicidal thoughts and self-harm are less common in Asian people than Caucasian people. Mental ill health is lower among Chinese people than in Caucasian people. The caveat to this is there may be underreporting from some communities, perhaps amongst other issues in relation to stigma and different cultural perceptions of mental illness.

COMMUNICATION

Working with these client groups requires an expert communicator, with high-level interpersonal skills. We have already touched on self-awareness and will now look at the basic principles of therapeutic communication and specific skills to think about in communicating with clients who have autism spectrum disorder (ASD) and/or LD or who are mentally unwell.

Therapeutic Communication

It can be difficult to define therapeutic communication precisely. Van Servellan (1997) defines therapeutic communication thus: 'interpersonal exchange, using verbal and non-verbal messages, that culminates in someone's being helped to overcome stress, anxiety, fear, or other emotional experiences that cause distress' (van Servallen 1997, p.30). This could describe any client in our service(s) so therapeutic communication should underpin all our communication in healthcare settings.

Fundamental Principles of Therapeutic Communication

Epstein et al. (2000) have suggested that all therapeutic communication is based on a therapeutic relationship with the client, which is determined by your therapeutic use of self Therapeutic use of self is the ability to use your personality consciously and in full awareness to establish a relationship with your client. Therapeutic communication always has a context. Things to be aware of in yourself and, if possible, your client are your/their values, attitudes and beliefs; culture and spirituality; gender, social status, age and developmental level (Epstein et al. 2000). These all determine how you both will interact and react to each other.

Some techniques for therapeutic communication include providing rationale, open-ended questioning, active listening techniques, non-verbal and verbal cues to continue the conversation, reflecting, exploring feeling tones, silence, clarification, non-verbal communication through expression, stance and gestures, summarising (Sharma and Gupta 2022).

Specific Issues in Communication Clients with ASD/LD

Communication is key when assessing an autistic person or a person with a learning disability. Where people use language, it is important to remember to keep our language simple and to slow down our speech. It is likely that the person you are communicating with is anxious, which will affect their ability to take in and understand information, even if they are usually able to. Easy-read guides, such as those available through EasyHealth, can help. These are free resources and mean that your patient can take information away with them to digest in their own time. Writing things down, drawing pictures or diagrams can also help, as can using any visual communication method. Body maps are a good example – these can help a person to point to a picture and show you where something hurts, rather than having to try and describe it. Some people may use a signing system such as Makaton or Signalong and may want to bring a supporter who can help them to communicate in this or any other way. Since this takes time, you may wish to consider double appointments, and appointments at the beginning of a clinic, where the person will not have to wait for so long, as waiting can increase anxiety. The most important thing is a willingness to communicate, to listen to behaviour and clinical signs and symptoms as well as words, and to adapt to meet that individual's needs.

CLINICAL INVESTIGATIONS

Mental Health Screening Tools

There are a multitude of screening tools that can be used in the assessment of mental health issues and as a pointer to further services, including specialist services if required. The two most used screening tools, which you may be familiar with, are the Generalised Anxiety Disorder 7 (GAD 7) and the Patient Health Questionnaire 9 (PHQ 9). The first screens for symptoms of anxiety and the second for depression. Depression is said to be the predominant mental health issue worldwide, followed by anxiety (Vos et al. 2013). If you or your service choose to use screening tools, you must ensure there is a clinical governance structure around them, including prescribed actions in relation to any score.

Holistic Mental Health Assessment

While we are focusing on holistic assessment in mental health, we would also like to suggest that all assessments should be/are holistic, as we work with an individual person and their systems, both internal and external, which impacts on their health presentation(s), hence the use of a biopsychosocial framework as a basis for assessment.

The biopsychosocial framework offers a basis for understanding the impact of an illness presentation, whether acute or chronic, on a person's life and how that may be expressed in the biological, psychological and social domains. This allows for a more in-depth understanding and synthesis of information gathered to inform the formulation of the person's difficulties and leads directly to a more targeted specific management plan. This use of the biopsychosocial model in mental health has more recently been supported in the proposed Research Domain Criteria (RDoC) by the National Institute of Mental Health (NIMH) as part of a framework for research into mental health which brings both physical and mental health together, rather than looking at them separately, which has been an issue in the past (Bolton and Gillett 2019).

To undertake holistic assessments in mental health within a biopsychosocial framework, it is necessary to consider the following.

- Interpersonal skills and therapeutic communication, which we have looked at in more detail earlier in the chapter.
- The purpose of the assessment and any limitations to what you and your service can offer.

Some useful questions to think about before undertaking a mental health assessment are contained in this short precis from Garlick and Rhodes (2011) below.

WHY

This is usually based on information from the referrer and/or carers or other agencies. Consider whether the person knows they have been referred. Why have they been referred now? Triggers? What is the level of risk? Do they have a communication issue?

WHAT

What is the aim of the assessment? Is it an emergency? Are you assessing whether the person can be treated at your service or for treatment elsewhere?

WHERE?

Where will the assessment take place? Your service, home, online? Risk in relation to environment should be considered here.

WHO?

Who should undertake the assessment? Should it be a joint assessment? Should parents/carers be there? Do you need an interpreter?

WHEN?

This is based on local definitions of timelines for emergencies: is this an emergency; is it urgent; is it routine?

Other issues to consider in a mental health assessment include the following.

- Whether your service has a local protocol for conducting a mental health assessment.
- The reason for referral, including the perception of the person being referred and the referrer/carer perception of the referral as appropriate, particularly in relation to how much you involve a carer.
- Individual information including personal history, spiritual beliefs and cultural practices.
- Mental and physical health history past and current, including medication.
- Substance use.
- Current social circumstances.
- Synthesis and formulation.

All mental health assessments must include a mental state examination (MSE).

Ten-point Guide to Mental State Examination

Examples of what to look for in each category from Hufton et al. (2022).

- *Appearance*: posture, gait, dress, self-care, physical health
- *Behaviour*: facial expression, eye contact
- *Speech*: rate and flow, volume
- *Mood*: how does the patient describe how they are feeling?
- *Affect*: patient's expression, what you observe
- *Thoughts*: what does the patient talk about? Any abnormalities?
- *Perception*: consider the presence of hallucinations
- *Cognition*: an awareness of self and environment; do they know what day it is, etc.?
- *Insight*: do they recognise and understand their experiences? What is their understanding of the problem?
- *Clinical judgement and risk assessment*: summarise your findings, including an assessment of risk.

Risk Assessment in Mental Health

Risk assessment is an essential and intrinsic component of any mental health assessment. There are three primary risks to consider in a mental health assessment.

- Risk to self (self-harm, suicidality, neglect, substance use, etc.)
- Risk to others (violence)
- Risk from others (safeguarding). This is the risk that is most often overlooked in a mental health presentation. It needs to be remembered that these are vulnerable adults and safeguarding must always be considered.

RED FLAGS

Taken from the UK Mental Health Triage Scale

Emergency

- Current actions endangering self or others
- Overdose/suicide attempt/violent aggression
- Possession of a weapon
- Suicide

Very high risk

- Acute suicidal ideation or risk of harm to others with clear plan or means
- Ongoing history of self-harm or aggression with intent
- Very high-risk behaviour associated with perceptual or thought disturbance, delirium, dementia or impaired impulse control

High risk

- Suicidal ideation with no plan or ongoing history of suicidal ideas with possible intent
- Rapidly increasing symptoms of psychosis and/or severe mood disorder
- High-risk behaviour associated with perceptual or thought disturbance, delirium, dementia or impaired impulse control
- Overt/unprovoked aggression in care home or hospital ward setting
- Wandering at night (community)
- Vulnerable isolation or abuse

Moderate risk

- Significant patient/carer distress associated with severe mental illness (but not suicidal)/absent insight/early symptoms of psychosis
- Resistive aggression/obstructed care delivery
- Wandering (hospital) or during the day (community)
- Isolation/failing carer or known situation requiring priority intervention or assessment (Sands et al. 2016).

Assessing Different Groups

Assessing Children and Young People

It is not within the scope of this chapter to go into detail here, but you should always assess a young person in the context of their wider systems (family, school, etc.) and genograms are a very useful way to obtain a history and identify patterns. A genogram is a diagram outlining the history of the behaviour patterns (e.g. divorce or suicide) of a family over several generations (Merriam Webster 2022). It is a useful tool to engage the family with their story and to highlight both mental and physical health issues generationally.

Assessing People with Autism

Autism is a lifelong condition believed to be caused by a diverse range of neurological differences, which result in characteristic social interaction and communication difficulties, as well as restricted and repetitive behaviours. We often hear autism described as a 'spectrum', meaning that there are wide-ranging severities and symptoms, characterised by social communication deficits and restricted, repetitive and inflexible patterns of behaviour, interests or activities. Sensory processing issues are also a recognised part of the condition (Fernandez-Prieto et al. 2021). This can make carrying out a clinical assessment and history taking more complex. It should be borne in mind that some, though not all, autistic people also have a learning disability (see below), which will also affect their understanding and communication skills.

People with autism experience the full range of physical and mental illnesses as the general population, and although research into the health of autistic people is limited, there is evidence that there is a greater prevalence of physical and mental health co-morbidity in this group (Sala et al. 2020; Cashin et al. 2018). Autistic children seem to be more likely to be overweight and obese than their neurotypical peers, and have higher rates of CNS anomalies, bowel disease, diabetes mellitus and epilepsy than their neurotypical peers (Kohane 2012). The autistic adult population shows increased prevalence of constipation, epilepsy, sleep disorders and psychiatric disorders. Rates of hyperlipidaemia and hypertension are also increased; however, this group receives less treatment for these conditions (Cashin et al. 2018). Some studies also show increased hospitalisations and surgeries (Jones 2015), which could indicate that symptoms have been overlooked in the earlier stages, due to communication difficulties and/or diagnostic overshadowing, which we have addressed earlier in the chapter. People with autism often live with anxiety (Spain et al. 2018) and are more likely to live with some mental health conditions such as anxiety disorders, depression and schizophrenia (Hollocks et al. 2019; Zeng et al. 2021; Cashin et al. 2018; Kohane 2012).

Although the range of physical and mental conditions experienced by people with autism are the same as in the general population, albeit with differing prevalence in some cases, symptoms may present atypically. Evidence suggests that people with autism respond to pain atypically, being hyposensitive in some instances and not recognising or responding to illness or injury, and hypersensitive in others, experiencing extreme pain in response to a stimulus that would not cause such a response in a neurotypical person (Liu et al. 2020). The combination of these atypical responses and difficulties in communication can make it problematic for a clinician to assess pain accurately.

Clinical observation is key – an autistic person may respond to being asked 'How are you feeling?' by saying that they are OK, but appear pale and clammy and have a resting pulse rate of 120. In this instance, clearly, further investigation is required. Asking more direct questions, such as 'Do you have pain?' and 'Where is the pain?' may help if the patient communicates verbally. If they do not, then attention needs to be paid to their behaviour, and observed behaviour change. Family and carers are a good source of information, and their input should be sought. Stereotypical and self-injurious behaviours can also be a sign of an underlying physical health problem (Summers et al. 2017).

Unfortunately, these behaviours are sometimes erroneously attributed solely to the person having autism, and they are left with untreated illness or pain. Whether or not it is because of hyposensitivity to pain, atypical pain expression or issues with social skills and communicating pain, the fact remains that this can impede diagnosis and lead to poorer health outcomes for this group. One of the ways in which this can be addressed is by expanding clinicians' knowledge and understanding of autism, so that they are prepared for these issues. Various pain assessment tools are available to support practitioners in assessing pain and discomfort. These use clinician or carer reports to observe and assess behavioural manifestations of pain, such as facial expressions, vocalisations, body movements, etc. The Non-communicating Children's Pain Checklist is one such tool which has been validated for children with autism (Courtemanche et al. 2016). The revised Face, Legs, Activity, Cry, Consolability Scale is another (Dubois et al. 2017).

Although at the time of writing, there is no validated tool specifically for children with autism, these tools can still be effective inasmuch as they focus the clinician on the need to look for more than verbal confirmation of pain or illness, and to consider behaviour as well as description in their assessment.

For adults, the Non-communcating Adults Pain Checklist has been used effectively (Garcia-Villamisar et al. 2019); this too uses non-verbal pain responses to gauge the patient's pain. Clinical observations of physiological responses to pain and distress, such as heart rate, blood pressure, O_2 saturation and respiratory rate, should be combined with this information to support a thorough assessment (Liu et al. 2020).

The effect of anxiety on the individual's ability to engage with assessment should not be underrated. As well as exacerbating pain, anxiety can further limit any individual's ability to communicate effectively. This effect is amplified for people with autism, who are likely to find the events before and during a clinical assessment difficult. Small considerations and changes can be very useful in relieving some of this anxiety. For instance, familiarising people with the room, with a visit, photos or videos before the assessment, meeting the clinician beforehand, ensuring that waiting time is limited (the first appointment of the day or after lunch perhaps), and holding the assessment in a quiet, calm environment can all contribute to a successful outcome.

The use of alternative communication methods, such as socials stories and simple (perhaps easy read for some) written information to prepare for a visit can be helpful.

In the assessment, using pictures, signs and symbols can help people who have a learning disability as well as autism. Body maps are a useful tool to aid people in pinpointing and communicating pain. These are simple strategies but require the clinician to understand the individual and to make reasonable adjustments to their practice that are suitable to that person. Again, information from carers and family can be particularly useful here.

Mental health also needs consideration when assessing an autistic individual. The Psychiatric Autism Checklist (Helverschou et al. 2009) has been found to be useful in identifying autistic adults who need psychiatric services. This again relies on carers and family members providing reports on which the clinicians base their assessment.

Finally, the environment in which the assessment is undertaken should be carefully considered in relation to the sensory processing issues that autistic people experience. Busy, noisy, smelly, cluttered, bright environments are likely to be overwhelming and lead to additional stress, making assessment harder for the clinician and very unpleasant or even painful for the patient. Consider making simple changes to the environment, such as shutting doors or blinds to eliminate noise or glare, or find a quiet spot. Double appointments to allow extra time, and appointments at the beginning of a clinic where there will be little waiting could be arranged. All these things would be considered reasonable adjustments under the Equality Act (2010).

Assessing People with Learning Disability

There is considerable overlap between autism and learning disability, although the exact prevalence rates are hard to establish (Dunn et al. 2019). As such, many of the considerations discussed above for autistic people will also apply to those with a learning disability. Information about the specific health issues of people with autism is relatively new, but decades of research have highlighted the health inequalities and premature deaths experienced by people with a learning disability (Perera et al. 2020).

The most recent information at the time of this publication from the Learning Disability Mortality Review (LEDER) suggests that the median age at death for people with learning disabilities is 23 years younger for males and 27 years younger for females, and that preventable deaths are more prevalent (LEDER 2020). The 2019 Action from Learning LEDER report (NHS England 2019) cites sepsis, cancer, constipation and dysphagia as focus areas, so it makes sense to be particularly aware of the signs and symptoms associated with these conditions when assessing people with a learning disability.

Various early warning tools have been developed in recent years to flag sepsis. The NEWS 2 is one of the more widely used scales, providing a risk score based on clinical observations. However, the data required to assess risk may be difficult to assess in people with a learning disability, particularly those with a more severe disability. It is also difficult to assess the level of consciousness if the person's normal level of communication and cognitive abilities are not known, and any monitoring of oxygen saturation may be skewed if the patient with learning disabilities is not able to use an oxygen enrichment device consistently. As a result, the 'STOP AnD WATCH' tool was developed to monitor 'soft signs' of sepsis. This tool recognises that most people with a learning disability are supported by social care staff or family, who may not have the medical knowledge to use an early warning scale such as the NEWS 2 but are likely to know the person well, and know that something is not right (Table 15.1).

Cancer rates are still lower than in the general population, although there is suggestion that this could be due to underdiagnosis or late diagnosis, or relatively lower rates of smoking and drinking (Perera et al. 2020; Will et al. 2018). Gastrointestinal disorders, including GI cancers, however, seem to have a higher prevalence in this group, and this should be borne in mind when assessing people with a learning disability, especially if they present with GI symptoms. There is currently a national focus on the early detection of cancers in the general population, and this must be extended to those with a learning disability. This can be challenging when assessing a person with a more severe learning disability where we cannot rely on self-report. The concerns of families and carers should be listened too and their concerns regarding behaviour change or a 'feeling that something is wrong' should be taken seriously. There is a tendency in the medical professions to assume that people with learning disabilities will not be compliant with tests or investigations when this need not be the case. With the right support from the local learning disability nursing team, this can be overcome to ensure that people with learning disabilities are able to access health investigations and treatments equitably.

Constipation is a significant issue for people with learning disabilities, and is particularly associated with cerebral palsy and immobility, as well as poor diet and fluid intake, particularly for those with dysphagia (Robertson et al. 2018; Maslen et al. 2022). It is a cause of preventable hospitalisation, and if not treated can lead, and has led, to death (LEDER 2020). Once more, when assessing a person with a learning disability, non-verbal signs and symptoms of discomfort should be considered as well as clinical signs. Some of these will be more obvious, such as infrequent bowel movements, hard, dry stools, discomfort or pain on passing a stool, abdominal bloating, pain or discomfort. In a person who does not

TABLE 15.1 'Soft signs' of sepsis – STOP AnD WATCH

- Seems different from usual
- Talks or communicates less than usual
- Overall needs more help than usual
- Participates in activities less than usual
- Ate less than usual (not because of dislike of food)
- N . . .
- Drinks less than usual
- Weight change
- Agitated or nervous more than usual
- Tired, weak, confused or drowsy
- Change in skin colour or condition
- Help with walking, transferring or toileting more than usual

use words to communicate, there may be behaviour change or they may try to remove faeces from the rectum manually, so faeces under the fingernails or wiped in unusual places should also be considered a potential symptom.

RED FLAGS

Dysphagia is linked to constipation, as it may contribute to suboptimal dietary and fluid intake. It is also implicated in aspiration pneumonia, which is a significant cause of death in the learning-disabled population (LEDER 2020). There is an increased prevalence of eating, drinking and swallowing difficulties in the LD population. More severe LD, cerebral palsy and Down syndrome are associated with increased rates of dysphagia (Roberston et al. 2017). Dysphagia has long been acknowledged as a health risk for people with learning disabilities, leading to choking and death (PHE 2016). It is also a significant contributing factor to deaths caused by aspiration pneumonia – a leading cause of death among people with learning disabilities. It is therefore important to recognise and act on symptoms and involve speech and language professionals for assessment and support as necessary. Some common symptoms can be seen in Table 15.2.

Failure to recognise and act upon these symptoms can lead to serious health issues and death, so knowledge of them is crucial. For example, respiratory conditions remain a leading cause of death and, more importantly, a leading cause of preventable death in the LD population. This links with the higher dysphagia rate, since aspiration pneumonia is a notable contributing factor in respiratory deaths, and some notable serious case reviews. Practitioners need to be aware of the potential seriousness of respiratory conditions for this group, and to look for underlying causes, rather than simply treating the pneumonia/infection.

Additionally, diabetes mellitus is estimated to be twice as common in people with learning disabilities compared to the general population. People with learning disabilities are also more likely to be admitted to hospital with complications of diabetes. This is likely to be linked to higher obesity rates and the prescription of antipsychotic medications, poor diet and poor self-management skills (House et al. 2018). It is important to recognise that patients who are mentally unwell, are autistic or have a learning disability may not be able to self-report symptoms verbally, so clinicians need to be aware of behaviour changes and physical observations that could indicate diabetes, such as increased fatigue/lethargy or changes to drinking and toileting patterns.

TABLE 15.2   Some common symptoms.

- Inability to swallow
- Pain on swallowing
- Regurgitating food
- A sensation that food is stuck in the throat or chest
- Unexplained weight loss
- Developing repeated and frequent lung infections
- Frequent chest infections
- Change in colour when eating and drinking
- Watering eyes when eating and drinking
- Breathlessness after swallowing
- Vomiting regularly after eating/drinking
- Refusing food/drink
- Distress when eating/drinking

A Note on Challenging Behaviour

The pain or discomfort caused by physical conditions, injury or ill health is recognised in the literature as being expressed through behaviour, and sometimes as challenging behaviour (de Winter et al. 2011; de Knegt et al. 2013). Unfortunately, this is sometimes misunderstood or ignored, attributed to being 'just what people with learning disabilities do'. This of course is not the case and can be dangerous. This is termed 'diagnostic overshadowing' and has been acknowledged as a contributory factor in health inequality and the premature deaths of people with learning and intellectual disabilities (Doody and Bailey 2019; Mencap 2007, 2012). This has also been discussed in relation to mental health earlier in the chapter. As such, it is vital that behaviour change or exacerbated challenging behaviour is seen as a potential indicator of pain or ill health (Doody and Bailey 2019; Breau and Camfield 2011; Findlay et al. 2015), and a full physical health assessment should be carried out to rule out any physical cause.

Evidence suggests that mental illness is more common in people with learning and intellectual disabilities, with some studies suggesting that it is twice as prevalent (Cooper et al. 2007; Hatton et al. 2017; Dunn et al. 2019). Symptoms of mental ill health can be difficult to spot in people with learning disabilities, and autistic people, especially where people do not use speech or there are communication issues. It is easy for mental illness to be overlooked or for diagnostic overshadowing to come into play. For this reason, mental health checking should be integral to overall health assessment and should also be considered as part of the plan to support individuals with challenging behaviour, particularly if there has been behaviour change.

PHARMACOLOGICAL PRINCIPLES

The same universal principles that apply for all patients should also be followed in relation to pharmacology for both these client groups. Most psychiatric disorders use both psychosocial and pharmacological interventions. In relation specifically to mental health patients who use medication to help manage their illness, concordance may be an issue, especially for those whose symptoms are severe. Not taking a prescribed medication can lead to worsening of the illness, further interventions and admission to hospital. The input and expertise of a pharmacist is said to be good practice when prescribing and monitoring a medication for severe mental health conditions (RPS 2022).

There are four primary types of medication for mental health problems (MIND 2022).

- *Hypnotics and anxiolytics* – these medications can be prescribed for severe anxiety or insomnia (difficulty getting to sleep or staying asleep).
- *Antidepressants* – usually for moderate to severe depression. Some are also licensed to treat anxiety, phobias, bulimia and some physical conditions, including managing severe pain.
- *Antipsychotics* – to reduce the symptoms of schizophrenia, schizoaffective disorder, psychosis and sometimes severe anxiety or bipolar disorder, as well as the psychotic symptoms of a personality disorder. Some are also licensed to treat physical problems, such as persistent hiccups, problems with balance and nausea (feeling sick), agitation and psychotic experiences in dementia. This is only recommended if there is a risk to self or others, or in severe distress.
- *Lithium and other mood stabilisers* – licensed to be used as part of the treatment for bipolar disorder, mania and hypomania, recurrent, severe depression and schizoaffective disorder. Lithium, anticonvulsants and antipsychotics are the three main types of medication which are used as mood stabilisers.

When working with people with learning disabilities, it is important to consider their ability to take oral medications, particularly in tablet form, as some may have dysphagia or other musculoskeletal or sensory issues that make swallowing tablets problematic. Liquid forms of medications can be considered, or patches. Since it is known that autistic adults and those with a learning disability are more likely to be both over- and underweight than the general population, this should be considered when considering dosage.

The overmedication of people with learning disabilities and/or autism has been an issue for many years (Branford et al. 2018), including the use of psychotropic drugs without a clear association with their primary indication. Prescribing such medicines as an intervention for challenging behaviour, without considering physical and environmental/contextual causes for the behaviour, is also an ongoing problem. The STOMP campaign was set up to address this as part of the Transforming Care agenda. Practitioners need to be aware of the issue of overmedication and other available interventions to ensure that questions are asked before medication is prescribed as a default, and to make sure that people receive holistic, high-quality care.

Case Studies

Mental health

M is a 30-year-old single woman who lives alone. She works as a secretary. She was admitted to an acute psychiatric ward after being found singing loudly in a neighbour's garden dressed only in her night clothes. Her neighbours reported that she had not been herself since breaking up with her boyfriend two weeks ago. She had become verbally aggressive and started asking them to join her plan to save the world. She had also started playing loud music during the night which had led to a visit by the police. She was admitted to a psychiatric unit two years ago following an overdose of an antidepressant. She was seen by a psychiatrist in the community 10 months ago when she was reported to be 'very happy and overfamiliar with strangers in the street'. She was prescribed lithium but did not take it regularly. Her mother, who committed suicide when M was 15 years old, according to her father, experienced similar problems to M.

- What are the risks relating to violence, self-harm/suicide and self-neglect in this case?
- What factors may increase the risk of violence, self-harm/suicide and self-neglect?
- What are the current and potential risks?
- What would a risk management plan look like?

LEARNING DISABILITY

Lydia is a 47-year-old white British woman who is autistic and has a severe learning disability. She does not use words to communicate, but will lead staff to what she wants, and make sounds to indicate her mood.

Lydia has no family supporting her, but lives with two other people with learning disabilities and is supported by a team of social care support workers.

Her team have been worried about her for some time, as she has seemed 'out of sorts' for some months. They have taken her to the GP, who has not ordered any tests, and has said she probably has had a virus.

Lydia's symptoms are as follows.

- Increased unhappy/distressed sounds.
- Reluctance/refusal to engage with preferred activities.
- Decreased appetite and weight loss.
- Abdominal bloating.
- Increased incontinence of urine.
- Irregular periods.

What might be the potential causes of her symptoms?
What should happen next?

RESOURCES

Learning Disability Learning Event

Look at the following resource about supporting people with learning disability and diabetes:

- Diabetes UK – How to make reasonable adjustments to diabetes care for adults with a learning disability. www.diabetes.org.uk/resources-s3/2018-02/Diabetes%20UK%20-%20How%20to%20make%20reasonable%20adjustments%20to%20diabetes%20care%20for%20adults%20with%20a%20learning%20disability.pdf

Do you know if any of these adjustments are in place at your local diabetes service? Would the reasonable adjustments they describe apply to your place of work? What would a similar guide for your place of work look like?

Mental Health Learning Event

World Mental Health Day is run by the World Federation for Mental Health. It occurs with a different theme each October. The theme for 2022 was: 'Make mental health and wellbeing for all a global priority'.

Mental Health UK are partnering with ITN Productions Industry News to produce Play Your Part, a digital news-style programme highlighting how everyone has a role to play when it comes to the future of mental health.

Mental Health UK states

'The programme will raise awareness around the cost-of-living crisis and the affect this has on mental health, highlight the positive stories surrounding the recovery phase of the pandemic and showcase the changing conversations around mental health in the workplace. Showing how prevention is key, the programme will also explore the importance of educating the digital first generation at an early age, provide information to empower individuals to understand and manage their own mental health and will highlight the role of the NHS and local community initiatives'.

Please watch this programme: www.youtube.com/watch?v=mQT26jD4AZg

CONCLUSION

Working with people who are mentally unwell, have a learning disability or are autistic requires a high degree of self-awareness, enhanced and advanced communication skills, as well as a deep understanding of the conditions. This chapter cannot possibly cover the depth or breadth of information that is really required to fully appreciate the needs and complexities of these populations. However, we hope that by highlighting the principles that underpin the work, such as parity of esteem, diagnostic overshadowing, including unconscious bias, some of the risks, red flags and providing information on what to look out for along with some suggestions for resources and interventions, this chapter will encourage clinicians to consider the needs of these groups and focus more attention on their needs. There are, of course, experts in the fields of mental health, autism and learning disability who can and should be consulted, and often a multidisciplinary approach is called for when working with individuals who are mentally unwell, have a learning disability or are autistic.

Good-quality care for these groups hinges upon a commitment to therapeutic communication, holism, making reasonable adjustments and providing person-centred care, as well as an appreciation of the value of all individuals. Only then will we begin to address the huge health inequalities that still exist for these individuals and achieve true parity of esteem.

Take Home Points

- Advanced-level practitioners must understand the importance of their own mental health and be aware of diagnostic overshadowing and potential unconscious/cognitive bias.

- Communication skills must be effectively tailored to the client's needs. Adaptive communication is encouraged within clinical practice and offers enhanced interaction and patient safety.

- Underpinning evidence-based practice remains imperative and should be used by all advanced practitioners inclusive of the use of frameworks. A patient-centred, individualised and therapeutic approach enhances the quality of care that is offered.

REFERENCES

Baker, C and Gheera, M. (2020). Mental Health: Achieving 'parity of esteem'. House of Commons Library. https://commonslibrary.parliament.uk/mental-health-achieving-parity-of-esteem/

Bolton, D. and Gillett, G. (2019). The Biopsychosocial Model of Health and Disease: New Philosophical and Scientific Developments. www.ncbi.nlm.nih.gov/books/NBK552028

Branford, D., Gerrard, D., Saleem, N. et al. (2018). Stopping over-medication of people with an intellectual disability, autism or both (STOMP) in England part 2 – the story so far. *Advances in Mental Health and Intellectual Disabilities* 13 (1): 41–51.

Breau, L.M. and Camfield, C.S. (2011). The relation between children's pain behaviour and developmental characteristics: a cross-sectional study. *Developmental Medicine and Child Neurology* 53 (2): e1–e7.

Cashin, A., Buckley, T., Trollor, J.N., and Lennox, N. (2018). A scoping review of what is known of the physical health of adults with autism spectrum disorder. *Journal of Intellectual Disabilities* 22 (1): 96–108.

Centre for Mental Health (2013). Parity of esteem: a briefing note. www.centreformentalhealth.org.uk/publications/parity-esteem-briefing-note

Cooper, S.A., Smiley, E., Morrison, J. et al. (2007). Mental ill-health in adults with intellectual disabilities: prevalence and associated factors. *British Journal of Psychiatry* 190 (1): 27–35.

Courtemanche, A.B., Black, W.R., and Reese, R.M. (2016). The relationship between pain, self-injury, and other problem behaviors in young children with autism and other developmental disabilities. *American Journal on Intellectual and Developmental Disabilities* 121 (3): 194–203.

Doody, O. and Bailey, M.E. (2019). Understanding pain physiology and its application to person with intellectual disability. *Journal of Intellectual Disabilities* 23 (1): 5–18.

Dubois, A., Michelon, C., Rattaz, C. et al. (2017). Daily living pain assessment in children with autism: exploratory study. *Research in Developmental Disabilities* 62: 238–246.

Dunn, K., Rydzewska, E., Macintyre, C. et al. (2019). The prevalence and general health status of people with intellectual disabilities and autism co-occurring together: a total population study. *Journal of Intellectual Disability Research* 63 (4): 277–285.

Epstein, R.M., Borrell, F., and Caterina, M. (2000). Communication and mental health in primary care. In: *New Oxford Textbook of Psychiatry* (ed. M.G. Gelder, J.J. López-Ibor, and N.C. Andreasen). Oxford: Oxford University Press.

Fernandez-Prieto, M., Moreira, C., Cruz, S. et al. (2021). Executive functioning: a mediator between sensory processing and behaviour in autism spectrum disorder. *Journal of Autism and Developmental Disorders* 51: 2091–2103.

Findlay, L., Williams, A., Baum, S., and Scior, K. (2015). Caregiver experiences of supporting adults with intellectual disabilities in pain. *Journal of Applied Research in Intellectual Disabilities* 28 (2): 111–120.

Garcia-Villamisar, D., Moore, D., and Garcia-Martínez, M. (2019). Internalizing symptoms mediate the relation between acute pain and autism in adults. *Journal of Autism and Developmental Disorders* 49 (1): 270–278.

Garlick, D. and Rhodes, L. (2011). *Holistic Adult Mental Health Assessment Tool*. Shoreham-by-Sea: Pavilion.

Hatton, C., Emerson, E., Robertson, J., and Baines, S. (2017). The mental health of British adults with intellectual impairments living in general households. *Journal of Applied Research in Intellectual Disabilities* 30 (1): 188–197.

Helverschou, S.B., Bakken, T.L., and Martinsen, H. (2009). The psychopathology in autism checklist (PAC): a pilot study. *Research in Autism Spectrum Disorders* 3 (1): 179–195.

Hollocks, M.J., Lerh, J.W., Magiati, I. et al. (2019). Anxiety and depression in adults with autism spectrum disorder: a systematic review and meta-analysis. *Psychological Medicine* 49 (4): 559–572.

House, A., Bryant, L., Russell, A.M. et al. (2018). Managing with learning disability and diabetes: OK-diabetes, a case-finding study and feasibility randomised controlled trial. *Health Technology Assessment* 22 (26): 1–328.

Hufton, F., Petch, J., and Rege, S. (2022). Ten Point Guide to Mental State Examination (MSE) in Psychiatry. www.psychscenehub.com

Jones, K.B. (2015). A description of medical conditions in adults with autism spectrum disorder: a follow-up of the 1980s Utah/UCLA autism epidemiologic study. *Autism* 20 (5): 551–561.

Jones, S., Howard, L., and Thornicroft, G. (2008). Diagnostic overshadowing: worse physical health care for people with mental illness. *Acta Psychiatric Scandinavica* 118: 169–171.

de Knegt, N.C., Pieper, M.J., Lobbezoo, F. et al. (2013). Behavioral pain indicators in people with intellectual disabilities: a systematic review. *Journal of Pain* 14 (9): 885–896.

Kohane, I.S. (2012). The co-morbidity burden of children and young adults with autism spectrum disorders. *PLoS One* 7 (4): e33224.

Lang, R. (2019). What is the difference between conscious and unconscious bias? Online course. https:// engageinlearning.com/faq/compliance/unconscious-bias/what-is-the-difference-between-conscious-and-unconscious-bias

LEDER (2020). The Learning Disability Mortality Review (LeDeR) programme Annual Report; University of Bristol.

Liu, J., Chen, L.L., Shen, S. et al. (2020). Challenges in the diagnosis and management of pain in individuals with autism spectrum disorder. *Review Journal of Autism and Developmental Disorders* 7 (4): 352–363.

Maslen, C., Hodge, R., Tie, K. et al. (2022). Constipation in autistic people and people with learning disabilities. *British Journal of General Practice* 72 (720): 348–351.

MENCAP (2007). *Death by Indifference*. London: MENCAP.

MENCAP (2012). *Death by Indifference: 74 Deaths and Counting*. London: MENCAP.

Merriam-Webster Dictionary. (2022). www.merriam-webster.com/dictionary/genogram

MIND (2021). www.mentalhealth.org.uk/explore-mental-health/a-z-topics/black-asian-and-minority-ethnic-bame-communities

MIND (2022). A to Z of psychiatric drugs. www.mind.org.uk/information-support/drugs-and-treatments/medication/drug-names-a-z/.

NHS England & NHS Improvement (2019). *Learning Disability Mortality Review (LeDeR) Programme: Action from Learning*. London: NHS England.

Perera, B., Audi, S., Solomou, S. et al. (2020). Mental and physical health conditions in people with intellectual disabilities: comparing local and national data. *British Journal of Learning Disabilities* 48 (1): 19–27.

Public Health England (2016). Dysphagia in people with learning difficulties: reasonable adjustments guidance. www.gov.uk/government/publications/dysphagia-and-people-with-learning-disabilities/dysphagia-in-people-with-learning-difficulties-reasonable-adjustments-guidance#:~:text=There%20are%20different%20causes%20and,process%20can%20be%20called%20dysphagia

Robertson, J., Chadwick, D., Baines, S. et al. (2017). Prevalence of dysphagia in people with intellectual disability: a systematic review. *Intellectual and Developmental Disabilities* 55 (6): 377–391.

Robertson, J., Baines, S., Emerson, E., and Hatton, C. (2018). Prevalence of constipation in people with intellectual disability: a systematic review. *Journal of Intellectual and Developmental Disability* 43 (4): 392–406.

Royal College of Nursing (2019). *Parity of Esteem – Delivering Physical Health Equality for those with Serious Mental Health Needs*. London: Royal College of Nursing.

Royal Pharmaceutical Society (2022). The role of pharmacy in mental health and wellbeing. www.rpharms.com/recognition/all-our-campaigns/policy-a-z/the-role-of-pharmacy-in-mental-health-and-wellbeing#:~:text=Identifying%20new%20symptoms&text=Through%20vigilance%20and%20rapport%20with,and%20substance%20or%20alcohol%20abuse.

Sala, R., Amet, L., Blagojevic-Stokic, N. et al. (2020). Bridging the gap between physical health and autism spectrum disorder. *Neuropsychiatric Disease and Treatment* 16: 1605.

Sands, N., Elsom, E., Colgate, R., and Haylor, H. (2016). Development and inter-rater reliability of the UK mental health triage scale. *International Journal of Mental Health Nursing* 25 (4): 330–336.

van Servellen, G. (1997). *Communication Skills for the Health Care Professional: Concepts and Techniques.* Gaithersburg.: Aspen.

Sharma, N. and Gupta, V. (2022). *Therapeutic Communication.* Treasure Island: StatPearls Publishing www.ncbi.nlm.nih.gov/books/NBK567775.

Spain, D., Sin, J., Linder, K.B. et al. (2018). Social anxiety in autism spectrum disorder: a systematic review. *Research in Autism Spectrum Disorders* 52: 51–68.

Summers, J., Shahrami, A., Cali, S. et al. (2017). Self-injury in autism Spectrum disorder and intellectual disability: exploring the role of reactivity to pain and sensory input. *Brain Science* 7 (11): 140.

Vos, T., Barber, R.M., Bell, B. et al. (2013). Global, regional, and national incidence, prevalence, and years lived with disability for 301 acute and chronic diseases and injuries in 188 countries, 1990–2013: a systematic analysis for the global burden of disease study. *Lancet* 386 (9995): 743–800.

Willis, D., Samalin, E., and Satgé, D. (2018). Colorectal cancer in people with intellectual disabilities. *Oncology* 95 (6): 323–336.

de Winter, C.F., Jansen, A.A.C., and Evenhuis, H.M. (2011). Physical conditions and challenging behaviour in people with intellectual disability: a systematic review. *Journal of Intellectual Disability Research* 55 (7): 675–698.

Zheng, S., Adams, R., Taylor, J. L., Pezzimenti, F., & Bishop, S. L. (2021). Depression in independent young adults on the autism spectrum: Demographic characteristics, service use, and barriers. *Autism*, 25 (7), 1960–1972.

FURTHER READING

Care Quality Commission (2020). Out of sight – who cares? Restraint, segregation and seclusion review. www.cqc.org.uk/publications/themed-work/rssreview

Health Education England (n.d.). Advanced Practice Mental Health Curriculum and Capabilities Framework. www.hee.nhs.uk/sites/default/files/documents/AP-MH%20Curriculum%20and%20 Capabilities%20Framework%201.2.pdf

Health Education England (2020). Advanced Clinical Practice: Capabilities framework when working with people who have a learning disability and/or autism. www.skillsforhealth.org.uk/wp-content/ uploads/2020/11/ACP-in-LDA-Framework.pdf

SELF-ASSESSMENT QUESTIONS

1. As a trainee AP, what are your learning needs in relation to providing care to people with mental health concerns, intellectual disability and autism?

2. How will you identify your additional needs for supervision and what documents and guidance will support this?

3. How will you evaluate and assess your clinical skills to prove your competency and capability in practice in the context of mental health and learning disabilities?

4. How can you ensure that you continue to develop your ability to refine your inclusive and holistic practice in the context of mental health and learning disability health and social care?

GLOSSARY

Autism   Autism is a lifelong developmental disability which affects how people communicate and interact with the world. Also known as autism spectrum disorder (ASD), it refers to a broad range of conditions characterised by challenges with social skills, repetitive behaviours, speech and non-verbal communication.

Learning disability   Learning disability includes the presence of:

- a significantly reduced ability to understand new or complex information, or to learn new skills (impaired intelligence)
- a reduced ability to cope independently (impaired social functioning), which started before adulthood, with a lasting effect on development.

Mental health   Mental health is a state of mental well-being that enables people to cope with the stresses of life, realise their abilities, learn well and work well, and contribute to their community. It is an integral component of health and well-being that underpins our individual and collective abilities to make decisions, build relationships and shape the world we live in. Mental health is a basic human right and it is crucial to personal, community and socioeconomic development.

Mental state examination   The mental state examination (MSE) is a structured way of observing and describing a patient's current state of mind, under the domains of appearance, attitude, behaviour, mood, affect, speech, thought process, thought content, perception, cognition, insight and judgement. The purpose of the MSE is to obtain a comprehensive cross-sectional description of the patient's mental state, which when combined with the biographical and historical information of the psychiatric history, allows the clinician to make an accurate diagnosis and formulation.

Patient-centred care   Providing care that is respectful of, and responsive to, individual patient preferences, needs and values, and ensuring that patient values guide all clinical decisions.

CHAPTER 16

Education and Learning

Joe Wood and Elizabeth Midwinter

Aim

The aim of this chapter is to discuss the theory underpinning teaching and learning.

LEARNING OUTCOMES

After reading this chapter the reader will:

1. have an underpinning knowledge of teaching and learning theory
2. be able to support learners in practice and understand the role of coaching and feedback
3. understand how safe learning environments are created and nurtured
4. be aware of how simulation and technology-enhanced learning can maximise learning opportunities

Multi-Professional Framework for Advanced Clinical Practice (HEE 2017)

Health care professionals working at the level of advanced clinical practice should be able to:

3.1 Critically assess and address own learning needs, negotiating a personal development plan that reflects the breadth of ongoing professional development across the four pillars of advanced clinical practice.
3.2 Engage in self-directed learning, critically reflecting to maximise clinical skills and knowledge, as well as own potential to lead and develop both care and services.

The Advanced Practitioner: A Framework for Practice, First Edition. Edited by Ian Peate, Sadie Diamond-Fox, and Barry Hill.
© 2024 John Wiley & Sons Ltd. Published 2024 by John Wiley & Sons Ltd.

3.3   Engage with, appraise, and respond to individuals' motivation, development stage, and capacity, working collaboratively to support health literacy and empower individuals to participate in decisions about their care and to maximise their health and well-being.

3.4   Advocate for and contribute to a culture of organisational learning to inspire future and existing staff.

3.5   Facilitate collaboration of the wider team and support peer review processes to identify individual and team learning.

3.6   Identify further developmental needs for the individual and the wider team and supporting them to address these.

3.7   Support the wider team to build capacity and capability through work-based and interprofessional learning, and the application of learning to practice.

3.8   Act as a role model, educator, supervisor, coach, and mentor, seeking to instil and develop the confidence of others.

Accreditation Considerations

- FICM ACCP Curriculum: 3.23 Teaching and training.
- RCEM ACP Curriculum: CC23 Teaching and Training

INTRODUCTION

The role of an advanced practitioners (AP) not only includes commitment to personal continuous professional development, but also contribution to the education and development of others, acting as a professional role model. Health Education England (HEE) states that 'It is now essential for education providers and institutions to demonstrate that those involved in the education and supervision of learners within their organisation have the necessary knowledge, skills and approaches to help develop and support all learner groups, across the healthcare professions' (HEE 2021). To do this, an understanding of the principles around learning, education and development is required.

PRINCIPLES OF TEACHING AND LEARNING

Understanding How We Learn

To be able to take control of one's own learning, and teach others, AP need to recognise how learning happens. While many theories exist (Table 16.1), there are several which particularly resonate with advanced practice. Cognitive behaviour theory focuses on helping learners discover how they think – by understanding their own thought processes, learners have greater control over their learning. In contrast, behaviourism theorises that learners are impacted by external forces rather than internal ones – bringing culture, mentorship and organisations into play. The theory of connectivism then focuses on how learners will grow and develop when they connect with things that excite and interest them.

TABLE 16.1 Key educational theories.

Theory	Main Theorists	Description
Experiential learning	Lewin (1951) Kolb (2014) Carver (1996) Yardley et al. (2012)	We learn more from experiences if those experiences are examined and reflected upon. Experience, reflect, conceptualise, experiment/plan. Ensure authenticity of material, actively involve learners, validate learner experiences, generalise learning to new situations.
Constructivism	Dewey et al. (1997) Vygotsky (1978)	Active participation and interaction with each other and the environment is key to construct meaning. Scaffolding – anchoring of understanding on past experience.
Deliberate practice	Ericsson et al. (1993) Ericsson (2004)	Deliberate, internally motivated repetitive practice with immediate expert feedback facilitates performance, reduces trial and error, and stops poor traits becoming habituated. Feedback and frequency are key.

Constructivism develops upon this, theorising that learners build new meaning and knowledge based on their prior experiences. This is fundamental to advanced clinical practice with clinicians building upon the underlying knowledge and skills they have gained whilst practising their base professions. Guiding learners to analyse their own thinking and build upon their past experiences helps to create learning which is uniquely relevant to the individual. This also promotes deep reflection – key for transformative learning. No two learners are alike and so may relate in varying degrees to any number of theories. Consequently, educators must have the ability to adapt their approach to match their audience and the situation.

Recognising Adult Learners

As senior clinicians, AP need to be recognised as adult learners, with competing interests and pressures. When planning learning, educators must consider the demands of clinical practice, as well as the impact of commitments outside the workplace. Ensuring that learning opportunities can be maximised is paramount. While undertaking advanced practice training, trainees should be given protected time to undertake learning. In the workplace, for both trainees and qualified AP, learning may take a variety of forms, from case-based discussions to deliberately planned teaching sessions.

Dual Coding Theory

Dual coding is the theory that imagery and verbal information, when provided together, improve the retention of knowledge – using poignant photographs or graphics alongside verbal lectures rather than having text-heavy presentation slides, for example. As visual and verbal information are processed through different pathways of the brain, a deeper, more rounded understanding is formed. Having appropriate images associated with key words allows learners to retain the information in their long-term memory as opposed to short-term, or working, memory (Figure 16.1).

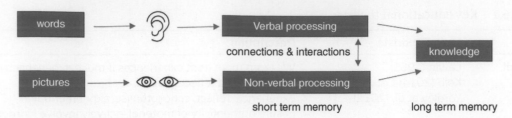

FIGURE 16.1 Dual coding theory.

Evidence-based Practice

When making decisions regarding patient treatment, the best available evidence should be used – incorporating professional judgement and the values of both the clinician and the patient. To this end, it is recommended that clinicians should receive education in how to critically appraise literature and establish how to implement best evidence in practice (see Chapter 18 for more details). When teaching others, it is important to distinguish between evidence-based knowledge and that which is experiential.

Self-directed Learning

Self-directed learning involves the student taking accountability for their own knowledge acquisition. It forms a large component of advanced practice training, with each specialty area often requiring more nuanced and focused learning in addition to the more generic advanced practice university programme. Consequently, the learner needs to be open to the fact that their development is their own responsibility, and subscribe to the idea that they will only get from the process what they put in. Self-reflection and the ability to identify gaps in knowledge are crucial to focus learning and formulate appropriate goals. This can be challenging for many learners and requires discipline and time management due to competing interests and priorities. Setting goals, making development plans and meeting regularly with supervisors, assessors and mentors can all help with keeping learning on track, along with regular re-evaluation of progress.

SUPPORTING OTHERS TO DEVELOP KNOWLEDGE AND SKILLS

Feedback

Feedback is defined as 'specific information about the comparison between an observed performance and a standard with the intent to improve performance' (Van de Ridder et al. 2008) and is often considered the most important aspect of learning (McGaghie et al. 2010). Unfortunately, in healthcare, this does not always happen in the ideal way, with research showing that clinicians are not effectively taught these skills (Burgess and Mellis 2015). Considering most people need five or more pieces of positive feedback to overcome one piece of negative feedback (Losada and Heaphey 2004), we must be mindful of the impact that poorly thought out and delivered feedback can have. Not giving feedback can also have detrimental effects. Those who are doing well are perhaps not aware of this, and may doubt themselves or feel they are underperforming. Conversely, those who are not meeting the expected standard may be oblivious to this fact, so that when formal or summative feedback is given, it comes as a surprise to them. In both cases, lack of feedback removes the opportunity for the learner to improve upon their current practice.

It is important to clarify that feedback is being given, as informal verbal feedback is often not recognised. By establishing that feedback is coming, the learner is prepared to receive the information and the educator delivering the feedback is also in the correct mindset. When giving feedback, it must be specific, targeted, timely and non-judgemental. Rather than a vague 'well done', let the learner know which aspect went particularly well (or poorly), doing so as soon after the event as possible. Feedback should then be constructive, informed by objective observations and related to future goals – be clear if any further development is needed and offer specific solutions to achieve this. Educators should also gather feedback from their learners to model a culture of improvement. Chapter 17 of this text discusses feedback and feedforward.

Appraisal Processes and Continuing Professional Development

The appraisal is a formal method of feedback, often scheduled at regular intervals – a facilitated review of practice and development. Good rapport must be established and mutual respect observed to ensure a successful two-way dialogue is opened from the outset of such meetings. Although the majority of appraisals should be self-facilitated, feedback from other sources is often a requirement. A well-rounded way of collating this is through 360° feedback from peers, supervisors and other colleagues of varying specialties and seniority. Appraisal should be undertaken by those who have been appropriately prepared and should give the opportunity for the individual to reflect on their own practice and compare this with the feedback given. The appraisal should offer the opportunity to set a professional development plan detailing goals for education and courses which may be undertaken in the coming timeframe, and any areas for improvement. This plan should specify how these objectives will be achieved and set an achievable timescale for this.

> **RED FLAG**
>
> Poor-quality feedback and debrief have the potential to detrimentally affect learning not only at the time but throughout future learning opportunities.

Learning from Mistakes: Safety I and Safety II

At the centre of learning and development in healthcare is a focus on patient safety. Safety is often measured by how many incidents have occurred – known as Safety I. Safety I focuses on mistakes and how we stop them from happening through modalities such as rapid incident review and audit. Conversely, safety II examines what goes right and why. This involves looking at how systems are already working and then building upon this. Assessment and measurement of safety II can be difficult in healthcare due to the fast-paced and dynamic clinical environment. Despite this, it is important for healthcare educators to promote a safety II mindset – framing teaching to emphasise how correct performance of a task will improve patient care, not simply the mistakes it will avoid.

Coaching, Mentoring and Role Modelling

Coaches and mentors are common in healthcare, and while they are often discussed together, the two are very different. Coaching is the practice of providing guidance, while allowing the learner to come to their own solutions. It relies on the learner applying their existing knowledge and skills to new learning opportunities. Mentoring, on the other hand, involves the mentor sharing their own knowledge and experience to help others develop, imparting their opinions and experiences to improve performance. Coaching and mentorship, especially in the case of advanced practice, may be interprofessional in nature.

Role modelling of behaviours is central to the pillar of education and development in advanced practice. Educators should be professional, credible, positive, supportive and motivational, and should, invest in, advise, challenge, push and empower – helping learners to reach their potential (Buck 2004). Role modelling may also simply be engaging in continual professional development or being open and honest in recognising good practice and challenging bad practice. Admitting fallibility and asking for help are also extremely helpful behaviours to role model. This demonstrates to learners that it is OK for them to not know all the answers – if the teachers feel safe showing vulnerability, so can the learners. This allows learners to raise concerns and feel comfortable in acknowledging their own limitations – promoting a culture of safe practice. Cultures that promote education and learning have also been shown to have higher retention of staff. By role modelling some of the above qualities, AP can positively influence those around them, making learners more likely to adopt good behaviours in their own clinical practice.

Developing a higher level of decision making is a large part of advanced clinical practice education, one which can be difficult to impart to new learners. The educator should take time to verbalise how they have reached their decision. By role modelling this transparent and 'out loud' approach to clinical reasoning, educators can help learners not only learn *what* to do, but *why*. If mirrored by the learner, this approach can also be useful in finding and addressing gaps in underpinning knowledge.

There may be times when educators are not able to provide the necessary education for the learner. In this situation, it is important that this is recognised and an appropriate solution identified. Learning goals could be achieved by visiting a different clinical area, spending time with other professionals or by directing the learner to further study or human resources. Allow the learner the opportunity to reflect on these different experiences, and encourage them to share their newfound knowledge, perhaps teaching others in the process. This promotes a culture of continual learning and sharing of knowledge while helping the learner to develop their own skills as an educator.

CREATING AN EFFECTIVE LEARNING ENVIRONMENT

In the healthcare setting, learning occurs in a wide range of environments, including clinical, non-clinical and virtual, and care must be taken to maximise learning opportunities while maintaining patient safety and effective caseload management. For each respective learning opportunity, consider how you will promote the ideal learner, teacher, process and space (Figure 16.2).

Optimise the Space

Physical

Consider the room set-up – what will maximise engagement? Ensure adequate temperature, lighting and accessibility of relevant teaching aids. In cases of learning in a direct patient-facing environment, a communal area away from the immediate learning event often allows discussion and debrief in a more relaxed space. Environments should ideally be quiet, free from distractions and accessible to all.

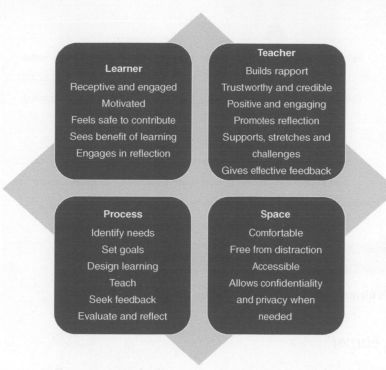

FIGURE 16.2   Learner, teacher, process, space.

Virtual

These may include 'face-to-face' lectures, discussions via virtual platforms, e-learning discussion forums or e-portfolios, amongst others. The teacher must ensure that the learner is able to access such platforms, considering how to guarantee access to up-to-date technology and sufficient internet speed, as well as how to improve computer literacy where necessary. The learner must be helped to recognise the benefits of virtual environments and feel safe in contributing to and engaging with these learning communities. Ground rules for both face-to-face and virtual communications must be set.

Ensure Learner-centredness

An effective learning environment must address a range of learner needs and motivations (Figure 16.3) and, where possible, promote a sense of belonging by including and consulting the learner in the planning of learning opportunities.

GREEN FLAG

Care must be taken to ensure that learning events and environments are inclusive to a diverse range of learners from varying socioeconomic and cultural backgrounds. Educators must work to guarantee equality of opportunity and accessibility of learning for all.

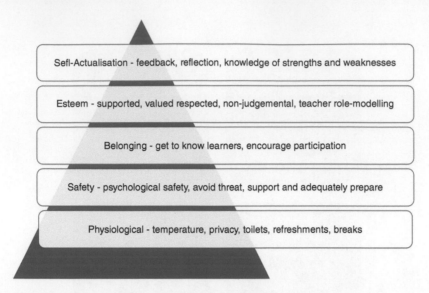

FIGURE 16.3　Maslow's hierarchy of needs. *Source*: Adapted from Maslow (1943).

Get to Know the Learner

The teacher should introduce themselves and get to know the learners on a first name basis, showing an enthusiastic and genuine interest in the learners' backgrounds and progress to date. This flattens hierarchy, promotes learner esteem and builds greater rapport.

Plan the Process

A learning needs assessment and setting of appropriate SMART (specific, measurable, achievable, realistic, timed) goals is key. The GROW acronym (Whitmore 1992) may help structure this process (Figure 16.4).

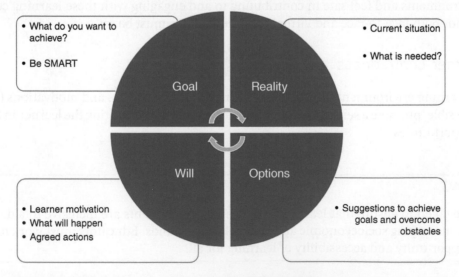

FIGURE 16.4　Planning teaching with goal, reality, options, will framework.

Acknowledge needs but take care to manage expectations (Riley 2016). Clearly communicate expected behaviours and ground rules, addressing confidentiality and non-judgemental peer feedback. When designing learning, it should be constructively aligned to the curriculum, pitched at the right level, well planned and accessible to all. Consider how each environment and teaching modality (lecture, simulation and so forth) will help or hinder achievement of desired learning outcomes.

Create Psychological Safety

Psychological safety is central to an effective learning environment and empowers the learner to express thoughts and feelings and participate without fear (Forrest and McKimm 2019). This encourages problem solving while protecting self-esteem. Psychological safety can, in part, be promoted by levelling the hierarchy between teacher and learners – especially important in the case of small group sessions and interprofessional learning. Other contributing factors are presented in Figure 16.5.

It is important to actively manage potential threats to psychological safety while ensuring the learner remains accountable for their actions and performance. A safe physical environment and graded increase in exposure, complexity and responsibility are also key to promoting psychological safety and maximising

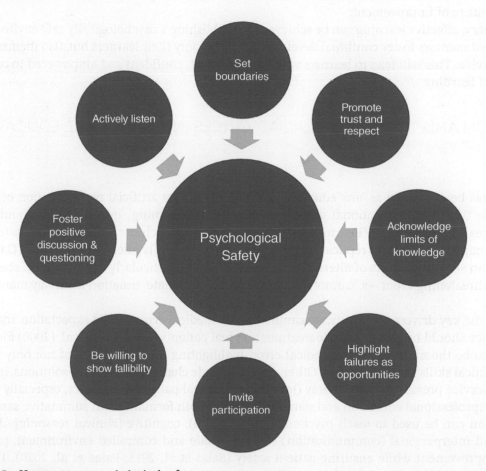

FIGURE 16.5 How to create psychological safety.

learner participation. If a psychologically safe ethos is promoted, clinicians are more likely to report and learn from error too – raising concerns to receptive colleagues (a learning process in itself).

ORANGE FLAG

Psychological safety and effective, non-judgemental debrief are key to minimising potential psychological trauma in clinical teaching and promoting honest reflection and incident reporting.

Promote Continual Improvement Via Reflection

Reflection fosters deep potential for learning and helps self-regulation (Bandura 2001). Robust mentorship allows open and honest discussion to promote reflection in, on and for action (Schon 1987; Thompson and Pascal 2012) and, given appropriate analysis, allows reframing of the learners' cognitive approach to problem solving (critical reflection – Mezirow 1990). Educators need to be prepared to challenge presuppositions to overcome barriers to such reflection (Boud and Walker 1993) and enable knowledge to be effectively assimilated (Moon 2000). For effective discussion and deep reflection to occur, psychological safety is essential. Educators should also embrace self-reflection and gather feedback from their learners to model a culture of improvement.

In summary, effective learning can be achieved by establishing a psychologically safe environment in which invested mentors foster continual development of not only their learners but also themselves and the wider service. This will lead to learners who are motivated, confident and empowered to contribute to a culture of learning.

SIMULATION AND TECHNOLOGICAL ADVANCES IN HEALTHCARE EDUCATION

Simulation

Simulation has been defined as 'any educational activity that uses artificial representation of the real-world process to achieve educational goals from experiential learning', importantly without the risk inherent in real-life experience (Bearman et al. 2013). This must achieve sufficient fidelity (discussed later in this chapter) to 'evoke or replicate real life experiences in a fully interactive manner' (Gaba 2007). Simulation can show the effects of alternative courses of action, particularly useful when a scenario is a rare but life-threatening event – a 'cannot intubate', 'cannot oxygenate' situation in airway management, for example.

Some of the key drivers for healthcare simulation are medical error, public expectation and safety – that experience should be gained prior to treatment on real patients. Donaldson et al. (2000) found communication to be the main source of medical error, highlighting the importance of not only technical but non-technical skills in patient safety. Other drivers include changing workforce solutions, improving technology, service pressures, reduced stay (less chance for real patient encounters, especially rare conditions), interprofessional education and standardisation of both formative and summative assessment.

Simulation can be used to teach psychomotor (technical), cognitive (clinical reasoning/decisions/attitudes) and interpersonal (communication) skills in a safe and controlled environment, promoting continual improvement while ensuring patient safety (Salas et al. 2015; Paige et al. 2020). Table 16.2 reflects the potential benefits of simulation to the patient, clinicians and the wider healthcare systems.

TABLE 16.2   Benefits of simulation in healthcare education.

	Benefits
Patient	Protects from inexperienced clinicians
Clinicians	Improves confidence (particularly in rare clinical cases)
	Improves proficiency in technical skills (Ericsson 2004; McGaghie et al. 2011)
	Improves non-technical skills (Konstantinidis et al. 2020; McGaghie et al. 2010)
	Improves communication (Hanson et al. 2004)
	Greater access to learning outside usual working hours (in cases of skills labs or computer-based programmes)
	Positive experience (Alinier et al. 2006)
	Adaptable to individual or group needs
	Teamwork
	Role transition (advanced practice)
Wider healthcare system	Evaluate new processes or protocols
	Establish if clinical area is fit for purpose
	Training after error (evaluating sources of error and implementing change)

Teaching Practical Skills – Reflections from Clinical Experience

Peyton's four-stage approach (Walker and Peyton 1998) can be particularly useful when teaching skills such as cannulation. The teacher first demonstrates the task at full speed without comment to give an exemplar. Then the process is performed more slowly, with the task deconstructed into its elements and rationale given for each step. Comprehension is then assessed by the student instructing the teacher to perform each step sequentially with feedback and correction given. The student then performs the task while describing each step. When used in a simulated environment, the repetition of this approach allows the steps of a task to become second nature, freeing up cognitive bandwidth to solve problems when applied to real-life practice.

Human Factors

Human factors (the interaction between humans and systems) are generally distinguished as cognitive (decision-making and situational awareness) and interpersonal (communication, teamwork and leadership). Simulation is often used to build a shared mental model, develop mutual trust and assess teamwork and may improve protocol design and resource allocation but this may need repeated simulations to be effective.

As for any simulation, teams-based simulation starts with a needs analysis (often coming from clinical incidents – loss of airway when repositioning an intubated patient, for example). Situational awareness includes the perception and comprehension of a situation and its components and the ability to project this into the future, allowing timely interventions. Simulation offers the unique capability to alter levels of complexity and add to cognitive load to assess such characteristics and is thus endorsed by education programmes in intensive care, surgery and emergency medicine (Brindley and Reynolds 2011). The Team STEPPS approach (Figure 16.6) may be useful when designing and assessing interventions (Brock et al. 2013; Weller et al. 2014). Table 16.3 gives some examples of how non-technical skills can be included in simulation scenarios.

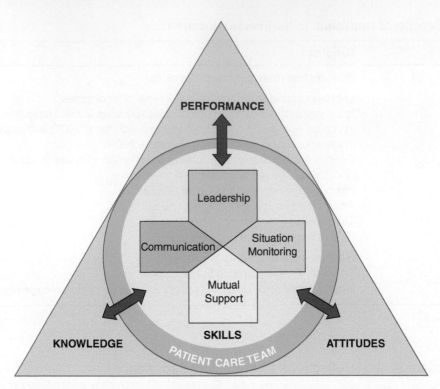

FIGURE 16.6 Team STEPPS – components of team performance. *Source*: Plonien C, Williams M (2015) Stepping up teamwork via Team STEPPS. AORN Journal 101(4): 465–470.

TABLE 16.3 How to incorporate non-technical skills into simulation.

Non-technical Skills Domain	Scenario Addition
Communication	Verbal handovers Taking referrals via phone MDT handovers in cases of interprofessional education
Fatigue and stress	Competing tasks or distractions
Decision making	Thinking out loud
Authority	Addition of a domineering character
Leadership	Advanced Life Support – leading an arrest Delegation of tasks Utilise SNAPPI tool (Weller et al. 2014)
Situational awareness	Tag relevant parts of scenario to help debrief Stipulate timings until critical incidents/action needed Adapt cognitive load, stress or time constraints to adjust challenge

Interprofessional Education

From a team perspective, simulation has also been used in interprofessional education (IPE) (Decker et al. 2015) – developing communication, teamwork (Weaver et al. 2014) and role identity via social learning (Bandura and Walters 1977). IPE improves interaction between, attitudes towards and knowledge of other professions (Paige et al. 2020) and has been shown to be useful in enhancing skills learning (Hughes et al. 2016). MDT simulation improves engagement and allows non-technical issues to be uncovered and thus has a sociological benefit too (Thomas and Reeves 2015). Practical considerations include funding and institutional support – particularly the ability to release clinical staff to attend these sessions.

Fields of Practice: Mental Health and Learning Difficulties

Education may focus on development of non-technical skills – particularly advanced communication skills. Learning and applying legislation related to informed consent may also be emphasised. Simulation may be difficult in these groups although programmes do exist (Maudsley Simulation).

Types of Simulation

Virtual patients involve use of computer software to explore decision pathways in case-based vignettes. These offer the learner a choice of how to proceed with history-taking questions, physical examinations or diagnostic test selection to reach a diagnosis. This method aims to develop clinical reasoning skills. Following on from this, game-based learning uses competitive problem solving to enhance learner engagement.

Simple role play may be considered simulation – breaking bad news, for instance. Simulated or standardised patients (SPs) are trained to portray a patient with a specific condition in a realistic, standardised and repeatable way. Although often actors or faculty, the role can also be fulfilled by patients with the condition. In all cases, the SP must be given appropriate instruction to ensure consistent and reliable response to learners' verbal and non-verbal interactions – realistic scripts and pre-brief are key (Riley 2016). SPs can give direct and constructive feedback on both technical and non-technical skills from the patient perspective (Kneebone et al. 2010) and offer a good conduit for deliberate practice, although adequate training may be time-consuming and certain conditions challenging to replicate.

Fields of Practice: Paediatrics

Simulation can be used to practise clinical skills such as cannulation and, via standardised patients, develop non-technical skills such as communication with concerned parents. Informed parental consent is crucial prior to direct patient-facing learning events and parental feedback should be incorporated into debrief and reflective practice.

Part-task trainers are also commonplace – the most recognisable being Resusci Anne and subsequent iterations used for basic life support training. Hybrid simulation (Kneebone 2003) describes the combination of a task trainer with a simulated patient, the most common example being a cannulation arm taking the place of an actor's arm. In this case, the clinician can practise both practical and non-technical skills such as communication.

Human patient simulators are computerised full-body manikins that aim to d reliably represent patient clinical signs and symptoms (Maran and Glavin 2003). The most complex can replicate pupillary reaction, heart and lung sounds and even allow selected practical interventions such as needle decompression or intubation. Such manikins can also provide a wealth of feedback, whether that be through voice (controlled by faculty) or data on adequacy of depth of chest compressions, for example. Specialist high-fidelity simulators may also offer haptic feedback (physical feedback/the feeling of instruments through skin). Most have physiological modelling with observations which deteriorate over time, as a patients would. Human patient simulators are becoming more portable, allowing training to take place in a wider variety of environments. Entirely portable self-contained immersive environments are also available, described as distributed simulation.

Virtual reality, including inertial sensors and wearable technology, is becoming increasingly popular and offers a means of interactive, problem-based learning. Virtual and augmented reality increases learner engagement and motivation (Akcayir and Akcayir 2017) and shortens the learning curve (Zhu et al. 2014) but does not necessarily improve performance or test scores (Stepan et al. 2017; Moro et al. 2021). Problems with refresh rates, lag and ability to import data from other systems (imaging and so forth) are common but potentially surmountable problems in this field. Virtual worlds have also been used in education as collaborative forums, where avatars can discuss cases, co-create content and even interview patients from around the world.

Case Study

During the first wave of the COVID-19 pandemic, access to patients was limited to ensure minimal exposure of staff. This meant that supernumerary AP had limited opportunities to perform physical clinical examination. A number of simulated patients were produced to allow practical examination skills to be undertaken. These could then be reproduced to allow all trainees equal exposure. A virtual reality programme was also used to allow trainees to practise their clinical reasoning and decision-making skills. This promoted accessibility, equity of opportunity and learning in a safe environment.

The Concept of Fidelity

Fidelity has many definitions but can be thought of as how 'true to life' a simulation is (Forrest and McKimm 2019). Common facets include the following.

- *Psychological fidelity:* the degree of immersion and accuracy of emotional response, including perception of, and reaction to, cognitive load.
- *Physical fidelity:* includes equipment (ventilators, phone to contact colleagues and so forth), people you would expect in the environment (also known as sociological fidelity), notes, charts, smells, sights and appearances. Enhanced physical fidelity is linked to enhanced learning (Roberts and Roberts 2014). Manikin fidelity also falls under this category. With low to medium fidelity manikins, the facilitator will often have to 'fill gaps' with verbal cues as to changing clinical condition and these therefore require proactivity to ensure 'reality' is maintained.

Traditionally, low fidelity refers to non-computerised manikins (often task trainers), mid-fidelity to SPs, computer programs and video games, and high fidelity to computerised human patient simulators that respond to treatment (Konstantinidis et al. 2020). There is no convincing or consistent evidence that greater fidelity manikins lead to greater learning (Forrest and McKimm 2019) and thus fidelity should be considered 'a means to optimise learning, not a goal in itself' (Kneebone et al. 2010). Also, manikin fidelity is dynamic, depending on learning outcome (Hamstra et al. 2014) – a so-called high-fidelity manikin has little utility in assessment of history taking and the nuanced response to non-verbal cues, for instance. Here, although technologically advanced, the manikin provides very poor overall fidelity for the clinical situation.

In Situ Simulation

In situ simulation is performed in a functional clinical environment, offering the chance of enhanced authenticity (Sorenson et al. 2017). These sessions can be run with a manikin or SP. Environmental and psychological fidelity is high, with layout, location of equipment, noise and distractions adding to realism. This form of simulation is particularly useful in identifying systems-based problems in health-care delivery and associated team and space readiness for clinical practice. This is most reflected in assessment of new treatment protocols with in situ simulation which can identify 'latent threats' before these affect patient care (Riley 2016). It has also been widely used in team-based training with utility in practising role identification, MDT communication and non-technical skills.

In situ simulation does represent a risk to psychological safety, however, with potentially poor performance witnessed by the learner's team and in the learner's subsequent working environment inducing significant anxiety and risking learner disengagement. Also, these sessions are often completed near to real patients, raising the risk of impacted patient care and loss of confidentiality/privacy (particularly if sessions are recorded). This risk extends to clinical staff and impact on non-participants must always be considered. Logistical problems surrounding transfer of audiovisual equipment, manikins and connecting these to respective software/networks must also be considered. Thus, despite its potential benefits, in situ simulation necessitates significant risk assessment and planning.

Designing Simulated Learning

When designing learning, action learning cycles can help structure the process (Figure 16.7). Establish the reason for simulation – is it to learn existing algorithms, repeat critical incidents, test new protocols, learn specific technical skills or develop non-technical skills in a team?

Identifying the learning needs of the intended audience and formulating learning outcomes is essential before proceeding with scenario design. Needs may be viewed in terms of highlighted areas of poor performance or clinical incident, or constructively aligned to core competencies, professional

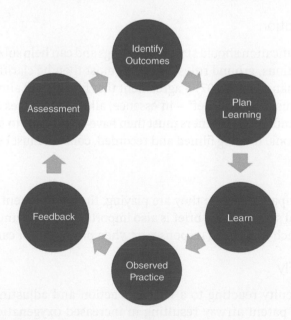

FIGURE 16.7 Action learning cycle.

standards or curricula. Outcomes generally include both technical and non-technical skills with expected demonstrable knowledge, skills and behaviours. It must be established at this stage how you expect learners to demonstrate achievement of learning outcomes. Outcomes must be matched to fidelity, assessable, clear, future-orientated, achievable and lend themselves to the environment and modality chosen (Popenici and Millar 2015).

Scenario Writing

The scenario must be relevant to the participants and as detailed as possible, encouraging evidence-based and deliberate practice. Pitching the simulation at the right level is key to ensuring self-efficacy (Bandura 2001) and thus knowing your audience is essential. The scenario must reflect the hospital/community in which the staff will be practising after the session. Baseline characteristics must be given along with changes based on timings or anticipated learner actions (known as triggers). Many templates exist to aid scenario design – TEACH Sim is one example (Benishek et al. 2015). Constant reflection on and evaluation of scenarios are essential to ensure they become as polished and realistic as possible and address the learning outcomes as intended.

Practical Considerations

Before the day, consider room booking, environment (preparation, fire exits and so on), equipment needs, cost and acquisition of consumables and refreshments. To ensure adequate time and resources are allocated, faculty should discuss scenarios and running of the day well in advance, ideally with a real-time 'dry run' (Riley 2016). This should inform any changes to the scenario and highlight any additional needs, including faculty skill mix and training requirements. Robust continual professional development and training is recommended for faculty (Forrest and McKimm 2019), particularly around debrief. The Association for Simulated Practice in Healthcare and the International Nursing Association for Clinical Simulation and Learning can help identify appropriate courses. In the case of IPE, faculty should represent the range of professions attending the simulation (Paige et al. 2020).

Introductions and Orientation

Introductions with role identification should start proceedings and can help subsequent team performance (Cooke et al. 2000). Expectations, ground rules and goals must then be clarified. Here, fiction contracts must be established (Dieckmann et al. 2007) – agreement that faculty will aim to ensure the best fidelity possible, and learners will 'suspend disbelief' – in essence, allow themselves to be as fully immersed as possible and 'buy in' to the simulation. Learners must then have ample time to familiarise themselves with the simulator and its limitations. If being filmed and recorded, consent must be gained from participants.

Pre-brief

Set the stage – tell the participants the role they are playing, the environment they are in, the team they can call upon and the clinical scenario. Pre-brief is also important for any simulated patients and faculty, providing key information such as scripted responses or when prompting of candidates may be necessary.

Programmed vs On the Fly

On the fly describes the faculty reacting to a learner's action and adjusting variables accordingly – for example, establishing a patent airway resulting in increased oxygenation. Programmed refers to a scenario which follows strict timings – if a particular action is not taken in x amount of time, the patient will deteriorate in a predefined way. On the fly is often better when the learners are likely to depart from a planned course or are more novice, although this places greater responsibility on faculty to observe and respond in a timely manner. This also requires a trained clinician to be in the control room, unlike the programmed scenario which can be run by a technician without the need for clinical knowledge. In either, using an earpiece to communicate with faculty during the simulation may be useful to ensure the scenario progresses in a productive and timely way or is paused to allow skills practice or introduce another team member. Once a predefined endpoint is reached, the session proceeds to debrief.

Debrief

Defined as 'a conversation held after an event aimed at sustaining or improving performance' (Riley 2016), the quality of debrief has been reported as one of the biggest determinants of extent of learning in simulation (Tannenbaum and Cerasoli 2013). It also reduces the potential for psychological trauma, especially when the ethos of psychological safety is actively promoted.

Debrief should occur as soon after the event as possible, in a positive, non-threatening environment away from the simulated environment (Fanning and Gaba 2007), and be afforded at least as much time as the simulation itself. Most of the talking should come from participants (Cantrell 2008) with careful investigation of emotion and accompanying perspectives to maximise the affective component of learning (Knowles 1978; Riley 2016). Performance gaps should be identified and feedback provided to move to a new understanding of the simulated events and underlying cognitive processes. Observer checklists aligned to main learning outcomes and video playback may facilitate structured debrief and promote postsession reflection. Other key aspects are presented in Table 16.4.

TABLE 16.4   The do's and don'ts of debrief.

Do	Establish learner agenda
	Actively listen, use open-ended questions to encourage dialogue
	Clarify and summarise expectations/gold standard
	Empathise – recognise emotions and opinions
	Build rapport – be honest, fair, sincere and compassionate
	Establish intention and contrast with effect – explore assumptions underlying decision making
	Distinguish between person and performance
	Reflect questions back to group to promote collaboration
	Avoid interruptions; be fluid but keep to time
	Support and challenge
	Use confluent body language to ensure questions perceived as genuine
	Be polite and non-judgemental, and encourage engagement
	Remind of learning outcomes, allow all to contribute, establish solutions
	Facilitate and guide reflection
	Show credibility – apply theory to clinical content
	Be non-threatening – safe environment, flattened hierarchy
Do not	Forget emotional response
	Criticise without recommending
	Comment on personal attributes
	Neglect body language
	Be dishonestly kind

Although approaches to debrief are varied (Table 16.5), key concepts include assessing candidate reaction (active listening), the candidate or an observer describing the narrative timeline of events (limit to minimum), setting the agenda for discussion (focus points related to learning), analysing events objectively, and concluding application to future practice. Debrief in IPE should include role identity issues (particularly if these overlap traditional roles as for advanced practitioners) and exploration of individual and professional mental models or signature pedagogies.

Reflections from Clinical Practice

Following clinical events, particularly those in emergency situations, it is often helpful to perform a debrief as soon as practicable. These so-called 'hot debriefs' can identify strong emotions and opinions from team members which can then be recognised and appropriately addressed. This helps improve team working and, importantly, promotes staff well-being by identifying where further support may be needed. This can be applied to trainee AP experiencing critical events for the first time. This is then reinforced by a 'cold' debrief further down the line, usually at 3–4 weeks post incident. The purpose of the cold debrief is to ensure the psychological well-being of those involved, as 'normal' stress responses such as anxiety or sleep disturbance should have begun to ease at this point. This form of critical incident debrief should only be attended by those who were involved in the case, as inappropriate attendance or facilitation can cause further psychological harm to attendees.

TABLE 16.5 Core models for debrief.

Debrief	Author	Key Elements
Advocacy and enquiry	Rudolph et al. (2006)	Focus on insight into thoughts behind actions. Debriefing with good judgement describes a non-judgemental approach to debrief underpinned by a genuine desire to understand performance.
Diamond	Jaye et al. (2015)	Describe events, analyse (how and why), apply (learning and course of action).
SHARP	Ahmed et al. (2013)	Set learning objectives, how did it go, address concerns, review learning points, plan ahead.
Pendleton's Rules	Pendleton et al. (2003)	Learner what went well, teacher what went well, learner what could be better, teacher what could be better.

Debriefing requires organisational skills, group process skills, communication skills, conflict resolution and aspects of counselling (Pearson and Smith 1985) and is thus difficult to master. Designated courses are available for this very reason and tools such as the debriefing assessment for simulation in healthcare (DASH) are available to assess and continually develop the quality of debrief (Brett-Fleegler et al. 2012).

Case Study
Following the death of a paediatric trauma patient, a 'hot' debrief was held to ensure psychological well-being, allow the team to 'decompress', ensure they could continue their shift and establish if further support was needed. A cold debrief was held four weeks later, where it was ascertained that several staff were suffering from flashbacks and were thus referred to the Trust psychological well-being service. The cold debrief also found that communication between the emergency department and theatre teams could be improved in future cases.

Despite its many potential benefits, simulation should not be used for the sake of it. Simulation should be thought of as a pedagogical technique, not a technology (Gaba 2004), and must always be carefully devised to align appropriately to curricula and learning outcomes.

Technology-enhanced Learning

The 'flipped' classroom or blended approach is the concept of allowing asynchronous on-demand access to learning at a time which suits the learner (Shahoumian et al. 2014). This has been shown to reduce class time, enhance self-directed learning and reduce facility needs (Perkins et al. 2012). Although this seems beneficial, learners are often not given set time to access this learning, meaning extra work in their own time. There is also no guarantee of acquisition of the necessary prior knowledge. Often, a summary lecture is included at the start of the follow-up session to combat this. Care must be taken to ensure content is peer reviewed, constructively aligned to set standards and up to date. Establish how, where and on what devices the material will be accessed and whether content is available online only or can be downloaded.

Social media has the potential to share tailored information, increase interaction, widen access and provide valuable peer and social support with often immediate response to questions posed by learners. Educators should make students aware of the limitations of information gathered via social media – lack of peer review, for example (Ventola 2014; Moorhead et al. 2013). Each regulatory body offers guidance on social media which should be followed by respective professions. Other resources include video streaming, webinars, podcasts, massive open online courses (MOOCs) and smart phone applications. Some of these applications may be useful within a simulation – offering immediate access to risk stratification tools to inform management options. As learners will inevitably access such resources, signposting the most reliable and peer-reviewed content is a must, as is role modelling of digital professionalism.

Use of video recordings to assist feedback has received some interest in the literature, with software now available to tag notable moments in real-time and link these to specific domains (for example, communication or teamwork). Although potentially useful, medicolegal and ethical issues of consent for filming, storage, right of access and subsequent usage must be robustly addressed. Furthermore, nervous candidates may find filming worsens performance and thus fears must be well allayed in the pre-brief.

Artificial intelligence and learning analytics have a huge role to play in future education, with modalities such as virtual patients, serious games and quizzes able to adapt and tailor future scenarios based on the user's past performances or common mistakes. In doing so, a learner's weaker areas are preferentially targeted for improvement.

Technology-enhanced learning, although not without its drawbacks, is likely to continue to grow in both complexity and popularity and has the potential to provide tailored, easily accessible education to a wide audience.

CONCLUSION

Through creation of a suitable and psychologically safe learning environment, consideration of appropriate learning design and effective mentorship, APs can provide and benefit from a huge range of learning opportunities. With a greater understanding of learning theories and exploration of the impact of prior experience on thought processes, these can become truly transformational. APs have a vital role to play in education and must role model effective feedback, deep reflection and professionalism – promoting an ethos of continual development.

Take Home Points

As a teacher

- Know your audience and identify learning needs.
- Align learning outcomes to curricula.
- Choose an appropriate modality.
- Give effective feedback.
- Provide robust mentorship.
- Encourage regular in-depth reflection.
- Optimise the learning environment – ensure psychological safety.
- Consider how technology can make learning more effective and accessible.
- Reflect on and evaluate your interventions.

As a learner

- Engage with the learning process.
- Contribute to discussions and learning design.
- Reflect on thought processes, learning styles and reactions to learning events.
- Be motivated and self-directed.
- Be responsive to feedback.

REFERENCES

Ahmed, M., Arora, S., Russ, S. et al. (2013). Operation debrief: a SHARP improvement in performance feedback in the operating room. *Annals of Surgery* 258 (6): 958–963.

Akçayır, M. and Akçayır, G. (2017). Advantages and challenges associated with augmented reality for education: a systematic review of the literature. *Educational Research Review* 20: 1–11.

Alinier, G., Hunt, B., Gordon, R., and Harwood, C. (2006). Effectiveness of intermediate-fidelity simulation training technology in undergraduate nursing education. *Journal of Advanced Nursing* 54 (3): 359–369.

Bandura, A. (2001). Social cognitive theory: an agentic perspective. *Annual Review of Psychology* 52 (1): 1–26.

Bandura, A. and Walters, R.H. (1977). *Social Learning Theory*, vol. 1. Englewood Cliffs: Prentice Hall.

Bearman, M., Nestel, D., and Andreatta, P. (2013). Simulation-based medical education. In: *Oxford Textbook of Medical Education* (ed. K. Walsh), 186–197. Oxford: Oxford University Press.

Benishek, L.E., Lazzara, E.H., Gaught, W.L. et al. (2015). The template of events for applied and critical health-care simulation (TEACH Sim): a tool for systematic simulation scenario design. *Simulation in Healthcare* 10 (1): 21–30.

Boud, D. and Walker, D. (1993). Barriers to reflection on experience. In: *Using Experience for Learning* (ed. D. Boud, R. Cohen, and D. Walker), 73–86. New York: McGraw-Hill.

Brett-Fleegler, M., Rudolph, J., Eppich, W. et al. (2012). Debriefing assessment for simulation in healthcare: development and psychometric properties. *Simulation in Healthcare* 7 (5): 288–294.

Brindley, P.G. and Reynolds, S.F. (2011). Improving verbal communication in critical care medicine. *Journal of Critical Care* 26 (2): 155–159.

Brock, D., Abu-Rish, E., Chiu, C.R. et al. (2013). Republished: interprofessional education in team communication: working together to improve patient safety. *Postgraduate Medical Journal* 89 (1057): 642–651.

Buck, M.A. (2004). Mentoring: a promising strategy for creating and sustaining a learning organization. *Adult Learning* 15 (3–4): 8–11.

Burgess, A. and Mellis, C. (2015). Feedback and assessment for clinical placements: achieving the right balance. *Advances in Medical Education and Practice* 6: 373–381.

Cantrell, M.A. (2008). The importance of debriefing in clinical simulations. *Clinical Simulation in Nursing* 4 (2): e19–e23.

Carver, R. (1996). Theory for practice: a framework for thinking about experiential education. *Journal of Experimental Education* 19 (1): 8–13.

Cooke, N.J., Cannon-Bowers, J.A., Kiekel, P.A. et al. (2000). Improving teams' interpositional knowledge through cross training. *Proceedings of the Human Factors and Ergonomics Society Annual Meeting* 44: 390–393.

Decker, S.I., Anderson, M., Boese, T. et al. (2015). Standards of best practice: simulation standard VIII: simulation-enhanced interprofessional education (Sim-IPE). *Clinical Simulation in Nursing* 11 (6): 293–297.

Dewey, J., Montessori, M., Strzemiński, W. et al. (1997). Constructivism (learning theory). *Journal of Social Sciences, Literature and Languages* 9–16.

Dieckmann, P., Gaba, D., and Rall, M. (2007). Deepening the theoretical foundations of patient simulation as social practice. *Simulation in Healthcare* 2 (3): 183–193.

Donaldson, M.S., Corrigan, J.M., and Kohn, L.T. (ed.) (2000). To err is human: building a safer health system. In:. https://nap.nationalacademies.org/catalog/9728/to-err-is-human-building-a-safer-health-system.

Ericsson, K.A. (2004). Deliberate practice and the acquisition and maintenance of expert performance in medicine and related domains. *Academic Medicine* 79 (10): S70–S81.

Ericsson, K.A., Krampe, R.T., and Tesch-Römer, C. (1993). The role of deliberate practice in the acquisition of expert performance. *Psychological Review* 100 (3): 363.

Fanning, R.M. and Gaba, D.M. (2007). The role of debriefing in simulation-based learning. *Simulation in Healthcare* 2 (2): 115–125.

Forrest, K. and McKimm, J. (ed.) (2019). *Healthcare Simulation at a Glance*. Chichester: Wiley.

Gaba, D.M. (2004). The future vision of simulation in health care. *BMJ Quality and Safety* 13 (suppl 1): i2–i10.

Gaba, D.M. (2007). The future vision of simulation in healthcare. *Simulation in Healthcare* 2 (2): 126–135.

Hamstra, S.J., Brydges, R., Hatala, R. et al. (2014). Reconsidering fidelity in simulation-based training. *Academic Medicine* 89 (3): 387–392.

Hanson, J., Smith, C., Luthra, P. et al. (2004). An assessment of the educational value of the Laerdal SimMan in improving the assessment and treatment of critically ill patients. *Emergency Medicine Australasia* 16.

Health Education England (2017). Multi-professional Framework for Advanced Clinical Practice in England. www.hee.nhs.uk/sites/default/files/docuemtns/HEE%20ACP%20Framework.pdf

Health Education England (2021) Professional Development Framework for Educators. https://london.hee.nhs.uk/sites/default/files/professional_development_framework_for_educators_2022.pdf

Hughes, A.M., Gregory, M.E., Joseph, D.L. et al. (2016). Saving lives: a meta-analysis of team training in healthcare. *Journal of Applied Psychology* 101 (9): 1266.

Jaye, P., Thomas, L., and Reedy, G. (2015). 'The diamond': a structure for simulation debrief. *Clinical Teacher* 12 (3): 171–175.

Kneebone, R. (2003). Simulation in surgical training: educational issues and practical implications. *Medical Education* 37 (3): 267–277.

Kneebone, R., Arora, S., King, D. et al. (2010). Distributed simulation – accessible immersive training. *Medical Teacher* 32 (1): 65–70.

Knowles, M.S. (1978). Andragogy: adult learning theory in perspective. *Community College Review* 5 (3): 9–20.

Kolb, D.A. (2014). *Experiential Learning: Experience as the Source of Learning and Development*. Upper Saddle River: Pearson Education.

Konstantinidis, S., Bamidis, P.D., and Zary, N. (ed.) (2020). *Digital Innovations in Healthcare Education and Training*. New York: Academic Press.

Lewin, K. (1951). Field Theory in Social Science: Selected Theoretical Papers. In: (ed. D. Cartwright). New York: Harper & Bros.

Losada, M. and Heaphy, E. (2004). The role of positivity and connectivity in the performance of business teams. *American Behavioral Scientist* 47 (6): 740–765.

Maran, N.J. and Glavin, R.J. (2003). Low-to high-fidelity simulation – a continuum of medical education? *Medical Education* 37: 22–28.

Maslow, A. (1943). A theory of human motivation. *Psychological Review* 50 (4): 370–396.

McGaghie, W.C., Issenberg, S.B., Petrusa, E.R., and Scalese, R.J. (2010). A critical review of simulation-based medical education research: 2003–2009. *Medical Education* 44 (1): 50–63.

McGaghie, W.C., Draycott, T.J., Dunn, W.F. et al. (2011). Evaluating the impact of simulation on translational patient outcomes. *Simulation in Healthcare* 6 (Suppl): S42.

Mezirow, J. (1990). *Fostering Critical Reflection in Adulthood*, 1–20. San Francisco: Jossey-Bass.

Moon, J. (2000). *Facilitating Reflective Learning in Higher Education*. London: McGraw-Hill Education.

Moorhead, S.A., Hazlett, D.E., Harrison, L. et al. (2013). A new dimension of health care: systematic review of the uses, benefits, and limitations of social media for health communication. *Journal of Medical Internet Research* 15 (4): e1933.

Moro, C., Birt, J., Stromberga, Z. et al. (2021). Virtual and augmented reality enhancements to medical and science student physiology and anatomy test performance: a systematic review and meta-analysis. *Anatomical Sciences Education* 14 (3): 368–376.

Paige, J.T., Sonesh, S.C., Garbee, D.D. et al. (2020). *Comprehensive Healthcare Simulation: InterProfessional Team Training and Simulation*. Cham: Springer Nature.

Pearson, M. and Smith, D. (1985). Debriefing in experience-based learning. In: *Reflection*, 69–84. Cambridge: Routledge.

Pendleton, D., Schofield, T., Tate, P., and Havelock, P. (2003). Learning and teaching about the consultation. In: *The New Consultation: Developing Doctor–Patient Communication* (ed. D. Pendleton). Oxford: Oxford University Press.

Perkins, G.D., Kimani, P.K., Bullock, I. et al. for the Electronic Advanced Life Support Collaborators (2012). Improving the efficiency of advanced life support training: a randomized, controlled trial. *Annals of Internal Medicine* 157 (1): 19–28.

Popenici, S. and Millar, V. (2015). *Writing Learning Outcomes: A Practical Guide for Academics*. Melbourne: University of Melbourne.

Riley, R.H. (ed.) (2016). *Manual of Simulation in Healthcare*. New York: Oxford University Press.

Roberts, D. and Roberts, N.J. (2014). Maximising sensory learning through immersive education. *Journal of Nursing Education and Practice* 4 (10): 74–79.

Rudolph, J.W., Simon, R., Dufresne, R.L., and Raemer, D.B. (2006). There's no such thing as "nonjudgmental" debriefing. In:. https://thedebriefingacademy.com/wp-content/uploads/2019/01/Rudolph_DebriefGoodJudgment_SIH_2006.pdf.

Salas, E., Shuffler, M.L., Thayer, A.L. et al. (2015). Understanding and improving teamwork in organizations: a scientifically based practical guide. *Human Resource Management* 54 (4): 599–622.

Schön, D.A. (1987). *Educating the Reflective Practitioner: Toward a New Design for Teaching and Learning in the Professions*. San Francisco: Jossey-Bass.

Shahoumian, A., Saunders, M., Zenios, M. et al. (2014). Blended simulation based medical education: a complex learning/training opportunity. In: *Presented at the International Conference on Learning and Collaboration Technologies*, 478–485. Cham: Springer.

Sørensen, J.L., Østergaard, D., LeBlanc, V. et al. (2017). Design of simulation-based medical education and advantages and disadvantages of in situ simulation versus off-site simulation. *BMC Medical Education* 17 (1): 1–9.

Stepan, K., Zeiger, J., Hanchuk, S. et al. (2017). Immersive virtual reality as a teaching tool for neuroanatomy. *International Forum of Allergy and Rhinology* 7 (10): 1006–1013.

Tannenbaum, S.I. and Cerasoli, C.P. (2013). Do team and individual debriefs enhance performance? A meta-analysis. *Human Factors* 55 (1): 231–245.

Thomas, L. and Reeves, S. (2015). Sociological fidelity: keeping the patient at the heart of interprofessional learning. *Journal of Interprofessional Care* 29 (3): 177–178.

Thompson, N. and Pascal, J. (2012). Developing critically reflective practice. *Reflective Practice* 13 (2): 311–325.

Van De Ridder, J.M., Stokking, K.M., McGaghie, W.C., and Ten Cate, O.T.J. (2008). What is feedback in clinical education? *Medical Education* 42 (2): 189–197.

Ventola, C.L. (2014). Social media and health care professionals: benefits, risks, and best practices. *Pharmacy and Therapeutics* 39 (7): 491.

Vygotsky, L. (1978). Social constructivism. In: *Mind in Society*. Cambridge: Harvard University Press.

Walker, M. and Peyton, J.W.R. (1998). Teaching in theatre. In: *Teaching and Learning in Medical Practice* (ed. J.W.R. Peyton), 171–180. Rickmansworth: Manticore Publishers Europe.

Weaver, S.J., Dy, S.M., and Rosen, M.A. (2014). Team-training in healthcare: a narrative synthesis of the literature. *BMJ Quality and Safety* 23 (5): 359–372.

Weller, J.M., Torrie, J., Boyd, M. et al. (2014). Improving team information sharing with a structured call-out in anaesthetic emergencies: a randomized controlled trial. *British Journal of Anaesthesia* 112 (6): 1042–1049.

Whitmore, J. (1992). *Coaching for Performance*. London: Nicholas Brealey.

Yardley, S., Teunissen, P.W., and Dornan, T. (2012). Experiential learning: AMEE guide no. 63. *Medical Teacher* 34 (2): e102–e115.

Zhu, E., Hadadgar, A., Masiello, I., and Zary, N. (2014). Augmented reality in healthcare education: an integrative review. *PeerJ* 2: e469.

FURTHER READING

ASPIH Standards for simulation-based education in healthcare. `https://aspih.org.uk/`

IPEC Core Competencies. Recommendations and IPE competencies. `www.ipecollaborative.org/`

Stone, D. and Heen, S. (2014). *Thanks for the Feedback: The Science and Art of Receiving Feedback Well*. New York: Penguin.

Weinstein, Y., Sumeraki, M., and Caviglioli, O. (2018). *Understanding How We Learn: A Visual Guide*. Cambridge: Routledge.

SELF-ASSESSMENT QUESTIONS

1. Describe five educational theories.
2. How is psychological safety established for learners?
3. What are five benefits of using simulation-based education?
4. What are five dos and don'ts of debriefing?

GLOSSARY

Appraisal   A formal method of feedback, often scheduled at regular intervals.

Debrief   A conversation held after an event aimed at sustaining or improving performance.

Dual coding theory   The theory that imagery and verbal information, when provided together, improve the retention of knowledge.

Feedback   Specific information about the comparison between an observed performance and a standard with the intent to improve performance.

Self-directed learning   The student taking accountability for their own knowledge acquisition.

Simulation   An educational activity that uses artificial representation of the real-world process to achieve educational goals from experiential learning in a safe environment.

CHAPTER 17

The Advanced Practitioner as Educator

Phil Broadhurst

> ## Aim
> The aim of this chapter is to provide the advanced clinical practitioner with an understanding of clinical education.

LEARNING OUTCOMES

After reading this chapter the reader will:

1. be able to use effective teaching and assessment strategies in healthcare
2. understand the importance of effective feedback and the models used to facilitate it
3. be able to consider the importance of behaviour in managing change
4. demonstrate an ability to facilitate effective clinical learning in a busy environment.

INTRODUCTION

Clinical and workplace education is a key component of the advanced practitioner's (AP) role, with Health Education England (2017) recognising it as one of the four pillars. Whether supporting colleagues in practice or empowering patients to make informed lifestyle choices and healthcare decisions, APs are well placed to facilitate professional and service user learning across the entire healthcare spectrum.

The Advanced Practitioner: A Framework for Practice, First Edition. Edited by Ian Peate,
Sadie Diamond-Fox, and Barry Hill.
© 2024 John Wiley & Sons Ltd. Published 2024 by John Wiley & Sons Ltd.

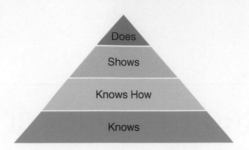

FIGURE 17.1   Miller's pyramid. *Source*: Adapted from Al-Eraky and Marei (2016).

To facilitate effective professional learning opportunities, it is often a helpful starting point to consider taxonomy scales and how they can be used to influence and guide strategies when providing teaching and supervision for colleagues. Miller's pyramid (Miller 1990) (Figure 17.1) proposes a structure through which learners progress as their competence increases. At the pyramid's base, the learner can demonstrate the ability to recall information. At its peak, however, the learner has progressed beyond the theoretical and simulated learning environments and into the workplace, where their competence is validated within authentic clinical practice as part of their ongoing professional role. Examples of effective workplace-based assessments include Direct Observation of Procedural Skills (DOPS), Mini Clinical Exercises (Mini-CEX) and case-based discussions (Liu 2012), as well as peer review processes, including multi-source feedback, that focus upon both technical and non-technical skills, the clinician's medical knowledge, professionalism, outcomes, problem-solving ability and patient satisfaction (Norcini 2003).

Arguably, one of the most valuable aspects of clinical assessment and supervision is the opportunity it affords clinicians to utilise feedback as part of the learning process, and studies into the processes of feedback have reinforced the importance that feedback and feedforward hold in professional development (McConnell et al. 2016). Research has also demonstrated a direct correlation between feedback and performance, finding that where feedback processes encourage learners to participate in self-assessment, performance and skills can be enhanced (Egan et al. 2020). Models of feedback will be explored later in this chapter.

Another learning domain in which AP play a key role is patient education. By advocating for lifestyle changes such as smoking cessation or postoperative self-care in an Enhanced Recovery After Surgery (ERAS) programme (ERAS Society 2022), healthcare professionals can help to grow a partnership approach to decision making, therefore facilitating behaviour change and ownership of a person's own health journey and condition management (Haskell and Lord 2017). The COM-B model of behaviour change (Figure 17.2) (Michie et al. 2011) helps educators to consider priorities when designing and delivering programmes to patients by ensuring that the programme provides sufficient opportunity and motivation for patients and is appropriate in its expectation of what patients can achieve both physically and emotionally.

For behaviour change to be effective, clinicians should consider the four key steps that patients will need to pass through for successful achievement (Box 17.1) (Cullen et al. 2001). Furthermore, the wider concepts of andragogy (the theory underlying adult learning) propose that adults learn what they want to learn, based upon its perceived personal value (Knowles 1984). Therefore, patient and service user education needs to consider not just what we want them to understand, but also their recognition of the need for change and desire to do so.

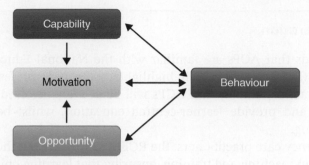

FIGURE 17.2 COM-B. *Source*: Adapted from Whitehead (2017).

Box 17.1 Four Steps to Behaviour Change.

1. Recognising the need for change *(Motivation)*
2. Establishing an achievable goal *(Capability)*
3. Monitoring activity related to the goal *(Opportunity)*
4. Self-reward for achieving the goal *(Behaviour has changed)*

Source: Adapted from Cullen et al. (2001).

Multi-Professional Framework for Advanced Clinical Practice (HEE 2017)

1.5 Demonstrate effective communication skills, supporting people in making decisions, planning care or seeking to make positive changes, using Health Education England's framework to promote person-centred approaches in health and care.

2.1 Pro-actively initiate and develop effective relationships, fostering clarity of roles within teams, to encourage productive working.

2.4 Actively engage in peer review to inform own and others' practice, formulating and implementing strategies to act on learning and make improvements.

2.7 Critically apply advanced clinical expertise in appropriate facilitatory ways to provide consultancy across professional and service boundaries, influencing clinical practice to enhance quality, reduce unwarranted variation and promote the sharing and adoption of best practice.

3.3 Engage with, appraise and respond to individuals' motivation, development stage and capacity, working collaboratively to support health literacy and empower individuals to participate in decisions about their care and to maximise their health and well-being.

3.4 Advocate for and contribute to a culture of organisational learning to inspire future and existing staff.

3.7 Supporting the wider team to build capacity and capability through work-based and interprofessional learning, and the application of learning to practice.

3.8 Act as a role model, educator, supervisor, coach and mentor, seeking to instil and develop the confidence of others.

Accreditation Considerations

FICM (2022) recommends that ACPs are familiar with the National Education and Competence Framework for ACCPs (DOH 2008), which highlights some core professional expectations in advanced critical care practice, namely that ACPs will be actively involved in teaching across the multidisciplinary team, and provide learner-centred education, whilst being aware of the key principles of adult learning.

For advanced emergency care practitioners, the RCEM (2019) sets out the expectation that ACPs will be actively involved in teaching and training, ensuring that learning objectives are set and met, feedback processes are used and appraisals are carried out for junior colleagues. It also recognises the importance of the ACP in patient education strategies.

The RCGP (2020) outlines that primary care ACPs should be actively involved in feedback processes and peer review, whilst actively encouraging shared learning and facilitating interprofessional learning.

The Royal Pharmaceutical Society's Advanced Practice Framework (RPS 2013) dedicates section 5 of its framework to education, highlighting the requirements of role modelling, mentorship and development of training within the descriptors of its expectations for advanced clinical practice. Section 1 also recommends that advanced practitioners in pharmaceutical settings are able to provide effective care programmes for patients.

Fields of Practice – Mental Health

There is an ongoing recognition that parity of esteem needs to be realised within mental health, with a much needed focus on creating equality with physical health needs (Kirkbride and Jones 2014). For this to be realised, healthcare professionals should be proactive in helping service users to understand the need to access services and developing behaviours that promote their health, as well as addressing stigma amongst the wider population, with healthcare education integrating mental health considerations into the wider format of curricula (Mitchell et al. 2017).

There is a growing emphasis on mindfulness as the subject of training and well-being, and a growing acceptance that patients often want to take ownership of their mental health and related learning (Groves 2016). Indeed, a recent large RCT found that mindfulness training can help to reduce levels of stress and anxiety in the older population who are experiencing cognitive decline when compared to traditional educational strategies (Marchant et al. 2018). Mindfulness-based intervention is based around a series of core skills that can help the learner to process their thoughts and feelings in a more desirable way through attention and awareness, and accepting and letting go (Hick and Chan 2010).

PROVIDING FEEDBACK

Advanced clinical practitioners often find themselves involved in the clinical supervision and education of multidisciplinary peers. One example where the AP can be routinely involved is in the teaching of clinical skills, and there are numerous resources available to assist with this. The use of DOPS is widely accepted within medical and healthcare education (Hengameh et al. 2015; Lagoo and Joshi 2021).

For such a learning encounter to be effective, however, there needs to be some consideration of the context in which the assessment is used.

Fields of Practice – Paediatrics

Patient education within the paediatric sector has two key considerations: that of the child and that of the parent or caregiver.

One strategy that has proved effective in empowering new parents to manage the health of their children is parental education groups. These groups exist to provide a bridge between healthcare professionals and children's caregivers by offering a social learning environment for parents to share experiences and access supported learning and key information (Frykedal et al. 2021). Although key to promoting healthcare change within the paediatric population, it can often be seen as challenging for some healthcare professionals to provide leadership for these groups as they are often working in isolation away from peer support and peer review. One possible solution to this is to look at building up service user understanding by using the Dreyfus skills model, where the learner progresses from being a novice through the stages of advanced beginner, competent and proficient (Benner 2004). Evidence has shown that these groups can be effective learning environments for parents in a variety of contexts, from antenatal classes to helping them to manage childhood asthma (Agusala et al. 2018; Berlin et al. 2016).

For parental education classes to be effective, APs should ensure that the content of classes is relevant and worthwhile, with plenty of opportunity for discussion and peer support and a leader who is engaged and knowledgeable (Berlin et al. 2016).

Feeding Back and Feeding Forward

There is increasing recognition amongst clinical educators that formative assessment on its own is limited in enhancing a learner's development, and that in order to progress, the processes of *feedback* and *feedforward* are key elements within learning (Sadler 2010). The purpose of feedback and feedforward is to allow learners to reflect on their performance and identify points which can help them to improve and develop their skills (Henderson et al. 2005). Furthermore, feedback is proven to work best when it is objective, addressing specific tasks in order to improve the process of self-regulation, with studies demonstrating that feedback is often more focused when used alongside scheduled observational activities (Pelgrim et al. 2012). There are many feedback models that have been validated for use in medical education, but the Pendleton model (Figure 17.3) (Pendleton et al. 2008) and the Agenda-Led Outcome-Based Analysis (ALOBA) model (Figure 17.4) (Silverman et al. 1996) are often seen as the most accessible.

The Pendleton feedback model allows the learner to reflect on their performance, discussing what they did well and how they could improve next time. The educator is also able to reinforce the learning points identified by the learner and add their own perspectives. This combined feedback and feedforward is then used to create an action plan to help the learner develop the areas identified. It is believed that the Pendleton model is particularly valuable as it allows the learner to play an active part in the learning conversation (Archer 2009), and research has further demonstrated that when a learning conversation is used to also provide feedforward, in which the assessor provides points to help inform future practice, learners can deem the feedback to be of a useful quality, especially when they have already been encouraged to reflect on the area in which they need to improve (Hewson and Little 1998).

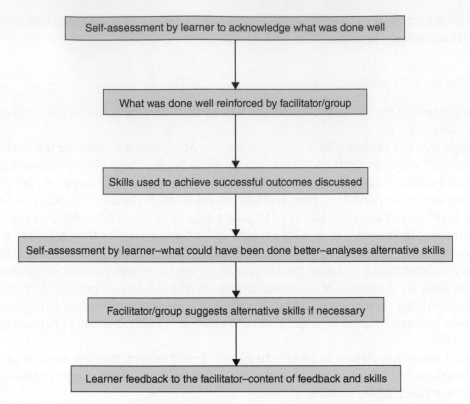

FIGURE 17.3 Pendleton's model for feedback. *Source*: Chowdhury and Kalu (2004)/Royal College of Obstetricians and Gynaecologists.

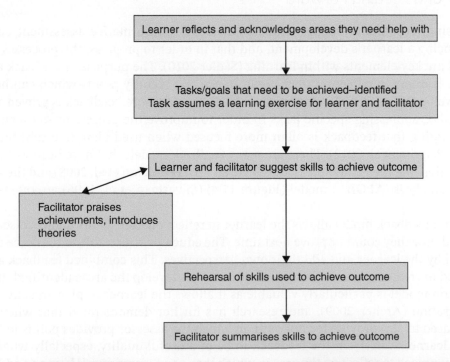

FIGURE 17.4 ALOBA model for feedback. *Source*: Chowdhury and Kalu (2004)/Royal College of Obstetricians and Gynaecologists.

Fields of Practice – Learning Disabilities

In a report, the UK Department of Health (DOH 2010) found that people with learning disabilities were often not empowered to exercise choice over their lifestyle. This places a burden of responsibility on clinicians to ensure that educational materials are as accessible as possible, and consideration should be given to enabling people with learning disabilities to access information that allows them to take ownership of their health needs in a way that is appropriate for them. For example, when providing written information, is the person able to read? Maybe they are partially sighted or blind and require Braille, large-print or spoken information, or maybe their learning difficulty prevented them from learning to read and their information needs to be given via other media. Other tools that could be used in patient education include pictures and drawings, recordings or electronic devices that provide prompts for patients (Rossignol and Paasche-Orlow 2013).

A key principle in empowering people with learning disabilities to learn is the concept of positive reinforcement, where behaviour change is realised via reward for implementing new understanding; in other words, reward becomes the motivation for learning (Wills 2014). This can often come in the form of praise or physical reward and the AP needs to consider how these can complement the desired outcomes.

Sometimes the Pendleton model has been criticised for being too rigid and not empowering learners and assessors to be able to discuss the required improvements and the deficits of which they are unaware (Cantillon and Sargeant 2008; Chowdhury and Kalu 2004). The ALOBA model provides an alternative structure that can be used for feedback. It differs from Pendleton in that it offers a learner-centred approach where the learner focuses on what they want to learn, with the emphasis being on problem solving rather than highlighting the problem, thus avoiding the learning discussion becoming an educator-led diagnosis of problems (Archer 2009).

The ALOBA model comprises three key areas, beginning with the learner reflecting and clarifying which area they would like to focus on before agreeing what they want to achieve. The assessor and learner then engage in discussion in order to clarify what skills may be required in order to achieve the desired outcome, as well as agreeing the learning goal for future development of the skill. Finally, the assessor provides a summary of the feedback encounter to ensure there is clarity around what has been agreed. It is argued that ALOBA empowers learners to self-assess and provides ownership of the discussion, thus motivating them to improve (Cantillon and Sargeant 2008).

THE ONE-MINUTE PRECEPTOR

The AP role often creates demand on available time. When working in busy healthcare settings with high clinical need, it can often feel that teaching and learning opportunities are scarce due to the pace and pressure of work. When working with healthcare learners, it can be easy to feel overwhelmed by the need to support learning and balance it against the requirements for patient care. An easy structure that practitioners can use to assist learners in their development is the one-minute preceptor (OMP) (Neher 2003), which provides a simple, five-step model to help clinicians provide a quality learning encounter for learners without detracting from clinical needs (Gallagher et al. 2012) (Box 17.2).

The OMP process works by asking the learner open-ended questions and encourages them to consider their reasoning before allowing the preceptor to input into the process to help connect the points and

> **Box 17.2   The One-Minute Preceptor**
>
> 1. Get a commitment from the learner (for example, ask them for a diagnosis).
> 2. Probe for their underlying understanding and reasoning (why did they come to that conclusion?).
> 3. Teach a general rule (offer a core concept they can remember for the future).
> 4. Offer feedback (what did the learner do well?).
> 5. Correct mistakes (highlight points for improvement).
>
> *Source*: Adapted from Gallagher (2012) and Rashid et al. (2017).

offer additional considerations in the process (Rashid et al. 2017). Several studies have validated the OMP as an effective teaching tool within clinical education, demonstrating improvements in the performance and understanding of learners within the healthcare sector. However, some research suggests that the tool works best when preceptors have a strong understanding of feedback processes and an ability to consider the needs of individual learners to which they can adapt accordingly (Furney et al. 2001; Seki et al. 2016). As is the case with feedback models, when used flexibly the OMP empowers learners to take ownership by challenging their clinical reasoning and opens the encounter up to a productive feedback conversation (Swartz 2016).

ORANGE FLAGS – PSYCHOLOGICAL CONSIDERATIONS

Self-awareness

1. Being self-aware can help you understand why you feel like you do and why you behave as you do.
2. Having this awareness helps you make changes to the things that you would like to change, therefore making your life better.
3. Self-awareness is at the core of professional development.
4. Being self-aware helps you understand how you can affect others.

GREEN FLAGS – SOCIAL AND CULTURAL CONSIDERATIONS

Decolonisation of the Curriculum

Patient populations are growing increasingly diverse and complex, APs and learners should be provided with the skills and knowledge to treat patients from minority groups equitably and non-judgementally. Diversity-related topics increase confidence in communication and have the potential to improve patient care.

CONCLUSION

The responsibilities of APs in relation to education and supervision are well defined within the four pillars of advanced practice and the framework for advanced practice (HEE 2017). Through understanding taxonomies of competence, support for junior multidisciplinary colleagues can be provided to help them grow and develop their clinical abilities, using feedback and feedforward as validated methods of providing guidance and support as they reflect on their skills.

While providing care to patients, APs should consider the ways in which they provide education and lifestyle advice, underpinned by behaviour change models to ensure that patient information is provided in an accessible manner that empowers them to achieve their goals and embrace ownership of their healthcare needs.

Take Home Points

- Miller's taxonomy can help learners and supervisors to consider the context in which skills are learnt and demonstrated, encouraging appropriate use of assessment tools to guide development.

- The processes of feedback and feedforward have been demonstrated to be the most valuable aspects of assessment within skills acquisition, and the use of Pendleton's model or ALOBA can help supervisors to encourage reflection on learning.

- COM-B helps clinicians to consider the capability, opportunity and motivation for patients to engage in behaviour change to empower them with their health needs.

REFERENCES

Agasula, V., Vij, P., Agusala, V. et al. (2018). Can interactive parental education impact health care utilization in pediatric asthma: a study in rural Texas. *Journal of International Medical Research* 46 (8): 3172–3182.

Al-Eraky, M. and Marei, H. (2016). A fresh look at Miller's pyramid: assessment at the 'is' and 'do' levels. *Medical Education* 50 (12): 1253–1257.

Archer, J.C. (2009). State of the science in health professional education: effective feedback. *Medical Education* 44 (1): 101–108.

Benner, S. (2004). Using the Dreyfus model of skill acquisition to describe and interpret skill acquisition and clinical judgement in nursing practice and education. *Bulletin of Science Technology Society* 24 (3): 188–199.

Berlin, A., Törnkvist, L., and Barimani, M. (2016). Content and presentation of content in parental education groups in Sweden. *Journal of Perinatal Education.* 25 (2): 87–96.

Cantillon, P. and Sargeant, J. (2008). Giving feedback in clinical settings. *BMJ* 337 (7681): a1961.

Chowdhury, R.R. and Kalu, G. (2004). Learning to give feedback in medical education. *Obstetrician and Gynaecologist* 6 (4): 243–247.

Cullen, K.W., Baranowski, T., and Smith, S.P. (2001). Using goal-setting as a strategy for dietary behaviour change. *Journal of the American Dietetic Association* 101 (5): 562–566.

Department of Health (2008) The National Education and Competence Framework for Advanced Critical Care Practitioners. www.ficm.ac.uk/sites/ficm/files/documents/2021-10/National%20Education%20%26%20Competence%20Framework%20for%20ACCPs.pdf

Department of Health (2010) Valuing People Now – Summary Report March 2009 – September 2010. https://assets.publishing.service.gov.uk/government/uploads/system/uploads/attachment_data/file/215891/dh_122387.pdf

Egan, R., Chaplin, T., Szulewski, A. et al. (2020). A case for feedback and monitoring assessment in competency-based medical education. *Journal of Evaluation in Clinical Practice* 26 (4): 1105–1113.

ERAS Society (2022) Guidelines. https://erassociety.org/guidelines

FICM (2022) ACCPs. www.ficm.ac.uk/careersworkforce/accps

Frykedal, K.F., Rosander, M., and Barimani, M. and Belin, A. (2021). Cooperative learning in parental education groups – child healthcare nurses' views on their work as leaders and on the groups. *Children's Health Care* 51 (1): 20–36.

Furney, S.L., Orsini, A.N., Orsetti, K.E. et al. (2001). Teaching the one-minute preceptor. A randomized controlled trial. *Journal of General Internal Medicine* 16 (9): 620–624.

Gallagher, P., Tweed, M., Hanna, S. et al. (2012). Developing the one-minute preceptor. *Clinical Teacher* 9 (6): 358–362.

Groves, P. (2016). Mindfulness in psychiatry – where are we now? *BJPsych Bulletin.* 40 (6): 289–292.

Haskell, H. and Lord, T. (2017). Patient and families as coproducers of safe and reliable outcomes. In: *Surgical Patient Care: Improving Safety, Quality and Value* (ed. J.A. Sanchez, P. Barach, J.K. Johnson, et al.). Cham: Springer.

Health Education England (2017). Multi-professional Framework for Advanced Clinical Practice in England. www.hee.nhs.uk

Henderson, P., Fersuson-Smith, A.C., and Johnson, M.H. (2005). Developing essential professional skills: a framework for teaching and learning about feedback. *BMC Medical Education* 5 (1): 111–116.

Hengameh, H., Afsaneh, R., Morteza, K. et al. (2015). The effect of applying direct observation of procedural skills (DOPS) on nursing students' clinical skills: a randomized clinical trial. *Global Journal of Health Science* 7 (7): 17–21.

Hewson, M.G. and Little, M.L. (1998). Giving feedback in medical education: verification of recommended techniques. *Journal of General Internal Medicine* 13 (2): 111–116.

Hick, S.F. and Chan, L. (2010). Mindfulness-based cognitive therapy for depression: effectiveness and limitations. *Social Work in Mental Health* 8 (3): 225–237.

Kirkbride, J.B. and Jones, P.B. (2014). Parity of esteem begins at home: translating psychiatric research into effective public mental health. *Psychological Medicine* 44 (8): 1569–1576.

Knowles, M. (1984). *Andragogy in Action: Applying Modern Principles of Adult Learning.* London: Jossey-Bass.

Lagoo, J. and Joshi, S. (2021). Introduction of direct observation of proceduaral skillsn (DOPS) as a formative assessment tool during postgraduate training in anaesthesiology: exploration and perceptions. *Indian Journal of Anaesthesia* 65 (3): 202–209.

Liu, C. (2012). An introduction to workplace-based discussions. *Gastroenterology and Hepatology from Bed to Bench* 5 (1): 24–28.

Marchant, N. L., Barnhofer, T., Klimecki, O. M. et al. for the SCD-WELL Medit-Ageing Research Group (2018) The SCD-well randomized controlled trial: effects of a mindfulness-based intervention versus health education on mental health in patients with subjective cognitive decline. *Alzheimer's and Dementia* 4(1), 737–745.

McConnell, M.M., Harms, S., and Saperson, K. (2016). Meaningful feedback in medical education: challenging the "failure to fail" using narrative methodology. *Academic Psychiatry* 40 (7): 377–379.

Michie, S., Van Stralen, M.M., and West, R. (2011). The behaviour change wheel: A new method for character-ising and designing behaviour change interventions. *Implementation Science* 6 (42): 42.

Miller, G.E. (1990). The assessment of clinical skills/competence/performance. *Academic Medicine* 65 (9): S63–S67.

Mitchell, A.J., Hardy, S., and Shiers, D. (2017). Parity of esteem: addressing the inequalities between mental and physical healthcare. *BJPsych Advances* 23 (3): 196–205.

Neher, J.O. (2003). The one-minute preceptor: shaping the teaching conversation. *Family Medicine* 6: 391–393.

Norcini, J.J. (2003). Work based assessment. *BMJ* 326 (7392): 753–755.

Pelgrim, E.A.M., Kramer, A.W.M., Mokkink, H.G.A., and van der Vleuten, C.P.M. (2012). The process of feed-back in workplace-based assessment: organisation, delivery, continuity. *Medical Education* 46 (6): 604–612.

Pendleton, D., Schofield, T., Tate, P., and Havelock, P. (2008). *The New Consultation: Developing Doctor-Patient Communication*. Oxford: Oxford University Press.

Rashid, P., Churchill, J.A., and Gendy, R. (2017). Improving clinical teaching for busy clinicians: integration of the one-minute preceptor into mini-clinical examination. *ANZ Journal of Surgery* 87 (7-8): 535–536.

Rossignol, L.N. and Paasche-Orlow, M.K. (2013). Empowering patients who have specific learning difficulties. *Journal of the American Medical Association* 310 (14): 1445–1446.

Royal College of Emergency Medicine (2019) Advanced Clinical Practitioner Curriculum and Assessment (v.2). `https://rcem.ac.uk/wp-content/uploads/2021/10/EC_ACP_Curriculum_2017_Adult_and_Paediatric-for_publication-Last_Edit_14-03-2019.pdf`

Royal College of General Practitioners (2020) Core Capabilities Framework for Advanced Clinical Practice (Nurses) Working in General Practice/Primary Care in England. `www.hee.nhs.uk/sites/default/files/documents/ACP%20Primary%20Care%20Nurse%20Fwk%202020.pdf`

Royal Pharmaceutical Society (2013) The RPS Advanced Pharmacy Framework. `www.rpharms.com/Portals/0/RPS%20document%20library/Open%20access/Frameworks/RPS%20Advanced%20Pharmacy%20Framework.pdf`

Sadler, D.R. (2010). Beyond feedback: developing student capability in complex appraisal. *Assessment and Evaluation in Higher Education* 35 (5): 535–550.

Seki, M., Otaki, J., Breugelmans, R. et al. (2016). How do case presentation teaching methods affect learning outcomes? SNAPPS and the one-minute preceptor. *BMC Medical Education* 16 (1): 12.

Silverman, J.D., Kurtz, S.M., and Draper, J. (1996). The Calgary-Cambridge approach to communication teach-ing skills teaching 1: agenda-led outcome-based analysis of the consultation. *Education for General Practice* 4: 288–299.

Swartz, M.K. (2016). Revisiting "the one-minute preceptor". *Journal of Pediatric Health Care* 30 (2): 95–96.

Whitehead, K. (2017). Behaviour change. In: *How to Facilitate Lifestyle Change: Applying Group Education in Healthcare* (ed. A. Avery, K. Whitehead, and V. Halliday). London: Wiley.

Wills, J. (ed.) (2014). *Fundamentals of Health Promotion for Nurses*, 2e. Chichester: Wiley Blackwell.

FURTHER READING

Avery, A., Whitehead, K., and Halliday, V. (2017). *How to Facilitate Lifestyle Change: Applying Group Education in Healthcare*. London: Wiley.

Chowdhury, R.R. and Kalu, G. (2004). Learning to give feedback in medical education. *Obstetrician and Gynaecologist* 6 (4): 243–247.

Ende, J. (1983). Feedback in clinical medical education. *Journal of the American Medical Association* 250 (6): 777–781.

Michie, S., Van Stralen, M.M., and West, R. (2011). The behaviour change wheel: a new method for characterising and designing behaviour change interventions. *Implementation Science* 6 (42): 42.

Neher, J.O. (2003). The one-minute preceptor: shaping the teaching conversation. *Family Medicine* 6: 391–393.

SELF-ASSESSMENT QUESTIONS

1. What are the stages of Pendleton's feedback model? How do they differ from the ALOBA model?
2. What assessment tools are appropriate for work-based assessment and how can they be effectively used?
3. What are the key elements of the COM-B model and how can this help with developing patient education programmes?
4. How can the One-Minute Preceptor be used in practice to support learning?

GLOSSARY

Andragogy   The theory of adult learning.

Braille   A tactile alphabet that allows people who are visually impaired to read.

Competence   The ability to complete a task or demonstrate a skill independently and knowledgeably.

Curriculum   The total course of individual components of study.

Feedback   The process of providing reflection and observations on previous performance.

Feedforward   The process of providing action plans and advice for future performance and improvement.

Mindfulness   The ability to consider and evaluate one's thoughts and emotions.

Parental education group   Facilitated group to support parents in promoting their child's health and well-being.

Parity of esteem   The valuing of mental health equally to physical health.

Self-awareness   An awareness of our character and traits that allows us to evaluate our choices and actions.

Taxonomy   Scale that allows practitioners to qualify their competence.

CHAPTER 18

Research Principles

Brigitta Fazzini and Roberta Borg

Aim

This chapter offers an overview of research methods and principles and demonstrates how research should encompass the advanced practice role and inform clinical practice.

LEARNING OUTCOMES

After reading this chapter the reader will:

1. understand why research is part of the advanced clinical practice framework and how it helps incorporate evidence-based practice in advanced practice roles
2. appreciate the hierarchy of evidence and be able to appraise it
3. master the research process
4. discern the different types of research methods
5. be aware of the ethics surrounding healthcare research
6. recognise the value of quality improvement projects.

WHY RESEARCH IS IMPORTANT

Medical and healthcare advances can only be possible through research designed to understand population needs and disease processes and evaluate and enhance treatment options.

Healthcare professionals have a duty to provide the best and safest clinical practice by keeping up to date with knowledge and skills, using evidence-based practices, educating and sharing our knowledge. For this reason, Health Education England (HEE 2017) recognises research as one of the four pillars

The Advanced Practitioner: A Framework for Practice, First Edition. Edited by Ian Peate,
Sadie Diamond-Fox, and Barry Hill.
© 2024 John Wiley & Sons Ltd. Published 2024 by John Wiley & Sons Ltd.

that underpin advanced clinical practice. Box 18.1 highlights some of the capabilities expected of the advanced clinical practitioner in relation to research.

Box 18.1   Research Capabilities for Advanced Clinical Practice in England.

4.1   Critically engage in research activity, adhering to good research practice guidance, so that evidence-based strategies are developed and applied to enhance quality, safety, productivity, and value for money.

4.2   Evaluate and audit own and others' clinical practice, selecting and applying valid, reliable methods, then acting on the findings.

4.3   Critically appraise and synthesise the outcome of relevant research, evaluation and audit, using the results to underpin own practice and to inform that of others.

4.4   Take a critical approach to identify gaps in the evidence base and its application to practice, alerting appropriate individuals and organisations to these and how they might be addressed in a safe and pragmatic way.

Source: Adapted from HEE (2017)

The Research Process

An understanding of the research process (Figure 18.1) is required by all advanced practitioners, using healthcare literature to inform their evidence-based practice.

Learning Event

Reflect on your current clinical practice: Can you identify any gaps in the evidence on which you base your practice?

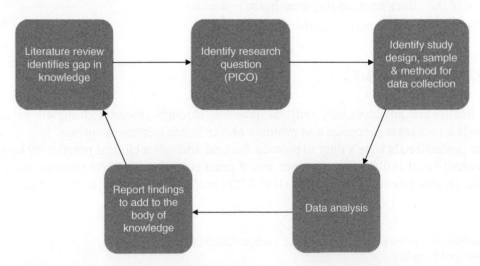

FIGURE 18.1   The research process. *Source*: Roberta Borg.

CRITICAL APPRAISAL AND THE HIERARCHY OF EVIDENCE

Critical appraisal skills and an understanding of the hierarchy of evidence are also crucial skills for the advanced clinical practitioner. There are several critiquing tools that can be used, such as the Cochrane tool, the Critical Appraisal Skill Programme (CASP) checklist and the National Institutes of Health quality assessment tool, amongst others. The purpose of an appraisal tool is to guide the practitioner to systematically assess the trustworthiness, relevance and results of published papers. The critique should also consider the risk of bias in the results and ultimately help the practitioner decide whether the evidence or conclusion presented in the study is robust enough to incorporate into practice.

The hierarchy of evidence pyramid provided by the National Health and Medical Research Council (Figure 18.2) is used to rank the relative strength of results obtained from scientific research, by using the notion that the study design and the endpoints measured affect the strength of the evidence. The higher the study is positioned, the more rigorous is the methodology and minimal the effect of bias on the results.

The GRADE approach (Grading of Recommendations, Assessment, Development and Evaluations) is another widely endorsed method of assessing the quality of evidence and the strength of recommendations (Table 18.1).

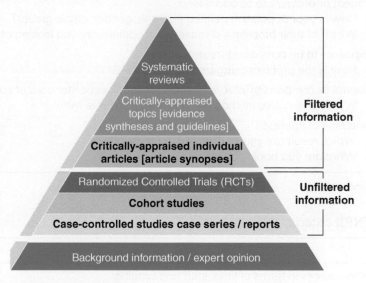

FIGURE 18.2   The evidence hierarchy pyramid.

TABLE 18.1   GRADE rating for quality of evidence from the Cochrane Handbook.

High	There is a lot of confidence that the true effect lies close to that of the estimated effect
Moderate	There is moderate confidence in the estimated effect: the true effect is likely to be close to the estimated effect, but there is a possibility that it is substantially different
Low	There is limited confidence in the estimated effect: the true effect might be substantially different from the estimated effect
Very low	There is very little confidence in the estimated effect: the true effect is likely to be substantially different from the estimated effect

DESIGNING A RESEARCH PROJECT

The research design is the plan made to answer a research question, while the research method is the strategy used to implement that plan.

Every Research Project Starts with a Question

The research question refers to a problem that can be evaluated and analysed to provide information. A successful research project starts with a well-formulated research question, often based on a background which may be a clinical problem or a specific disease.

The PICO (population, intervention, control, outcomes) format (Table 18.2) is a widely used strategy which facilitates formulation of research questions. In addition, the FINER criteria (Table 18.3) ensure that the research question is relevant, researchable and significant.

TABLE 18.2   The PICO framework.

PICO	
P: Population or Problem of interest	Patient or problem to be addressed: • How is your population defined (e.g. age, gender, ethnic group)? • Which of their problems, diseases or conditions are you looking at?
I: Intervention	Exposure to be considered/treatment/test • How is the problem being treated?
C: Comparator	Control or comparison intervention treatment/placebo/standard of care • Which alternative method are you comparing this with?
O: Outcome	Outcome of interest • Which result are you focusing on or measuring? • What are you hoping to improve?

Source: Adapted from Haynes (2006).

TABLE 18.3   The FINER criteria.

FINER	
F: Feasibility	Sufficient resources in terms of time, staff and funding Appropriate study design Manageable in scope Adequate sample size
I: Interesting	Interesting for researcher, collaborators, stakeholders Investigator's motivation to make it interesting and relevant
N: Novel	Is this a new finding or extension of previous findings? A thorough literature search and guidance from mentors and experts is key
E: Ethical	Following ethical guidelines Regulatory approval from Institutional Review Board
R: Relevant	Influences clinical practice Encourages further research and shapes health policy

Source: Adapted from Hulley et al. (2007).

Learning Event

Think back to the gap in evidence you identified earlier. Formulate a research question using the PICO model. Can you apply the FINER criteria to this research project?

TABLE 18.4 Type of research and the question it aims to answer.

Type of Research	Type of Question the Research Attempts to Answer
Exploratory	'What?'
Descriptive	'What?' and 'How?'
Explanatory	'What?', 'How?' and 'Why?'
Evaluation	Reviewing the effectiveness of an intervention
Conclusive	Generate findings that can be practically useful for decision-making

Research Methods

The method used depends upon the research question, the aim and what subjects (or who) the study will focus on (Table 18.4).

Scientific Hypothesis

A scientific hypothesis is a testable explanation for a phenomenon in the natural world.

It is a tentative answer to your research question that has not yet been tested and it is not a 'guess' or a 'random prediction', but is based on existing knowledge, theories and observations.

Hypotheses propose a relationship between two or more variables.

- An *independent variable* is something the researcher changes or controls.
- A *dependent variable* is something the researcher observes and measures.

The hypothesis is generally generated in two ways.

- The *null hypothesis* predicts that there will be no relationship between the variables tested, or no difference between the experimental groups.
- The *alternative hypothesis* predicts the opposite: that there will be a difference between the experimental groups.

Refer to the following case study for a practical example.

Case Study 18.1   Developing a Hypothesis

Step 1. Writing a hypothesis begins with a research question that you want to answer. The question should be focused, specific and researchable within the constraints of your project.

Example: You are interested in understanding if critically ill patients receiving protein supplements have any change in muscle mass compared to those who did not receive it.

Step 2. The initial answer to the question should be based on what is already known about the topic.

Example: A literature search may identify theories and previous studies to help formulate assumptions about what your research will find.

Step 3. Formulate the hypothesis, ensuring this is specific and testable. The hypothesis should contain:

- the relevant variables
- the specific group being studied
- the predicted outcome of the experiment or analysis.

Step 4. Phrase your hypothesis.

- *Null hypothesis*: There will be no difference in the rate of muscle mass (growth or loss) between critically ill patients who had protein supplements and those who did not.
- *Positive hypothesis*: The rate of muscle mass will increase in critically ill patients who had protein supplements compared to those who did not.
- *Negative hypothesis*: The rate of muscle mass will decrease in critically ill patients who had protein supplements compared to those who did not.

QUANTITATIVE VERSUS QUALITATIVE RESEARCH METHODS

Quantitative and qualitative studies use different research methods to collect and analyse data, and they allow you to answer different kinds of research questions (Table 18.5).

TABLE 18.5   Quantitative and qualitative research: a comparison.

	Quantitative Research	Qualitative Research
Focus	To observe, measure and test theory and hypothesis	To explore ideas and understand a phenomenon with emphasis on the meaning, experiences and views of the participants
Analyses	Mathematical and statistical analysis expressed in numbers, graphs and tables	by summarising, categorising and interpreting; expressed in words
Advantages	Numerically reliable, mathematically accurate, replicable, can make predictions and test relationships, generalise results to wider populations	Flexibility, natural settings, meaningful insights, generation of new ideas
Disadvantages	Narrow focus on definition and population, may lack pragmatic approach, structural bias (i.e. missing data, inappropriate sampling), labour intensive	Unreliable, subjective, limited generalisability, labour intensive

Mixed-method research is a combination of some of the above, used to study a topic or a problem from different perspectives and ensure patient and participant involvement.

Refer to the following case study for a practical example.

Case Study 18.2   Planning a Research Project

You are interested in evaluating the educational and professional development of critical care nurses undertaking postgraduate studies.

PICO:

Population: Critical care nurses

Intervention/Exposure: Have undertaken postgraduate studies

Comparator: Critical care nurses without a degree

Outcome:

- Academic journey into postgraduate studies: postgraduate modules, MSc, PhD
- Professional development
- Research involvement
- Quality of patient care

Aim: To understand the educational and professional development of critical care nurses after they have undertaken postgraduate studies.

Subject: Educational and professional development of postgraduate critical care nurses.

Type of research: Mixed method (combination of quantitative and qualitative research).

Method used for data collection: Systematic literature review, surveys and interviews (retrospectively or prospective data collection).

Quantitative Research Method

The quantitative research method is generally used for descriptive, correlational or experimental research.

- *Descriptive* research: gives an overall summary of a study variables.
- *Correlational* research: investigates relationships between the study variables.
- *Experimental* research: systematically examine whether there is a cause-and-effect relationship between variables.

The types of study designs are summarised in Table 18.6.

The ability to draw conclusions with a reasonable amount of confidence relies on having an accurate sample size. Without this, results can be missed, biased or incorrect. A large sample size is beneficial in ensuring reliability and accuracy; however, a large sample size can put a huge strain on time and resources spent on recruiting and enrolling participants. To calculate a sample size, one can use a sample from a similar study, carry out a census or use a statistical calculator (i.e. power analysis).

TABLE 18.6   Summary of quantitative studies design.

Meta-analysis	A way of combining data and use of statistical processes to combine findings from different studies
Systematic review, narrative review	A rigorous method of locating, synthesising and critically evaluating a body of studies on a particular topic using a set of specific criteria. It typically includes a description of all the findings and may also include a quantitative pooling of data called meta-analysis
Randomised controlled studies	A controlled clinical trial that randomly assigns participants to two or more groups, generally to analyse a cause-and-effect relationship
Cohort study (prospective or retrospective observational study)	A study in which people who presently have a certain condition or receive a particular treatment are followed over time and compared with another group of people who are not affected by the condition
Case–control study	These are retrospective observational studies that begin with a known outcome. Researchers choose people with a particular result (e.g. disease present versus disease not present) and compare the groups to observe what experiences/exposures they had
Cross-sectional study	The observation of a defined population at a single point in time or time interval. Exposure and outcome are determined simultaneously
Case reports and series	A report on a series of patients with an outcome of interest. No control group is involved
Ideas, editorials, opinions	Commentaries put forth by experts in the field
Laboratory research	'Test tube' experiments conducted in a controlled laboratory setting
Animal research studies	Studies conducted using animal subjects

Data collection can be prospective or retrospective and may be collected through observation, experiments, surveys and/or interviews.

- *Prospective*: follows participants and outcomes during a predetermined period and relates this to factors such as a suspected risk or protective factor(s).
- *Retrospective:* individuals are sampled in a cohort and the data collected are about a specific period in the past.

Once data are collected, statistical analysis can be used to answer the research questions.

- *Descriptive statistics*: provide a summary of the data, including measures of averages and variability. Graphs, scatter plots and frequency tables are often used to present data and identify any trends or outliers.
- *Inferential or comparative statistics:* use mathematical/statistical tests to make predictions or generalisations based on the data. The hypothesis can be tested, or the sample data can be used to estimate the population parameter.

Qualitative Research Method

The qualitative research method is used to answer questions such as 'What is X; how does X vary in different circumstances, and why?' rather than 'How many Xs are there?'. Qualitative studies rely on personal accounts or documents that illustrate how people think or respond.

The qualitative research approaches are summarised in Table 18.7.

Data collection may use an unstructured or semi-structured format, allowing the researcher to pose open-ended questions and follow responses to explore varied or unexpected answers. Table 18.8 describes common data collection tools used in qualitative research studies.

Qualitative data can include texts, photos, videos and/or audio. There are several specific approaches to analysing qualitative data. Although these methods share similar processes, they emphasise different concepts (Table 18.9).

TABLE 18.7   Summary of qualitative research approach.

Approach	What it Entails
Grounded theory	Collecting rich data on a topic of interest and developing theories inductively
Ethnography	Immersion in groups or organisations to understand their cultures
Action research	Researchers and participants collaboratively link theory to practice, driving change
Phenomenological research	Investigating a phenomenon or event by describing and interpreting participants' lived experiences
Narrative research	Examining how stories are told to understand how participants perceive and make sense of their experiences

TABLE 18.8   Type of data collection for qualitative research.

Type of Data Collection	Process
Interviews	Use pre-set questions to shape a conversation with the purpose of exploring issues or topics in detail
Survey	Distribute a questionnaire with open-ended questions to participants
Focus groups	Leading a focused discussion among a group of people to gather opinions and generate data that can be used for further research
Observations	Participating in a community or organisation for an extended period of time to closely observe a culture or behaviour
Delphi method	A process used to arrive at a group opinion or decision by surveying a panel of experts. Experts respond to several rounds of questionnaires, and the responses are aggregated and shared with the group after each round. The experts can adjust their answers based on how they interpret the 'group response' provided to them. The ultimate result is meant to be a true consensus of what the group thinks
Literature review	Survey of published works by other authors

TABLE 18.9   Summary of approaches used to analyse qualitative research.

Approach	When to Use it	Example
Content analysis	To describe and categorise common words, phrases and ideas in qualitative data	To find out what kind of language is used by healthcare professionals when describing advanced clinical practitioners
Thematic analysis	To identify and interpret patterns and themes in qualitative data	Used in focused groups when exploring participants' perceptions, emotions or ideas
Textual analysis	To examine the content, structure and design of texts	To understand how concepts, perceptions or culture have changed over time
Discourse analysis	To study communication and how language is used to achieve effects in specific contexts	To study how patients generate trust in healthcare professionals

---

Learning Event

Review the research question you formulated earlier. Which research method and study design would be the best approach to answer the question?

HEALTHCARE RESEARCH ETHICS

Once the study design and methodology have been decided, the researcher must consider the ethical issues surrounding the study.

Medical and healthcare research often involves human subjects. For this reason, processes have been put in place to ensure that the rights, safety, dignity and well-being of participants are safeguarded. To ensure standards are met, studies involving human subjects are reviewed by an independent body such as an Ethics Review Committee.

The ethical principles for conducting research originate from the Nuremberg Code following the Second World War, setting out statements of moral, ethical and legal principles. The Declaration of Helsinki was first published by the World Medical Association in 1964, with several amendments since (World Medical Association 1964–2013). The Council for International Organisations of Medical Sciences (CIOMS) in collaboration with the World Health Organization (WHO) have issued guidelines on how ethical principles from the Declaration of Helsinki should be applied effectively in medical research; the most recent guidelines were published in 2016.

The four principles of Beauchamp and Childress (1989) – autonomy, non-maleficence, beneficence, justice – have been extremely influential in the field of medical ethics and remain very relevant in medical research (Avasthi et al. 2013). One of the principles stated by the UK Policy Framework for Health and Social Care Research (2022) stresses that: 'research projects are scientifically sound and guided by ethical principles *in all their aspects*'. Table 18.10 presents some ethical principles and how to apply these in different aspects of the research process.

TABLE 18.10   Ethics throughout the research process.

Ethical Principle	Relevance to the Research Process
Essential	Use expert opinion and literature to identify knowledge gaps and justify the research project
Beneficial	Conduct research aiming to promote patient and societal well-being A research question and unbiased analyses leading to meaningful conclusions Disseminate knowledge through scientific publications
Respects autonomy and includes informed consent	Recruitment process – voluntary participation after giving sufficient information and time to comprehend Participants can withdraw consent at any time
Non-exploitative Just	Population sampling – ensure it is just, representative with equal opportunities, non-coercive Equal distribution of benefits
Non-maleficent	Research conducted by competent practitioners using a research protocol reviewed by an independent body. Identify potential risks, take measures to minimise them and have mechanisms in place to identify undue harm and stop research if necessary
Private and confidential	Data collection – keep records safe, anonymised and confidential

Fields of Practice

Issues around informed consent often come up when doing research that involves children and/or other vulnerable groups. The principles contained in the Declaration of Helsinki and the International Ethical Guidance (CIOMS and WHO 2016) cover these issues.

Children and Young People

When the subject is a minor, incapable of giving informed consent, permission from the legally authorised representative should be sought in accordance with national legislation. Whenever the minor is able to give consent, the minor's consent must be obtained in addition to the consent of the minor's legal guardian.

Young people aged 16–18 are presumed to have sufficient understanding to give their consent to participate in research independently of their parents and guardians, unless there is significant evidence to suggest otherwise. Children under 16 can give their full consent providing they have been counselled, do not wish to involve their parents, and are believed to have enough intelligence, competence and understanding. This is known as being Gillick competent, and the Fraser guidelines exist to guide practitioners in such circumstances (NHS 2019a,b; NSPCC 2020).

Vulnerable Groups Who Lack Capacity Due to a Mental Illness or Learning Disability

These groups should only be included in research when it is of direct benefit to them, or research is necessary to promote the health of the population represented by them. In this case, the investigator must obtain informed consent from their legally authorised representative.

Institutionalised Persons

Residents of nursing homes, mental institutions and prisons are often considered vulnerable because in a confined setting, they have few options and are denied certain freedoms. For example, prisons have been described as 'inherently coercive environments', and care home residents may be in a dependent relationship with their caregivers or guardians. This may compromise the voluntariness of informed consent. In such circumstances, the research ethics committee may consider appointing an advocate to be present while signing consent.

A Note on Assent

This is the agreement given by a child/adult who is not legally empowered to give consent. Every effort should be made to explain the details of the study in a manner and at a level that can be understood by the potential participant to seek their assent. Their dissent (disagreement to be part of the study) should be respected.

Emergency Medicine

Research involving subjects who are incapable of giving consent (e.g. during cardiopulmonary resuscitation, collapsed or obtunded patients) may be done only if the condition is a necessary characteristic of the research group. The investigator must seek informed consent from the legally authorised representative. If they are not available and the research cannot be delayed, the study may proceed without informed consent provided that this allowance was stated in the research protocol and the study has been approved by a research ethics committee. Consent to remain in the research must be obtained as soon as possible from the participant or their legally authorised representative.

QUALITY IMPROVEMENT

Taking action to improve healthcare services is not new. There are many well-established approaches to evaluating and making changes to healthcare such as research, clinical audit and service evaluation (see Glossary). Quality improvement (QI) is a more recent approach with important differences in both intent and application. The term QI refers to the systematic use of methods and tools to try to *continuously* improve quality of care and outcomes for patients (Backhouse and Ogunlayi 2020). The key principles of QI are as follows.

- Aims to bring about a *measurable* change.
- *Training of staff* to have a *consistent use of an agreed methodology*.
- *Uses data* to understand variation (for example, data from research or clinical audit).
- *Empowers staff and service users* to contribute to improvement projects.
- Uses many *small-scale trials and tests* to understand 'what works'.
- Ensures a *continuous focus* on the needs and experience of the people served by the system.

There has been a big drive amongst healthcare providers to encourage QI, to improve quality and deliver better value care. This has been driven by patient safety reports as well as financial and operational

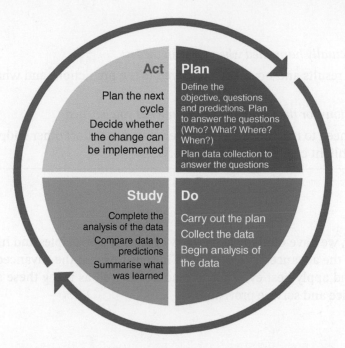

FIGURE 18.3   PDSA cycle. *Source*: NHS England and NHS Improvement (2021)/NHS/Public Domain.

pressures (The King's Fund 2017). NHS England (2021) provides a comprehensive list of improvement and redesign tools. There is no clear evidence that one approach is superior to others. Rather, it is the systematic approach and its consistent application that are important.

The following example of a QI project uses one of these tools, the Plan-Do-Study-Act (PDSA) cycle, to help explore this further (Figure 18.3).

Case Study 18.3   QI Project

Problem: The critical care outreach team (CCOT) has observed an increase in deteriorating patients being admitted to critical care at night.

Aim: *Questions you want answered with this test*

For example: Will the introduction of a CCOT at night reduce the critical care admissions?

Plan: *List the tasks needed to set up the test of change*

For example: Critical care outreach team implements a 24/7 rota for one week.

Data to collect:

- Number of deteriorating patients seen overnight
- Interventions done that avoided a potential admission
- Number of admissions to critical care and reason for admission

Do: *Run the test*

Study: *Describe what actually happened when you ran the test*

Describe the measured results and how they compared to the predictions and what you learned from the cycle.

Act: *Describe modifications for the next cycle based on what you learned*

For example: You may need to run the test for a longer period or collect other endpoints such as financial implications to highlight cost-effectiveness of service.

CONCLUSION

Throughout this chapter, we have offered an overview of research principles and highlighted the importance of research within the advanced practice role. This ensures that the advanced clinical practitioner can appraise research and apply best evidence to practice, as well as using these skills to evaluate and improve their own practice and service provision.

Take Home Points
- Effective research projects must be well designed, ethical and reviewed.
- Research and QI science should encompass the advanced practice role to continuously evaluate the quality of service provision and ensure that the best evidence-based practices are being used.

REFERENCES

Avasthi, A., Ghosh, A., Sarkar, S., and Grover, S. (2013). Ethics in medical research: general principles with special reference to psychiatry research. *Indian Journal of Psychiatry* 55 (1): 86–91.

Backhouse, A. and Ogunlayi, F. (2020). Quality improvement into practice. *BMJ* 368: m865.

Beauchamp, T.L. and Childress, J.F. (1989). *Principles of Biomedical Ethics*, 3e. New York: Oxford University Press.

Council for International Organizations of Medical Sciences (CIOMS), World Health Organization (WHO) (2016). International Ethical Guideline for Health-related Research Involving Humans. https://cioms.ch/publications/product/international-ethical-guidelines-for-health-related-research-involving-humans/#description

Haynes, R.B. (2006). Forming research questions. *Journal of Clinical Epidemiology* 59: 881–886.

Health Education England (2017). Multi-Professional Framework for Advanced Clinical Practice in England. www.hee.nhs.uk/our-work/advanced-clinical-practice/multi-professional-framework

Hulley, S., Cummings, S., Browner, W. et al. (2007). *Designing Clinical Research*, 3e. Philadelphia: Lippincott, Williams and Wilkins.

National Society for the Prevention of Cruelty to Children (2020). Gillick competency and Fraser guidelines. https://learning.nspcc.org.uk/child-protection-system/gillick-competence-fraser-guidelines

NHS (2019a). Children and young people. Consent to treatment. www.nhs.uk/conditions/consent-to-treatment/children

NHS (2019b). The Long Term Plan. www.longtermplan.nhs.uk

NHS England and NHS Improvement 2021. Quality, service improvement and redesign tools. www.england.nhs.uk/sustainableimprovement/qsir-programme/qsir-tools/

NHS Health Research Authority (2022). UK Policy Framework for Health and Social Care Research. www.hra.nhs.uk/planning-and-improving-research/policies-standards-legislation/uk-policy-framework-health-social-care-research/uk-policy-framework-health-and-social-care-research/#researchteams

The Kings Fund and The Health Foundation (2017). Making the case for quality improvement: lessons for NHS boards and leaders. www.kingsfund.org.uk/publications/making-case-quality-improvement

World Medical Association (1964–2013). Declaration of Helsinki – Ethical Principles for Medical Research Involving Human Subjects. www.wma.net/policies-post/wma-declaration-of-helsinki-ethical-principles-for-medical-research-involving-human-subjects

FURTHER READING

Armstrong, N., Herbert, G., Aveling, E.L. et al. (2013). Optimzing patient involvement in quality improvement. *Health Expectations* 16 (3): 36–47.

Bowling, B. (2014). *Research Methods in Health. Investigating Health and Health Services*, 4e. Buckingham: Open University Press.

Brignardello-Petersen, R., Izcovich, A., Rochwerg, B. et al. (2020). GRADE approach to drawing conclusions from a network meta-analysis using a partially contextualised framework. *BMJ* 371: m3907.

Crowl, A., Sharma, A., Sorge, L., and Sorensen, T. (2003). Accelerating quality improvement within your organization: applying the model for improvement. *Journal of the American Pharmaceutical Association* 55 (4): 364–376.

Cunningham, C., Weathington, B., and Pittenger, D. (2013). *Understanding and Conducting Research in the Health Sciences*. Wiley.

Etzioni, R., Mandel, M., and Gulati, R. (2021). *Statistics for Health Data Science. An Organic Approach.* New York: Springer International Publishing.

Gaglio, B., Henton, M., Barbeau, A. et al. (2020). Methodological standards for qualitative and mixed methods patient centered outcomes research. *BMJ* 371: m4435.

Health and Care Professions Council (2016). *Standards of Conduct, Performance and Ethics*. London: Health and Care Professions Council.

Higgins, P.T., Altman, D.G., Gøtzsche, P.C. et al. (2011). The Cochrane Collaboration's tool for assessing risk of bias in randomised trials. *BMJ* 343: d5928.

Hughes, R.G. (2008). Tools and strategies for quality improvement and patient safety. In: *Patient Safety and Quality: An Evidence-Based Handbook for Nurses* (ed. R.G. Hughes). Rockville: Agency for Healthcare Research and Quality.

International Council of Nurses (2020). *Guidelines on Advanced Practice Nursing*. Geneva: International Council of Nurses.

Jones, B. (2019). How to get started in quality improvement. *BMJ* 364: k5408.

Ma, L.L., Wang, Y.Y., Yang, Z.H. et al. (2020). Methodological quality (risk of bias) assessment tools for primary and secondary medical studies: what are they and which is better? *Military Medical Research* 7: 7.

Nee, P.A. and Griffiths R.D. (2022). Ethical considerations in accident and emergency research. https://emj.bmj.com/content/emermed/19/5/423.full.pdf

Nursing and Midwifery Council (2015). *Code of Professional Conduct*. London: Nursing and Midwifery Council.

Ogbeiwi, O. (2017). Why written objectives need to be really SMART. *British Journal of Healthcare Management* 23 (7): 324–336.

Page, M.J., McKenzie, J.E., Bossuyt, P.M. et al. (2021). The PRISMA 2020 statement: an updated guideline for reporting systematic reviews. *BMJ* 372: n71.

Pope, C. and Mays, N. (1995). Reaching the parts other methods cannot reach: an introduction to qualitative methods in health and health services research. *BMJ* 311 (6996): 42–45.

Riley, R.D., Ensor, J., Snell, K.I.E. et al. (2020). Calculating the sample size required for developing a clinical prediction model. *BMJ* 368: m441.

Skills for Health (2018). Advanced Clinical Practitioner (Integrated Degree) Standard. https://haso.skillsforhealth.org.uk/standards/#standard-355

UK Research and Innovation (2021). Framework for research ethics. www.ukri.org/councils/esrc/guidance-for-applicants/research-ethics-guidance/framework-for-research-ethics/our-core-principles/#contents-list

Wandersman, A., Alia, K.A., Cook, B., and Ramaswamy, R. (2015). Integrating empowerment evaluation and quality improvement to achieve healthcare improvement outcomes. *BMJ Quality and Safety* 24 (10): 645–652.

Yeung, Y, Couper K., Fritx Z. et al. (2021). Ethics Guidelines. www.resus.org.uk/library/2021-resuscitation-guidelines/ethics-guidelines

SELF-ASSESSMENT QUESTIONS

1. Are you involved in research activities?
2. Do you understand what research and quality improvement entail? What training and education would you need to be able to conduct research or quality improvement projects in your workplace?
3. Think about the benefit of research and quality improvement project in your workplace and reflect on how you can be involved, and would you be able to lead projects?
4. Think of the importance of sharing research and project results and outcomes: do you feel comfortable with academic writing, journal publication and public presentation at conferences? What education and training do you need?

GLOSSARY

Assent   The agreement of someone not able to give legal consent to participate in an activity.

Clinical audit   A way to find out if healthcare is being provided in line with standards and to let care providers and patients know where their service is doing well, and where there could be improvements.

Consent   Giving permission for something by someone who has the legal ability/right to do so.

Ethics Review Committee   A group of suitably qualified people who review research applications and give an opinion about whether the research meets ethical standards.

Quality improvement   A systematic continuous approach that aims to solve problems in healthcare, improve service provision and ultimately provide better outcomes for patients.

Research   The attempt to derive generalisable new knowledge by addressing clearly defined questions with systematic and rigorous methods.

Service evaluation   A process of investigating the effectiveness or efficiency of a service with the purpose of improving it.

CHAPTER 19

Leading Research in Advanced Practice

Leanne Dolman, Joanna De Souza, and Sara Stevenson-Baker

Aim

The aim of this chapter is to create an understanding of how advanced practitioners contribute to and lead a culture of research-driven high-quality care services that optimise health across care settings.

LEARNING OUTCOMES

After reading this chapter the reader will have an understanding of the value of using research:

1. to inform and improve clinical practice thorough evidence-based guideline, policy, protocol and procedure development
2. to harness the opportunities of digital capacity in using existing data to evaluate current models of care, including the efficacy of advanced practice roles
3. to identify patients and carers as a drivers for service development
4. to advance clinical and professional practice through the development of research to explore identified gaps in knowledge
5. to create organisational cultures that provide opportunities to release there search potential of all staff and users in a common goal of improving person-centred healthcare.

INTRODUCTION

Inspired by the NHS Long Term Plan (2019), the role of all healthcare professionals in leading and developing research to improve patient care has been embraced (Academy of Science 2020; Chief Nursing Officer 2021). As healthcare professionals with specific areas of expertise, advanced practitioners are well placed to lead on this ambition. Embedded in the role of an advanced practitioner is a raft of research capabilities (HEE 2017). For many advanced practitioners caught up in managing a busy clinical caseload, the ability to be involved in research seems difficult. A survey of advanced practitioners working in London demonstrated that they spend 73% of their time in direct clinical work with patients, 43% in management and leadership, leaving 14% of their time to devote to any kind of research activity (Stewart-Lord 2020). A wider survey found only 11% of advanced practitioners saw themselves as being involved in research (Fothergril et al. 2022), with few trusts seeing it as a priority. While far-reaching work has been done to develop advanced practice roles, limited work has been done to truly support the research pillar of practice (Bell and Colleran 2019; Whitehouse et al. 2022).

Working within a system in which evidence-based practice is deemed essential, delivering care that follows international, national or institutional protocols and guidelines is a core part of research involvement. While it is the responsibility of all healthcare professionals to be involved in developing and embedding professional knowledge in practice, practitioners working at an advanced level have a responsibility to lead on this activity. As advanced practice roles evolve and it becomes more mandatory for role holders to have developed Master's level research skills, this chapter explores ways in which this can be embedded in the role of any practitioner working at an advanced level (Figure 19.1).

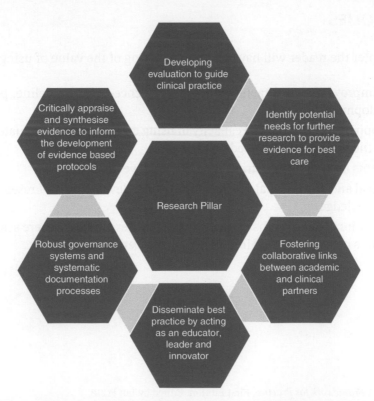

FIGURE 19.1   Research capabilities in the Multi-Professional Framework for Advanced Clinical Practice.
Source: Adapted from HEE (2017).

Accreditation Statements

4.1 Critically engage in research activity, adhering to good research practice guidance, so that evidence-based strategies are developed and applied to enhance quality, safety, productivity, and value for money.

4.2 Critically appraise and synthesise the outcome of relevant research, evaluation and audit, using the results to underpin own practice and to inform that of others.

4.3 Take a critical approach to identify gaps in the evidence base and its application to practice, alerting appropriate individuals and organisations to these and how they might be addressed in a safe and pragmatic way.

4.4 Actively identify potential need for further research to strengthen evidence for best practice. This may involve acting as an educator, leader, innovator and contributor to research activity and/or seeking out and applying for research funding.

4.5 Develop and implement robust governance systems and systematic documentation processes, keeping the need for modifications under critical review.

4.6 Disseminate best practice research findings and quality improvement projects through appropriate media and fora (e.g. presentations and peer review research publications).

4.7 Facilitate collaborative links between clinical practice and research through proactive engagement, networking with academic, clinical, and other active researchers.

ENABLING EVIDENCE-BASED PRACTICE

Advanced practice involves developing expertise in an aspect of practice or the delivery of a particular service. Advanced practitioners play a key role working alongside other professionals to ensure that care is informed by current evidence and processes exist that enable that care to be delivered at a consistently good standard. This is achieved by having systems in place to ensure that local policies, protocols and procedures are based on current guidelines and care being delivered is monitored using appropriate and effective methods of quality control. Guidelines within a health service are developed on a variety of levels, international, national and at unit level (Figure 19.2).

Policy, protocols, procedures and guidelines (PPPGs) provide guidance to enable consistent safe delivery of a service and a basis for a robust system of audit and continuous improvement. They can also be used to guide new staff on induction and as educational tools on an ongoing basis to maintain consistent standards of care (Table 19.1).

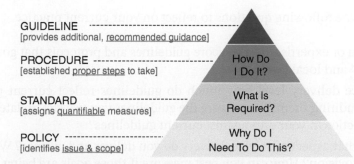

FIGURE 19.2   What is a policy, guideline, protocol. *Source*: Bahadur (2022).

TABLE 19.1   Core research skills.

• Analyse	1. Enabling evidence-based practice through guideline, protocol and procedure development and quality control
• Audit	
• Construct	2. Using machine learning to explore changing patterns in healthcare
• Create	3. Leading on quality improvement
• Cultivate	4. Dissemination of existing and new knowledge
• Design	5. Developing clinical academic roles
• Devise	6. Creating a culture of practice embedded in research
• Generate	
• Improve	
• Revise	

Using Local Procedures and Protocols – Role Modelling and Ensuring Continuity of Practice

Role modelling is an important influencing factor in creating a culture of evidence-based care delivery. Being explicit about the PPPGs that influence your expert care delivery as an advanced practitioner offers others a greater understanding of that care and ability to develop informed practice that is transferable to other settings. Ensuring the procedures you undertake are clearly documented in a procedural form, that is appropriate to your context and quality controlled, also enables other staff to learn and work to a similar standard when working alongside or covering your role.

Auditing Current Practice

As an advanced practitioner, it is important to be aware if the aims of care delivery are being successful or if there are aspects of care that are falling below an agreed standard. This helps to inform the development of your own practice as well as that of others. Many healthcare settings have existing audit systems, some of which may also inform national and international monitoring systems. Where these are built into the healthcare system, ensuring familiarity and understanding by all levels of staff and regular analysis of the outcomes is part of the leadership role of the advanced practitioner.

Learning Events

Take some time to use the following questions to reflect on your current practice.

1. What is your area of expertise? List the core guidelines and protocols that govern your area of care at a national and local level.

2. At a local service delivery level how much do guidelines reflect current practice? Who is responsible for auditing them? When were the guidelines you use last updated? What systems exist to audit practice in your area against current guidelines?

3. At a role level, what aspect of service delivery do you deliver and oversee? What are the goals of that service provision? How can you best measure if those goals are being achieved?

Utilising Clinical Audit

Clinical audit is a quality improvement process that seeks to improve patient care and outcomes through systematic review of care against explicit criteria (Burgess and Moorhead 2011) (Figure 19.3). Advanced practitioners are in a strong position to be able to analyse audit findings and explore solutions and implement change to embed alternative solutions.

Setting Standards and Developing New Protocols

When establishing a new standard, policy, procedure or protocol, it is important to undertake a scoping literature review to establish what work has already been done in this area. Being involved in national-level forums or scanning conference proceedings can also be a way of exploring others who may be working on PPPGs in your area. Collaborative working can save time and can result in more robust guideline development which can be utilised widely in your area of practice (Shannon and Maughan 2020).

A more detailed literature search of existing evidence is required in establishing the steps needed in your protocol/guideline. What is the evidence for what you do – does it exist? Developing the skills to be able to work with routinely collected data within the health service can offer an opportunity to identify bottlenecks and change opportunities (Kauch et al. 2021). In some instances, evidence has not yet been developed. It may in this case be appropriate to consider some kind of Delphi technique to draw together the opinions of other experts in the field to determine best practice.

Setting Intended Outcomes

As you develop your protocol, it is important to consider how a number of things can be audited and measured (Figure 19.4). First, what is the intended outcome of your protocol? What is it designed to achieve? How can this be measured over time? Building in essential elements of practice that can be observed and measured to explore the outcomes of utilising the new PPPG as part of the development process makes it easier to manage and more effective. Outcomes can be measured in a number of different ways, Are patients moving through the system more quickly? Is there any way of tracking patient outcomes such as length of stay, number of readmissions or functional ability improvements? Patient understanding

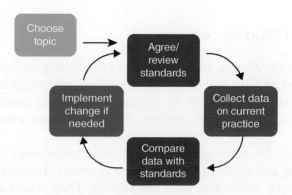

FIGURE 19.3 The audit cycle.

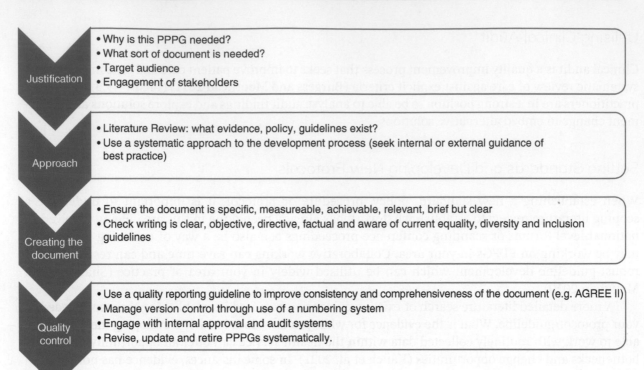

Justification
- Why is this PPPG needed?
- What sort of document is needed?
- Target audience
- Engagement of stakeholders

Approach
- Literature Review: what evidence, policy, guidelines exist?
- Use a systematic approach to the development process (seek internal or external guidance of best practice)

Creating the document
- Ensure the document is specific, measureable, achievable, relevant, brief but clear
- Check writing is clear, objective, directive, factual and aware of current equality, diversity and inclusion guidelines

Quality control
- Use a quality reporting guideline to improve consistency and comprehensiveness of the document (e.g. AGREE II)
- Manage version control through use of a numbering system
- Engage with internal approval and audit systems
- Revise, update and retire PPPGs systematically.

FIGURE 19.4   Steps in PPPG development.

of elements such as their medications, illness and clinical signs can also be used to demonstrate care effectiveness.

Patient-reported Outcome Measures

Patient-reported outcome measures (PROMs) measure a patient's perspective on their health status or health-related quality of life at a single point in time, and are collected through short, self-completed questionnaires. If written well, PROMs can be a helpful clinical tool to ensure users' needs are considered in ongoing PPPG development (Giolla et al. 2020).

Reviewing your Protocol (Quality Control)

Involving the quality team in developing your protocol or establishing an understanding of the way in which protocols are developed and quality controlled in your organisation is important.

What is the system in your place of work for organising policy reviews? Protocols and guidelines should have a system for review. In many organisations, this involves them being registered with a quality control number.

It may be helpful to assess the developing document using an external tool such as the AGREE II reporting guideline. Reporting guidelines are structured tools which provide a minimum list of features required in a document to make them clear, valid and reliable. They can be a useful reminder of what elements must be included in the protocol.

Learning Events

Take some time to use the following questions to reflect on your current practice.

1. What new ways of working or innovations have you implemented in practice?
2. What were your intended outcomes? How might you measure those outcomes?
3. Can you get service users involved in planning outcomes?

DEVELOPING GUIDELINES AT A NATIONAL/INTERNATIONAL LEVEL

Case Study 19.1   Developing Guidelines for the Management of Non-Malignant Chronic Pain

While working with patients using patient-controlled analgesia, RN Gillian Chumbley undertook a focus group study to develop an understanding of what patients wanted to know about being on patient-controlled analgesia. She used the findings of her study to inform the patient information leaflet produced, and to audit its usefulness over time. Gillian successfully obtained funding to conduct larger research studies into the use of ketamine for complex pain, the appropriate use of opioids for persistent pain and the safety of intravenous medication. During her career, Gillian has developed her knowledge and expertise through a combination of research, clinical practice and collaboration. Gillian has been on the development group of European guidelines on the management of non-malignant chronic pain (Häuser et al. 2021). Gillian continues her work in the pain service as a consultant nurse.

DEVELOPING NEW EVIDENCE FOR PRACTICE

Advance practitioner roles have been created to improve patient care. Many advanced practitioners are involved in developing new types of practice (Table 19.2). Quality improvement project methodology is designed to enable informed development of new project ideas.

TABLE 19.2   Sources of national/international evidence guidelines for clinical management.

National Institute for Health and Care Excellence (NICE)	www.nice.org.uk
Cochrane Library	www.cochranelibrary.com
Scottish Intercollegiate Guidelines Network (SIGN)	www.sign.ac.uk
York Centre for Reviews and Dissemination	www.york.ac.uk/inst/crd
Joanna Briggs Institute	https://jbi.global
World Health Organization	www.who.int

Leading on Quality Improvement

What sets quality improvement (QI) methodology apart from other approaches is that it uses the idea that we are system thinkers, full of curiosity, which allows us to be open to the idea that we never have the full answer to an issue, therefore leading to a willingness to explore different perspectives and next steps (Berwick 2013). Healthcare is and will continue to be a highly complex field and faces many significant challenges now and in the future, including an increase in the ageing population leading to patients being cared for in several settings and with multiple chronic conditions; waiting times increasing, staff shortages, rapid enhancement in technology, information access, medical innovations and costly treatments; the focus on person-centred care and providing value for money (Flynn et al. 2017).

Quality improvement aims to make a difference to patients by improving quality of care, safety, effectiveness and experience of care and improving financial efficiency by:

- using understanding of our complex healthcare environment
- applying a systematic approach
- designing, testing and implementing changes using real-time measurement for improvement.

The role of an advanced practitioner (AP) involves assessing, planning and evaluating patient care needs, advocating for patients, assuring their care is safe and that patients are satisfied with the care they receive. Consequently, they are in the ideal clinical leadership position to recognise aspects of care that require review and may have the potential for improvement. QI requires a combined effort, using a wide variety of tools and methods, to make changes that lead to better patient outcomes, better system performance and ongoing professional development (NHS Improvement 2016).

There are many QI methods and tools that can be used to implement the QI project and analyse the data as part of the measurement process. It has been highlighted that the step-by-step approach of improvement is more important than the specific approach, methods and tools chosen (The Health Foundation 2013). When QI efforts are less successful, it is rarely due to the approach, problem or tool but rather the human dynamics, the lack of team or leadership approach (NHS 2010). Therefore, the AP needs to understand the problem in the first instance and then use the local support and drivers, methods and tools that are applicable as the initial starting point.

The main starting point is identifying a problem, and the AP is in an ideal position to recognise potential problems that could benefit from improvement within practice (Table 19.3). Choosing a project area that aligns with the priorities of the organisation, clinical leads, other staff, patients, carers and other

TABLE 19.3   Underlying principles of quality improvement.

- Problem solving, continual learning and adaptation
- The starting point is to identify and understand the problem
- Form a team to look at the issue and develop a plan
- This plan would include understanding the processes and systems within your organisation
- Analysing the demand, capacity, and flow of the service
- Choosing the tools to bring about any change, including leadership and clinical engagement, skills development, and staff and patient participation
- Consider how you are going to evaluate and measure the impact of a change

Source: Adapted from NHS Improvement (2016).

service users is an ideal starting place (Kings Health Partners 2018, 2021). Having support from the organisation via potentially identifying aspects of care that require improvement, either through incentives like the Commissioning for Quality and Innovation framework of core clinical priority areas (NHS 2022) or through local initiatives and drivers, complaints/feedback and peer clinical feedback and interest in a given area of interest, increases the potential for success of the QI project.

> **Key Questions to Ask**
> - *What is the main thing to be achieved?*
>   Aims and objectives (Specific, Measurable, Achievable, Realistic, Timely) should be clear, relate to the problem, be consistent with current known policies/standards and evidence and have a clear time frame.
>
> - *What can be measured to demonstrate an improvement has occurred once the change has been implemented? Are these data available and accessible?*
>   Exploring what data are available and building a baseline of data and information, in order to be able to test the outcomes of the change by measuring this against the data throughout and at the end of the project.
>
> - *What changes can be made that will result in improvement?*

A key part of a successful project is the preparation and planning. Very often, it is too easy to dive straight in and start to implement potential solutions. Managing a successful project requires time spent in developing a clear project plan and therefore more likely to succeed (Kings Health Partners 2021). This involves identification of the project's aims and objectives, background and scope of the project, key timescales, risk analysis, collecting baseline data from the service and any knowledge already known about the problem, identifying stakeholders, including patients and carers, and appointing a core team within the project and collectively understanding what is going to be accomplished (NHS 2016).

Essential to a successful QI project is identifying and involving key groups and individuals who may be interested in or affected by the change. Involving others can increase the team's general knowledge of quality improvement methods leading to a problem solving approach being applied to the current problem but also to ongoing day to day practices (Latif et al. 2021). Within the project team, having the right people involved with the right expertise will encourage potential success from the start. Consider who may also provide project sponsorship from within the organisation, as they will provide potential strategic direction and support. Involving patients and service users is crucial as they will provide a different lived perspective to the problem and potential improvements. Sensitivity is needed on how this is approached and requires careful planning to ensure that it is handled well and incorporated clearly into the overall project plan.

Process mapping is a useful tool that enables the identification and visually interpretation of all the steps of the current process (NHS 2010). It allows the ability to review the complete process from beginning to end, enabling a better understanding of the system from both staff and patient perspectives. It enables further clarity of the problem and naturally starts to highlight potential solutions. Alongside this, assessing the factors within the current environment that will enable or hinder the improvement is a useful indicator of potential success. There are various tools that can be used to explore this within your project, including Lewis's force field analysis (NHS 2016). However, the main outcome is to discover the factors within the local environment that will enable or hinder the change or improvement from being successfully implemented. Engaging with stakeholders who may be able to provide a clear link to drivers including local and strategic initiatives but also the potential levers is a useful starting point.

The Model for Improvement provides a framework for developing, testing and implementing changes that lead to improvement, supported by testing change ideas using Plan, Do, Study, Act (PDSA) cycles (NHS 2016) (Figure 19.5). For large and small projects, it can be a useful way to test a range of potential changes before implementing the final change.

The value of doing this minimises the risks, reduces resistance to the change and enables the AP to learn from things that work and those that do not (NHS 2016). Understanding how people may react to change, both positively and negatively, is another important aspect of effectively implementing the change. Consider how the vision of the change will be shared, and how sharing the ownership of the problem rather than the solution may enable the team to engage in the process more fully (NHS Improvement 2014). Communication is key in managing change and it is an important element to consider throughout the process to allow engagement with the local and also the wider team that may be affected by the change.

An essential part of the project and within the PDSA cycle is the evaluation that the change has occurred or needs further review and adjustment. Whether the change was a success or not, it is one of the most important parts of the project (NHS 2016). Establishing a true baseline is key, and knowing the current state at the start helps to determine which aspects will need to be measured. Therefore, the importance of having clear, measurable data to support improvement work cannot be overstated. It is an important element of the project to be able to monitor and review key data throughout the project. These data will provide an understanding as to where the project is, where there might be problems and the impact the change is having. Take time at the beginning of the project to consider what data are required, where these data will come from, how often the data will be collected and by whom, and how the data will be analysed and shared (NHS 2016).

At the end of the QI project, a final key part is to share the learning, both good and bad, and celebrate the successes. This sustains the momentum but also helps colleagues and organisations learn

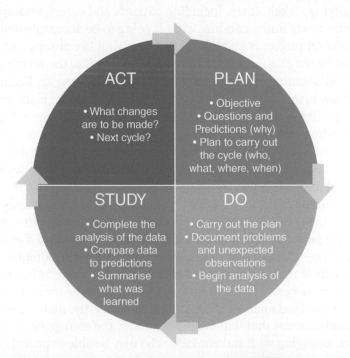

FIGURE 19.5   The PDSA cycle. *Source*: Adapted from NHS Improvement (2014).

from completed projects on a wider scale. Consider sharing the achievements both internally through your own organisation and externally, potentially through writing up the results into an article for publication.

There are many approaches and models that can support a QI project. However, the Model for Improvement (NHS 2016) highlights the three core stages: knowing what you are trying to achieve; considering how you will know that a change is an improvement; and what change will result in the improvement that is sought. The use of a systematic approach may require practice but incorporating quality improvement into daily work will improve clinical outcomes for patients.

DISSEMINATION OF EXISTING AND NEW KNOWLEDGE

Dissemination is one of the most important parts of research – for research to have an impact, it needs to reach a range of audiences. Dissemination should be part of the initial plan of any development work. Developing a team that crosses disciplinary boundaries increases opportunities for dissemination. Working as a team with artists, business colleagues and patients/carers and the general public offers an expansion of ways of communicating messages to diverse audiences of stakeholders. There are several ways of disseminating your guidelines and research within the healthcare field.

Local Dissemination

Presenting work to colleagues in unit meetings can be an excellent first stage for condensing work into a form accessible by others. New guidelines and protocols or QI work should be gathered together in a report format. This offers transparency on how the work was done and the results that were achieved. Presenting this to internal colleagues may be the first step in dissemination.

New methods such as lightning talks (presenting salient points of a project in five minutes) and three-minute theses are increasingly popular. These are designed for people to share work they have been doing using a short presentation format that may be limited to a five-minute presentation on their topic using one or two slides. They allow others to hear about your work in a focused way to raise awareness and prompt later networking to discuss further details. Increasingly hospitals, other healthcare organisations and academic partnerships hold local conferences for sharing work that is being done within the system. For projects involving policy development across departments, this can be a good platform to propose ideas and engage feedback.

Presenting at an External Conference

Finding a conference that is appropriate for your research is the first step. There are a range of conferences; some will be multiprofessional conferences specific to your clinical area such as State of the Art, a collaborative intensive care conference. Other conferences may be more generic. Engaging with clinical colleagues, professional journals or journals in your clinical area will raise your awareness of what conferences are good audiences for your work. Conferences have attendance costs even for presenters. Costs can be funded through project funding if your work is part of a project. Alternatively, local conference funding may be found but often is more forthcoming if some external funding as been sought, such as through professional organisations, charities and industrial partners.

Developing a Conference Abstract

Conferences call for abstracts, often a year prior to a conference taking place. Abstract submission dates are usually about six months prior to the conference. An abstract is a brief summary of the work you wish to present; it is similar to an abstract that you would write for a publication, highlighting all the keys parts of your work. After abstract submission, a team of healthcare professionals will screen the abstracts as a form of peer review and selection for appropriateness for the conference. Ensuring you have read the guidelines for abstract construction carefully, developed your submission and subjected it to local peer review will help in being selected. Your abstract becomes a potential template for a short talk or poster presentation as keeping detail limited while getting your keys ideas across is a major skill needed for successful idea dissemination. As an advanced practitioner, being involved in both journal and conference proceedings screening enhances your skills in reviewing evidence but also advances practice through the sharing of your expertise.

Developing a Poster

A poster is a visual representation of the research you have undertaken, a summary of your work presented in a clear manner. Posters are best created in slide presentation forms such as PowerPoint or Prezi. The important aspect of poster creation is focusing on the visual impact. The title needs to be clear and inviting, images conveying to a passing reader the nature of your topic of enquiry. Words need to be kept to a minimum, so use figures and tables where possible, with testing of font size for readability. Colour schemes need to be chosen carefully to enhance visibility but not distract from the content. Many healthcare institutions have online guidance, communications or IT teams who will assist with poster creation. For online conferences, or conferences with an accompanying online component, developing a lightning talk to attach to your poster enhances your dissemination reach.

Developing an Oral Presentation

Presentations can vary in length depending on where you are presenting. Oral presentations at conferences are chosen from abstracts that align explicitly with the conference's current focus, often illustrated by calls they make for papers on particular topics, and offer new knowledge or perspectives to subjects of interest to conference attendees. Conference presentations need to remain succinct with scope for stimulating discussion around findings and potential dissemination opportunities of the new knowledge being shared.

Writing for Publication

Writing for publication is a way of disseminating your work in a format that becomes a searchable, permanent account that can widen the impact of your work and offer a springboard to others in the area. Submitting work for publication engages academic scrutiny in the form of systematic peer review. Each publication has a guide for authors. Familiarising yourself with your chosen publication's expectations is crucial. Drawing on peer support or the support of a research office or dissemination office in your institution can be invaluable in getting your work published.

Joining a National Forum or Guideline Development Group

Taking your work into a forum of professionals who work in related areas can ensure your work is used to inform national guidelines and policy (Case Study 19.2).

DEVELOPING THE ADVANCED PRACTITIONER AS A CLINICAL ACADEMIC

Advances in modern medicine and healthcare have often been a product of collaborating expertise between a range of clinical professions with clinical practice and academia (Academy of Science 2020). There is currently a drive for there to be more clinical academics, who are health professionals who work in both clinical practice and academia (Bell and Colleran 2019). They work in a range of health and social care environments as clinicians to maintain, recover and improve health while also actively participating in research in new ways to deliver better outcomes for patients. They will also work in higher education institutions (HEIs) developing their scholarly activity. The duality of this role allows their research to be grounded to the day-to-day issues of the patients they see and the services they are part of. It stops people having to choose between the academic and clinical pathways and allows them to combine their skill sets. A successful clinical academic will be able to demonstrate not only that they are an excellent researcher but also that they can lead and inspire others in the clinical field.

The National Institute of Health Research (NIHR) suggests that a researcher immersed in a clinical setting is in an excellent position to identify what research questions really matter to the NHS, the profession, the patient and service user. They are able to ensure that the question being asked is really relevant to day-to-day practice and care, and to interpret the research in a way which is highly useful and applicable to the clinical setting. There is an increasing evidence base that research-active healthcare provider organisations use to provide better quality care, more treatment options and improved clinical outcomes (DoH 2021; NIHR 2018; Care Quality Commission 2018). Furthermore, research is becoming increasingly more important to patients and the public in general, who know the importance of research and want access to quality research so they are able to understand and be part of the decision making around their own treatment.

Within medicine and dentistry, there is a clear career pathway for clinical academics. However, for nurses, midwives and other allied health professionals (NMAHPs) this is still being developed and integrated throughout healthcare There is not one clear road to a clinical academic career, and not all staff should or will progress from the same starting point and finish at the same endpoint in a particular timescale. There is a range of different schemes available to aspiring clinical academics at both local and national level. The NIHR is funded by HEE to provide schemes to support aspiring clinical academics at different stages throughout their careers.

The HEE internship scheme is for individuals with minimal or no research experience and aims to engage the participant in a range of taught and academically supervised components of the research environment. It is an opportunity to gain the practical skills required to undertake a research project or develop a project idea with the support of an expert supervisor. The Pre-doctoral Clinical and Practitioner Academic Fellowship scheme offers candidates salaried time to produce a doctoral fellowship application and provides funded academic training which allows awardees to gain the skills and experience to access doctoral level funding. This scheme is available for researchers in the UK, early in their careers, who are committed to becoming clinical academics.

Doctoral schemes are also available through the NIHR such as the Doctoral Clinical Practitioner Academic Fellowship. This is a three-year full-time scheme or up to six years scheme part time, with approximately 80% of the time working academically and the other 20% of fellowship hours to spend on practice and professional development. There are further postdoctoral schemes available through the NIHR; the Advanced Clinical and Practitioner Academic Fellowship is a 2–5-year scheme which allows the awardee to develop their academic career whilst continuing their health or care career. Between 20% and 40% of the award must be dedicated to development of the awardee's clinical service or practice role.

As well as the NIHR, there is also funding available through charities, societies and local healthcare organisations. Therefore, when beginning on the clinical academic journey, it is vital to discuss with your organisation's research office what opportunities are available and to create a plan and get support to write your application.

However, the recognition of experience and expertise gained on completion of these models has often been noted to be lacking, with many NMAHPs stating they feel undervalued and undersupported within clinical practice (Trusson et al. 2019). However, the embedded researcher model has been proposed to make sustainable improvements that will embed research into practice (Whitehouse et al. 2022). It is proposed this will happen via three mechanisms.

- Introducing executive and departmental leaders who are committed to core funding for research focused roles or agreement for dedicated research time within existing/future NMAHP job roles on a permanent basis.
- A commitment to collaboration through formal clinical–academic partnerships in which all partner organisations recognise and value opportunities that enable authentic collaboration, knowledge-rich organisational and research evidence which informs decision making and integrated skill sets.
- A focus on research important to the local population.

The purpose of all the schemes mentioned is to increase the number of clinical academics in practice, as there are benefits not only for the individuals themselves but in developing relevant research and also improving patient care and implementing research into practice (Case study 19.2).

Case Study 19.2   Developing as a Clinical Academic

While Lisa Newington was a junior physiotherapist, she and her colleagues conducted a service evaluation to explore clinical outcomes and patients' experiences of those attending a group rehabilitation intervention (Adams and Newington 2012). This led to further refinement of their hand rehabilitation group. Lisa has continued to combine research and clinical practice through a series of research grants and fellowships, including an HEE research internship and later an NIHR doctoral research fellowship. Having completed her PhD, Lisa works as an AP hand therapist and research associate. Her research explores return to work after hand surgery/injury and the role and impact of clinical academics. Lisa is able to support her clinical team with research activities, including audit, service evaluation and the implementation of research findings (Newington et al. 2022).

CREATING A RESEARCH CULTURE AT ORGANISATIONAL LEVEL TO IMPROVE PERSON-CENTRED HEALTHCARE

There is a growing body of evidence which demonstrates that patients who receive care in research-active healthcare settings have better outcomes (Academy of Science 2020). This healthcare research embedded in clinical practice contributes to major advances in patient care. However, all the evidence about achieving a research culture in which NMAHPs can research in practice settings points to the need to develop an organisational culture that sees clinical researchers as an essential part of the workforce plan.

In the Chief Nursing Officer for England's strategic plan for research, Making Research Matter (2021), working alongside the NIHR, May lays out the five themes underpinning the strategy: aligning nurse-led research with public need, releasing nurses' research potential, building the best research system, developing future nurse leaders of research, and digitally enabled nurse-led research. When implemented, these themes will lay the foundations for creating organisations to build research-active staff across all levels and enable research lead by a range of health professional disciplines.

A range of models for creating research-active organisations exists. Ensuring research training and awareness is a core component of all preregistration training, with NMAHPs requiring a minimum of degree-level education to register. This was achieved in 2013 when nursing became an all-graduate profession, other professions having achieved this previously. Enhancing this with a requirement for Master's level study for advanced practice roles ensures that practitioners are equipped to engage with the research of others and to have an understanding of leading research themselves. However, maintaining the currency to develop that potential requires organisations to have clear operational links with other organisations that provide care along the patient journey and have a range of different forms of expertise, such as academic centres. Academic health partnerships have gone some way to doing this, but the involvement of NMAHPs has to date been limited. Partnerships with research bodies such as the NIHR and research priority setting organisations such as the James Lind Alliance offer opportunities to identify core research priorities and open funding streams which allow a wider range of practitioners to engage in person-centred research.

Providing roles and spaces for research-prepared staff with PhD level research skills to lead on research and involve others needs to be supported through the development of roles such as embedded researchers, continuing development of NMAMPs' research expertise and appropriate supervision support (Olive et al. 2022; Whitehouse et al. 2022; Newington et al. 2022; Van Dongen and Hafsteinsdóttir 2021; Harding 2020) (Case Study 19.3).

Case Study 19.3   Newcastle's NMAHP Researcher Development Institute Programme

The academic health sciences group in Newcastle created a developmental training institute designed to promote and support research development by NMAHPs. The institute is supported by a large grant from the Newcastle hospital charity. Ensuring NMAHPs have ongoing training and opportunities to develop their research has been identified as a major way of increasing research development within large healthcare institutions. This project hopes to do this by supporting a number of research training opportunities, like MScs and PhDs, as well as support to be a primary investigator on studies.

CONCLUSION

'The evolution of the landscape is encouraging; however, the pace of change is slow and the reality of developing, leading, and sustaining research for the benefit of others, while working in a busy clinical role as an NMAHP advanced practitioner remains challenging' (Tinkler 2022).

Take Home Points

- Understanding how the advanced practitioner can contribute and lead a culture of research-driven high-quality care services can optimise health across care settings.

- Clinical practice can be informed and improved through the application of evidence-based guidelines, policy, protocol and procedure development.

- Harnessing the opportunities that digital capacity brings in applying existing data for the evaluation of current models of care has the potential to develop further advanced practice roles.

- Patients and carers are key stakeholders as drivers for service development.

- Clinical and professional practice can be advanced through the development of research by exploring and identifying gaps in knowledge.

- The creation of organisational cultures provides opportunities to release the research potential of staff and those who use services with a common aim of improving person-centred healthcare.

REFERENCES

Academy of Medical Sciences (2020). *Transforming Health through Innovation: Integrating the NHS and Academia*. London: Academy of Medical Sciences.

Adams, Z., Newington, L., and Blakeway, M. (2012). Evaluation of outcomes for patients attending a rehabilitation group after complex hand injury. *Hand Therapy* 17 (3): 68–72.

Bahadur, A. (2022). HR Success Guide. www.hrsuccessguide.com/2014/01/Guideline-Procedure-Standard-Policy.html

Bell, C.A. and Colleran, V. (2019). Empowering nurses, midwives and allied health professionals to gain an academic, research and quality improvement experience within clinical practice. *International Journal of Practice-based Learning in Health and Social Care* 7 (2): 69–79.

Berwick, D (2013). A Promise to Learn – A Commitment to Act. https://assets.publishing.service.gov.uk/government/uploads/system/uploads/attachment_data/file/226703/Berwick_Report.pdf

Burgess, R. and Moorhead, J. (2011). *New Principles of Best Practice in Clinical Audit*. Oxford.: Radcliffe Publishing.

Care Quality Commission (2018). Trust-wide Well-Led Inspection Framework V6. www.cqc.org.uk/sites/default/files/20190412_trust_wide_well_led_inspection_framework_v6.pdf

Chief Nursing Officer for England (2021). *Making Research Matter: Strategic Plan for Research*. London.: NHS England and NHS Improvement.

Department of Health (2021). Saving and Improving Lives: The Future of UK Clinical Research Delivery. www.gov.uk/government/publications/the-future-of-uk-clinical-research-delivery/saving-and-improving-lives-the-future-of-uk-clinical-research-delivery

Flynn, R., Scott, S.D., Rotter, T., and Hartfield, D. (2017). The potential for nurses to contribute to and lead improvement science in health care. *Journal of Advanced Nursing* 73 (1): 97–107.

Fothergill, L.J., Al-Oraibi, A., Houdmont, J. et al. (2022). Nationwide evaluation of the advanced clinical practitioner role in England: a cross-sectional survey. *BMJ Open* 12 (1): e055475.

Giolla, Easpaig, B.N., Tran, Y. et al. (2020). What are the attitudes of health professionals regarding patient reported outcome measures (PROMs) in oncology practice? A mixed-method synthesis of the qualitative evidence. *BMC Health Service Research* 20: 102.

Harding, D. (2020). Workplace Supervision for Advanced Clinical Practice: an integrated multi-professional approach for practitioner development. https://www.hee.nhs.uk/sites/default/files/documents/Workplace%20Supervision%20for%20ACPs.pdf

Haüser, W., Morlion, B., Vowles, K. et al. (2021). European Pain Federation clinical practice recommendations Part 1: Role of opioids in the management of chronic noncancer pain. *European Journal of Pain* 25 (5): 949–968.

Health Education England (2017). Multi-Professional Framework for Advanced Clinical Practice in England. www.hee.nhs.uk/sites/default/files/documents/multi-professionalframeworkforadvancedclinicalpracticeinengland.pdf

Kausch, S.L., Moorman, J.R., Lake, D.E., and Keim-Malpass, J. (2021). Physiological machine learning models for prediction of sepsis in hospitalized adults: an integrative review. *Intensive and Critical Care Nursing* 65: 103035.

Kings Health Partners (2021). *Step 2 KIS Guidance for Deciding What to Improve and Assessing the Feasibility of a Quality Improvement Project*. London.: King's College London.

King's Health Partners (2018). King's Improvement Science – Step 1 KIS Introduction to Quality Improvement. https://kingsimprovementscience.org/cms-data/resources/KIS_QI_step_1_December_2018.pdf

Latif, A., Gulzar, N., Lowe, F. et al. (2021). Engaging community pharmacists in quality improvement (QI): a qualitative case study of a partnership between a higher education institute and local pharmaceutical committees. *BMJ Open Quality* 10: e001047.

National Institute for Health and Care Research (2018). *CQC Inspections to give more exposure to clinical research taking place in the NHS*. 2018. www.nihr.ac.uk/news/cqc-inspections-to-give-more-exposure-to-clinical-research-taking-place-in-nhs-trusts/11185.

Newington, L., Alexander, C.M., and Wells, M. (2022). What is a clinical academic? Qualitative interviews with healthcare managers, research-active nurses and other research-active healthcare professionals outside medicine. *Journal of Clinical Nursing* 31: 378–389.

NHS (2022) Commissioning for Quality and Innovation (CQUIN): 2022/23. www.england.nhs.uk/nhs-standard-contract/cquin/

NHS England (2019). The NHS Long Term Plan. www.longtermplan.nhs.uk

NHS Improvement (2014). Creating a vision for your change. www.england.nhs.uk/wp-content/uploads/2021/06/01-NHS104-Phase-2-Creating-a-vision-for-your-change-210817-A.pdf

NHS Improvement (2016). Developing People – Improving Care: A National Framework for Action on Improvement and Leadership Development in NHS-Funded Services. https://improvement.nhs.uk/resources/developing-people-improving-care

NHS Innovation and Improvement (2010). *Handbook of Quality and Service Improvement Tools*. London: NHS Institute of Innovation and Improvement.

Olive, P., Maxton, F., Bell, C.A. et al. (2022). Clinical academic research internships: what works for nurses and the wider nursing, midwifery and allied health professional workforce. *Journal of Clinical Nursing* 31 (3–4): 318–328.

Shannon, R.A. and Maughan, E.D. (2020). A model for developing evidence-based clinical practice guidelines for school nursing. *Journal of School Nursing* 36 (6): 415–422.

Stewart-Lord, A., Beanlands, C., Khine, R. et al. (2020). The role and development of advanced clinical practice within allied health professions: a mixed method study. *Journal of Multidisciplinary Healthcare* 13: 1705.

The Health Foundation (2013). *Quality Improvement Made Simple – What Everyone Should Know about Health Care Quality Improvement*. London: The Health Foundation.

Tinkler, L. (2022). Every organisation needs a sherpa. *British Journal of Nursing* 31 (9): 506–507.

Trusson, D., Rowley, E., and Bramley, L. (2019). A mixed-methods study of challenges and benefits of clinical academic careers for nurses, midwives and allied health professionals. *BMJ Open* 9 (10): e030595.

Van Dongen, L.J.C. and Hafsteinsdóttir, T.B. (2021). Leadership of PhD-prepared nurses working in hospitals and its influence on career development: a qualitative study. *Journal of Clinical Nursing* 31: 23–24.

Whitehouse, C.L., Tinkler, L., Jackson, C. et al. (2022). Embedding research (ER) led by nurses, midwives and allied health professionals (NMAHPs): the NMAHP-ER model. *BMJ Leader* 6: 323–326.

FURTHER READING

Lamb, A., Martin-Misener, R., Bryant-Lukosius, D., and Latimer, M. (2018). Describing the leadership capabilities of advanced practice nurses using a qualitative descriptive study. *Nursing Open* 5 (3): 400–413.

Montgomery, K.E., Ward, J., Raybin, L. et al. (2021). Building capacity through integration of advanced practice nurses in research. *Nursing Outlook.* 69 (6): 1030–1038.

NHS England National Quality Board (2021) A Shared Commitment to Quality for Those Working in Health and Care Systems. www.england.nhs.uk/wp-content/uploads/2021/04/nqb-refreshed-shared-commitment-to-quality.pdf

Ross-Hellauer, T., Tennant, J.P., Banelytė, V. et al. (2020). Ten simple rules for innovative dissemination of research. *PLoS Computational Biology* 16 (4): e1007704.

SELF-ASSESSMENT QUESTIONS

1. Why might the PDSA cycle be suitable for large and small projects?
2. Describe the three pillars that are associated with the embedded researcher model.
3. Identify the regulatory challenges and risks presented by registrants advancing practice and how regulators should respond, ensuring public protection.
4. There is no definition of advanced practice that is both standardised and accepted across the UK. What might your definition of advanced practice be?

GLOSSARY

Clinical audit   A quality improvement procedure seeking to enhance patient care and outcomes through systematic review of care against a specific set of criteria.

Clinical guidelines   Statements of good practice, recommendations on the appropriate treatment and care of patients with specific diseases and conditions. They permit deviation from a prescribed pathway according to individual circumstances and where reasons can be clearly demonstrated and documented.

Critical appraisal   The process whereby the appraiser systematically and meticulously examines the research, making a judgement about its credibility, value and significance in a specific context.

Embedded researcher   Defined as those who work inside host organisations as staff members, while also maintaining a relationship with an academic organisation.

Evidence synthesis   A way of combining information from multiple studies that have investigated the same thing, to arrive at an overall understanding of what they found, sometimes called systematic reviews.

Patient-reported Outcome Measures   These measures assess the quality of care delivered from a patient perspective.

Policy   A policy document is a formal document which is regarded as legally binding; therefore its purpose, definitions and responsibilities outlined in its content have to be upheld; it may be used to support an individual or the healthcare organisation during legal action.

Procedure   A procedure is a standardised series of actions taken to achieve a task so that everyone undertakes it in an agreed and consistent way in order to achieve a safe, effective outcome. The procedure is a formal document to be complied with; it may be used to support an individual or the organisation during legal action. Procedures are reviewed annually.

Protocol   This is a detailed description of the steps taken to deliver care or treatment to a patient, sometimes know as an 'integrated care pathway'. Designed at local level to implement national standards and determine care provision by using the best evidence. If national standards are not available, it can include recommendations or may detail competencies or delegation of authority. Protocols are less rigid than procedures.

CHAPTER 20

Innovations in Practice

Vanessa Taylor and Sarah Ashelford

Aim

This chapter explores the concept of innovation in advanced-level practice and applies this to the advanced practitioner role. Insights into the knowledge, facilitation skills and leadership strategies required by advanced practitioners as innovators at clinical team, organisation and system levels will be offered. The reader will be encouraged to reflect on and apply these to achieve and sustain the practice development, quality improvement, innovation and culture change associated with quality care in the workplace.

LEARNING OUTCOMES

After reading this chapter you will:

1. examine the concept of innovation and its relevance to advanced-level practice and the advanced practitioner role
2. evaluate the facilitation skills and leadership strategies required to develop practice, improve quality and innovate in advanced level practice
3. analyse the barriers and enablers influencing advanced-level practice development, quality improvement and innovation at team, organisation and systems levels
4. reflect on your own contribution as a facilitator and leader of quality care in the workplace, in practice development, quality improvement and leading culture change and innovation in practice.

INTRODUCTION

Innovation has significance for advanced practice and advanced practitioners. First, advanced practice is an example of a key systems innovation in global and national workforce transformation. Second, by focusing on the innovations that the advanced practitioner themselves may lead as part of their enactment

The Advanced Practitioner: A Framework for Practice, First Edition. Edited by Ian Peate, Sadie Diamond-Fox, and Barry Hill.
© 2024 John Wiley & Sons Ltd. Published 2024 by John Wiley & Sons Ltd.

as a clinical and professional leader facilitating and leading innovation at individual, team (micro), wider organisational (meso) and system (macro) levels.

A global workforce crisis, coupled with the increasing complexity of healthcare services in response to medical, technological and clinical knowledge development, an ageing population and escalating costs, is prompting countries to examine their healthcare workforce and skill mix (WHO 2016). The diversification and reconfiguration of the healthcare workforce, including the implementation of advanced practice roles for the nursing and allied health professional workforce, are part of a growing international trend in healthcare policy to redistribute the workforce aligned to professional accomplishment and patient outcomes, in contrast to historical workforce hierarchies and roles (Beech et al. 2019; Leary 2019; Leary and MacLaine 2019; de Bont et al. 2016).

In the UK, workforce transformation, quality improvement and service innovation are required to enable modern healthcare organisations and systems to meet the changing needs and expectations of the individuals and communities they serve (West 2021). Supporting innovation across the healthcare system is now more important than ever and is seen as central to securing transformation and improved patient outcomes (NHSE 2015). Key to the delivery of the NHS five-year forward view, the NHS Long Term Plan (NHSE 2019) and NHS People Plan (NHSE 2020), is creating the conditions and systems for collaborative approaches to innovation between health and social care sectors and related professional groups, enabling more efficient and innovative ways of working and facilitating the fast adoption of cost-effective new technologies (NHSE 2015, 2016, 2019, 2020). Enabling and supportive leadership and cultures for innovative and high-quality person-centred care are, therefore, essential for stimulating innovation and continuous quality improvement, ensuring innovation spreads within health and social care teams and becomes a cultural norm (West 2021; Manley and Jackson 2020).

Within this context of practice development, quality improvement and creating cultures for innovation at clinical team, organisation and systems levels, advanced practitioners are a growing part of the healthcare workforce worldwide, making valuable contributions to patient care, patient pathways, service and workforce transformation. Across the UK, health services are exploring the development and implementation of advanced-level roles to address workforce challenges. The advanced-level skills and extended scope of practice of the advanced practitioner are key to transforming the healthcare workforce and the development of new clinical roles to enable workforce expansion (NHSE 2019). As a relatively newly defined level of practice for the nursing and allied health professions workforce across the UK nations, practitioners at this advanced level are expected to deliver expert practice with a high degree of autonomy and complex decision making across four pillars of advanced clinical practice, including leading improvement and innovation at individual patient, client group and clinical team (micro) through to organisation (meso) and system (macro) levels (Lockwood et al. 2020; Manley and Jackson 2020; HEE 2017) (Tables 20.1 and 20.2). To achieve success as clinical and professional leaders focused on quality care in the workplace, advanced practitioners are expected to work collaboratively at all levels using their expert knowledge, skilled facilitation and leadership strategies, practice development, improvement skills and tools and culture change skills for transforming and sustaining cultures to ensure they support integrated health services that are person centred, safe and effective (Manley et al. 2011, 2014).

This chapter starts by examining what is meant by innovation, and then explores how innovation relates to advanced-level practice and the advanced practitioner. The enablers and barriers to innovation that advanced practitioners may experience resulting from historic and current system-wide changes are identified. Finally, the knowledge, facilitation and leadership skills required by advanced practitioners to create the conditions for practice development, quality improvement and innovation are examined.

TABLE 20.1   Links to Multi-professional Framework for Advanced Clinical Practice.

2.3 Evaluate own practice, and participate in multi-disciplinary service and team evaluation, demonstrating the impact of advanced clinical practice on service function and effectiveness, and quality (i.e. outcomes of care, experience and safety).

2.4 Actively engage in peer review to inform own and other's practice, formulating and implementing strategies to act on learning and make improvements.

2.5 Lead new practice and service redesign solutions in response to feedback, evaluation and need, working across boundaries and broadening sphere of influence.

2.6 Actively seek feedback and involvement from individuals, families, carers, communities, and colleagues in the co-production of service improvements.

4.7 Disseminate best practice research findings and quality improvement projects through appropriate media and for a (e.g. presentations and peer review research publications).

Source: Adapted from HEE (2017).

TABLE 20.2   Examples of area-specific/specialist accreditation considerations.

- Health Education England (2020) Advanced Clinical Practice: Capabilities Framework When Working with People who have a Learning Disability and/or Autism. www.skillsforhealth.org.uk/images/services/cstf/ACP%20in%20LDA%20Framework.pdf
- Health Education England (2022) Advanced Practice in Mental Health Curriculum and Capabilities Framework. https://healtheducationengland.sharepoint.com/:b:/s/APWC/EV18LBDz_PBGsbhePVPohAIBssOPOjPXvB3m0rAuZqVq8w?e=XrqpgY
- Faculty of Intensive Care Medicine (2019) Curriculum for Training for Advanced Critical Care Practitioners Part III Syllabus. www.ficm.ac.uk/sites/ficm/files/documents/2021-10/accp_curriculum_part_iii_-_syllabus_v1.1_2019_revision.pdf
- Royal College of Emergency Medicine (2019) Emergency Care Advanced Clinical Practitioner Curriculum and Assessment Adult and Paediatric Version 2.0. https://rcem.ac.uk/wp-content/uploads/2021/10/EC_ACP_Curriculum_2017_Adult_and_Paediatric-for_publication-Last_Edit_14-03-2019.pdf
- Royal College of General Practitioners (2020) Core Capabilities Framework for Advanced Clinical Practice (Nurses) Working in General Practice/Primary Care in England. www.hee.nhs.uk/sites/default/files/documents/ACP%20Primary%20Care%20Nurse%20Fwk%202020.pdf

INNOVATION, PRACTICE DEVELOPMENT AND SERVICE IMPROVEMENT

As highlighted in Table 20.2 the complexity of healthcare services, combined with the changing needs and expectations of patients and communities, and a global workforce crisis mean that innovation is needed to enable modern healthcare organisations and health systems to meet these demands (West 2021). Innovation involves new, better and more effective ways for solving challenges or problems that confront people, teams, organisations or communities in healthcare (The King's Fund 2017).

Innovation is described as different from improvement. The Health Foundation (2021), for example, suggests that improvement involves a systematic and co-ordinated approach to solving a problem using specific methods and tools with the aim of bringing about a measurable improvement in the quality of care, processes and outcomes for patients and service users in individual teams, services and care pathways in primary, secondary, community and social care settings. In contrast, innovation refers to both creativity – the generation of novel ideas – and implementation across the organisation and system

(West 2021; NHSIII 2007). Novel ideas, creativity and innovation are needed for the more significant changes required to deliver services and care differently in the health service (NHSIII 2007) with enabling leadership and cultures considered essential for ensuring innovation spreads and becomes a cultural norm. Similarly, McCormack et al. (1999) and Manley and Jackson (2020) reinforce that a transformative culture and context of care are also important for promoting the continuous process of improvement required for practice development by practitioners and clinical teams, not just at the wider organisational level.

This definition from West and Farr (1990) captures the three characteristics of innovation: (i) novelty (ii), an application component and (iii) an intended benefit:

> *. . . the intentional introduction and application within a role, group or organization of ideas, processes, products or procedures, new to the relevant unit of adoption, designed to significantly benefit the individual, the group, the organization or wider society.*

Within healthcare, the novelty and intended benefits of innovation have been further defined as:

> *. . . the introduction of a new concept, idea, service, process, or product aimed at improving treatment, diagnosis, education, outreach, prevention and research, and with the long-term goals of improving quality, safety, outcomes, efficiency and costs.*
>
> (Omachonu and Einspruch 2010, p. 5)

Similarly, the King's Fund (2017, p.5) defines innovation as: 'the introduction and application of processes, products, treatments or procedures, new to the team, department, ward, pathway, organisation, or system and intended to benefit patients, staff, the organisation or the wider society'.

Leighann and Massoud (2017) caution that the term 'innovation' has been too loosely applied in healthcare. Consistent with the definitions above, they emphasise that, in order for a solution to a healthcare problem to be an innovation, it must involve the introduction of something that is new or significantly different from other solutions in the field. The definitions from West and Farr (1990), Omanchonu and Einspruch (2010) and the King's Fund (2017) all emphasise 'new and improved' health policies, practices, services and delivery methods as innovations that can enhance healthcare. The innovation does not, however, have to be 'brand new'. The King's Fund, for example, identifies that the innovation can be the modification of an existing product or the redesign of an existing service implemented within a new context.

Innovations in healthcare are, therefore, novel and useful ideas which are implemented with the expectation of improving quality and outcomes for particular stakeholders. The main types of innovation are shown in Table 20.3 along with the main beneficiaries. As Table 20.3 illustrates, innovations typically improve the efficiency, effectiveness, quality, sustainability, safety and/or affordability of healthcare (World Health Organization 2016). The outcomes of innovation centre around the benefit to the patient and the receiver of care. Five key stakeholders are identified, namely healthcare professionals/teams, patients and service users, organisations, internal and external innovator companies, governments and regulatory agencies, each potentially benefiting from the innovation process, and with particular needs, wants and expectations (Table 20.3).

Ideally, innovations in healthcare should provide scalable solutions and enhancements in order to improve treatment, diagnosis, education, outreach, prevention, research quality and delivery, and access to healthcare. The characteristics of advanced practice as an innovation are illustrated in Table 20.4 and the expected contribution of advanced-level practice and the advanced practitioner role to these improvements is identified in Table 20.1.

TABLE 20.3 Types of innovation and key stakeholders.

Innovation Type	Example Applied to Advanced-Level Practice	Stakeholder: Needs, Wants and Expectations
Product innovation: introduction of a good or service that is new or significantly improved with respect to its characteristics or intended uses. For example: clinical procedure innovations	Extended scope of practice and capabilities for nursing and allied health professional as advanced practitioner	**Healthcare professionals:** improved clinical outcomes, improved diagnosis, treatment, management and care
Process innovation: implementation of a new or significantly improved production or delivery method including changes in techniques, equipment or software. In healthcare, this may include a novel change to delivering healthcare service increasing the value to or enhancing the experience of stakeholders	Developing and establishing the advanced practitioner role within a team or service to enhance care delivery and service user experiences	**Patients/service users:** improved experience, improved physiological and/or psychological well-being, reduced waiting time, reduced delay **Organisations:** Enhanced efficiency of internal operations, cost containment, increased productivity and quality and outcomes improvement
Structural/organisational innovation: implementation of new organisational method in practices, workplace organisation or external relations. A structural innovation may affect the internal and external infrastructure and create a new business model	Establishing AP-led services and new models of service delivery within an organisation and/or system	**Innovator companies:** profitability, improved outcomes **Government and regulatory agencies:** Reduced risks and improved patient safety

Source: Adapted from Varkey et al. (2008).

TABLE 20.4 Characteristics of advanced-level practice in England as an example of innovation.

Characteristic	Advanced-Level Practice and the Advanced Practitioner
Novelty	Nationally defined level of practice with education requirements and capabilities in practice, governance, clinical supervision and assessment requirements, area-specific/specialist credentials
Application	Across England, nursing and allied health professions, clinical pathways, specialties
Intended benefits	Clinical career pathway, retention and better use of experienced professionals, extended scope of practice, service transformation, patient-centred outcomes

While the novelty and scale of change within the healthcare system appear to be distinguishing features of innovation compared to improvement in the definitions above, it may be argued that innovation can also be a feature in a practice development approach at the level of a clinical team and organisation. Practice development is defined as a continuous process of improvement towards increased effectiveness in person-centred care achieved through the enabling of healthcare teams to transform the culture and context of care (McCormack et al. 1999, p.256). Practice development and quality improvement are about practitioners closest to the issues affecting care quality having the time, skills and resources they need to solve them using systematic and rigorous processes of change (The Health Foundation 2021; McCormack et al. 1999). McCormack et al. (1999) argue that a practice development approach links practitioner-led innovation to the context of the workplace with the potential for the organisation (local and wider) to adopt this approach as a means to improve 'practices' which will lead to the development and implementation of evidence-based policies and influence strategic vision.

The practice development approach offers practitioners the opportunity to critically evaluate and evolve their workplace practices and their practice culture while taking into account the organisational context of their work. Innovation, as defined above referring to both creativity – the generation of novel ideas – and their implementation across the organisation and system, suggests a 'top-down' approach where the novel ideas may come from a response to population data, external developments and policies in healthcare. However, novel ideas for clinical practice and service delivery may arise from a practice development approach, enabled and supported by facilitators committed to a systematic, rigorous, continuous process of emancipatory change (McCormack et al. 1999). Applying this practice development definition and its approach appears to align to the capabilities in Table 20.1 for change, improvement and innovation at different levels by the advanced practitioner.

Achieving improvement and innovation at micro, meso, and macro levels requires a culture for innovation and high-quality care. West (2021) identifies four fundamental elements of a culture for innovative and high quality: an inspiring vision and strategy; positive inclusion and participation; enthusiastic team and cross-boundary working; support and autonomy for staff to innovate with compassionate leaders playing a key role in nurturing each of these elements (West 2021). Similar elements are also identified for achieving a practice development approach (McCormack et al. 1999) and for building a workforce from micro to macro systems levels that is responsive, empowered and creative for supporting the complex change and transformation agenda across the healthcare system (Manley and Jackson 2020).

Barriers may, however, remain in place for an innovation to be recognised and taken up as the process of diffusion (Rogers 1983) is social and interactive. To be effective, therefore, innovation requires collaboration, communication and knowledge exchange between those involved in the healthcare system at all levels. Uptake requires stakeholders to see the advantage in adopting and implementing an innovation. Other considerations are capacity, compatibility, complexity, observability and risk. Evidence of barriers to the implementation of advanced practice as set out by the Health Education England (HEE 2017) Multi-professional Framework is emerging. Fothergill et al. (2022), for example, identifies a mismatch between organisations and individual advanced practitioners' knowledge of the Framework, alongside variability in knowledge between settings. Compliance with the four pillars of practice also poses challenges, with prioritisation of the 'clinical' pillar and barriers to engaging with the education, leadership and research pillars due to high workloads and limited time and resources (Higgins et al. 2014). Similarly, Gerrish et al. (2011) identified factors influencing advanced practitioners' ability to promote and facilitate evidence in practice, identifying that organisational culture should be conducive to enabling evidence-based practice with managers supportive of this aspect of the advanced practitioner role. Gerrish et al. (2011) also identified that organisational commitment at the highest level is key to advanced practitioners' ability to fulfil this aspect of their role.

Focusing on leadership, Elliott et al. (2016) identified organisation-level factors such as mentoring support from senior management, a lack of opportunity to participate at a strategic level and the absence of structural support for the role and size of caseload as barriers to advanced practitioners' ability to enact their leadership role.

The innovation process at clinical team (micro), organisation (meso) and system (macro) levels therefore involves problem solving, including problem identification and exploration; the generation of ideas; evaluation and implementation (West 2021; The King's Fund 2017). A culture of innovation requires compassionate leadership which is inclusive – ensuring all voices are heard in the process of delivering and improving care.

INNOVATION AND ADVANCED-LEVEL PRACTICE AND THE ADVANCED PRACTITIONER ROLE

Advanced-level Practice and Workforce Transformation: An Example of Healthcare Service Innovation

The development of new clinical roles with advanced-level knowledge and skill identified in the interim NHS People Plan to enable workforce expansion can be seen as an example of innovation (Table 20.4). The introduction and implementation of the Health Education England Multi-professional Framework for Advanced Clinical Practice (HEE 2017) and the establishment of the Centre for Advancing Practice offer consistency across advanced-level practice and the advanced practitioner workforce developments. The Multi-professional Framework for Advanced Clinical Practice (HEE 2017) in England and the equivalent advanced practice frameworks in Wales, Scotland and Northern Ireland are an important step forward, providing an overarching structure for creating greater consistency and governance for advanced practice workforce developments, in contrast to the former locally driven responses which resulted in lack of standardisation in role specifications, capabilities, education preparation and role title, posing challenges for scaling up and evaluating the implementation and demonstrating the benefits and impact of this innovation in workforce transformation.

Advanced practitioners are part of a workforce transformation innovation occurring globally (WHO 2016). While the advanced practitioner role is not new, the 'novelty' characteristic of this innovation can be related to the national development of this level of practice as part of the workforce transformation agenda, with the implementation being led by Health Education England, an executive non-departmental public arm of the Department of Health and Social Care. HEE's function is to provide national leadership and co-ordination for the education and training of the health and public health workforce in England. The implementation of the Multi-professional Framework for Advanced Clinical Practice in England provides a unifying national definition of advanced practice for a wide range of health and care professionals, alongside support for the implementation of advanced-level practice in health and care environments in order to ensure practitioners are supported in their role. The MPF and its equivalent frameworks in Wales, Northern Ireland and Scotland aim to create greater consistency across advanced clinical practice, including education requirements, the knowledge and skills essential to the level indicated in core capabilities across four pillars of advanced clinical practice: (i) clinical practice, (ii) leadership and management, (iii) education and (iv) research.

The ability to work autonomously, enabling healthcare professionals at this level to enhance capacity and capability within multiprofessional teams, is a key characteristic of practising at this level. By providing direct care and clinical leadership, enabling collaboration across the multidisciplinary team, advanced practitioners (APs) aim to improve clinical continuity and patient-focused care and contribute to the provision of safe, accessible and high-quality patient care (NHS Employers 2021).

While new models of care organisation and delivery are being rolled out, the need to invest in the development of new roles and advanced-level practice to enable workforce expansion also has two purposes – enabling experienced health and care professionals to work across professional boundaries and take on an extended scope of practice while also providing career development and opportunities to improve retention. These aims and purposes are relevant to the third characteristic of innovation of 'intended benefit'.

Evaluation of advanced practice as an innovation in workforce transformation since 2017 is needed and work to establish the evidence base focused on activity, outcomes, implementation challenges, retention and areas for future research around advanced practice in the UK is being reported (Evans et al. 2020a,b; Lawlor et al. 2020; Fothergill et al. 2022). Indeed, Evans et al. (2020a, p.3) emphasise that:

> ... there is an urgent need to understand more fully the current context of, and evidence around ACP across the specialities, sectors and the multiprofessional workforce in different roles across different care pathways to inform a baseline understanding of the contribution and challenges of ACP in the health service.

Guided by the Participatory Evidence-informed Patient-centred Process-Plus (PEPPA-Plus) framework developed by Bryant-Lukosius et al. (2016), Evans et al. (2020a) set out a proposal to undertake a scoping review to establish the current evidence base underpinning multiprofessional advanced-level practice from a workforce, clinical, patient and service perspective in the UK. The PEPPA-Plus framework (Figure 20.1) (Bryant-Lukosius et al. 2016) provides a comprehensive approach for advanced practice role evaluation, including implementation and outcomes. The framework is informed by the work of Donabedian and includes consideration of the structure, process and outcomes related to advanced practice roles across three stages of role development – introduction, implementation and long-term sustainability.

- *Structure*: factors which affect AP role implementation (title, remuneration, regulatory and governance frameworks, education preparation, setting).
- *Process*: tasks and activities undertaken by the AP, barriers and enablers to role implementation.
- *Outcomes*: (i) patient and family, (ii) quality of care, (iii) healthcare provider, team and stakeholder, (iv) organisation and (v) healthcare use and costs.

Recent examples of research related to evaluation of advanced practice include Lawler et al. (2020) who used a mixed-methods approach to evaluate the workforce experience of the implementation of the HEE Multi-professional Framework in England. Evans et al. (2020b) report the findings of a qualitative evaluation of nursing AP roles across general practices in one region of the UK. More recently, using a

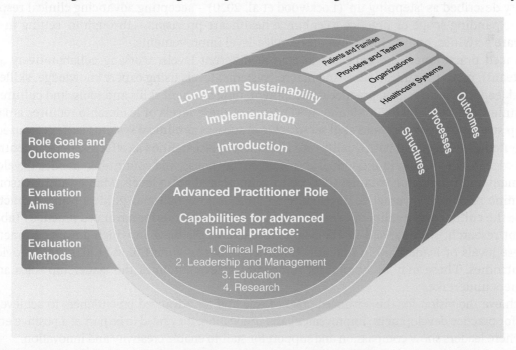

FIGURE 20.1 Participatory Evidence-informed Patient-centred Process-Plus (PEPPA-Plus) framework.
Source: Adapted from Bryant-Lukosius et al. (2016).

mixed-method online survey, Fothergill et al. (2022) published the first large-scale evaluation of the AP role across professions, geographical regions and settings to inform the development and improvement of policies relating to APs in the NHS in England.

These studies illustrate consideration of the range of aims for evaluation in terms of exploring, describing, understanding, assessing, explaining or predicting aspects of advanced practice and advanced practice roles using different research or evaluation methods. The 'evaluation methods' can include:

- qualitative research
- quantitative research
- mixed research methods
- programme evaluation
- quality improvement.

Findings from these studies indicate emerging themes around understanding the experiences of introducing and implementing advanced practice and the enablers and barriers in healthcare services.

Advanced Practitioner as Clinical (Practice Development/Improvement) and Professional (Service/System Development) Innovator

Leadership, as one of the four pillars of advanced practice, is a key activity for the advanced practitioner. The advanced practitioner role is complex, requiring autonomy and leadership within specific services and settings, in addition to performing and leading in teams with professionals from other specialties, services and organisations. Table 20.1 identifies the core capabilities for advanced practitioners in England focused on the clinical and professional leadership expectations with increasing scope of complexity described as 'stepping up' (Lockwood et al. 2020) – accepting advancing clinical responsibilities and expanding scope of practice to enhance healthcare provision – through to 'setting in motion' indirect care activities, quality initiatives and service-level improvements.

Advanced practitioners are expected to lead at different levels, working collaboratively at micro (clinical team), meso (organisational) and macro (systems) levels using expert knowledge, skilled facilitation and leadership strategies, practice development, improvement skills and tools, and culture change skills (Manley and Jackson 2020; Manley 1997). Each of these levels of leadership requires a particular leadership strategy, knowledge and skill set to achieve success as clinical systems leaders focused on the cultural outcomes associated with quality care in the workplace defined as effective person-centred care, empowered staff who maintain individual and team effectiveness, and continuing practice development, improvement and innovation (Manley 1997). At the micro and meso levels, Manley and Jackson (2020) describe nine principles of practice development (Table 20.5) which may guide advanced practitioners to achieve the culture and quality of care identified in the capabilities for advanced practice (Table 20.1).

Recent research, summarised in Table 20.6, focused on the ways in which advanced practitioners enact these levels of leadership in practice (Elliott et al. 2012) while Elliott et al. (2014) provide leadership outcomes. These may be helpful for informing an evaluation of the leadership roles advanced practitioners undertake.

To achieve the vision for the advanced practice role and for advanced practitioners to achieve the full potential for practice development, improvement and innovation, they need to be part of a positive emotional climate where leaders show compassion and support for staff to enable creativity and innovation.

The King's Fund (2017), West (2021), Manley and Jackson (2020) and McCormack et al. (1999) variously describe compassionate, transformative or emancipatory leadership as an enabling factor that

TABLE 20.5   Principles of practice development.

1. Develop person-centred care, evidence-based care demonstrated by human flourishing and an effective healthy workplace culture
2. Focus on relationships at the microsystem level where care is provided and experienced at the frontline of practice
3. Facilitate active learning and formal systems and learning processes to enable real-time learning and care transformation
4. Enable use of evidence generated in, through and from practice to transform and improve care delivery and outcomes
5. Enable creativity through promoting the importance of free thinking by blending creativity with more formal learning approaches
6. Select from a range of practice development methods in an intentional and systematic way to help people learn, change and develop their practice in a sustainable and effective way
7. Ensure these practice development methods accord with methodological principles and the stated objectives of the project/research/activity
8. Use processes which can be translated into specific skills required for any context including 1:1, team, organisational and systems leadership
9. Integrate evaluation approaches that are collaborative, inclusive and participative between key stakeholders

Source: Adapted from Manley and Jackson (2020).

will create a culture of improvement and innovation among individuals, in teams, in the process of inter-teamworking, at the level of organisational functioning as a whole, and in cross-boundary systems working across health and social care. A culture of innovation is described as the most important aspect to address if sustainable transformation is to be achieved and having the skills to achieve culture change at every level of the system is important alongside recognising the enablers that need to be in place at each level (Manley and Jackson 2020).

West (2021) identifies four key elements of culture that must be in place within teams, organisations and across systems to create strong cultures for innovation (Table 20.7).

The King's Fund (2017) describe compassionate leadership as promoting a culture of learning, with risk taking encouraged within safe boundaries and an acceptance that not all innovation will be successful. Compassion creates an effective workplace culture of psychological safety, where staff feel empowered and supported to develop and implement ideas for new and improved ways of delivering services (West 2021). Similarly, Manley and Jackson (2020) describe creating culture change in frontline teams as involving integrating values about effective care with being person centred in all relationships and ways of working that build effective teams through:

- individual enablers (skilled facilitation, transformational leadership and role clarity)
- embedding values in systems of evaluation, learning, development and improvement and stakeholder participation
- organisational enablers (collaborative and authentic senior leadership, focus on supporting 'bottom-up' change)
- embedding values in organisational systems for learning, development and improvement based on an appreciation of what works and growing organisational capacity and capability in leadership and facilitation.

TABLE 20.6   Enacting levels of leadership in advanced practice.

Levels of Leadership (Elliot et al. 2012)		Leadership Outcomes (Elliott et al. 2014)
Clinical leadership activities – involves promoting change in the organisation or microsystem Acting as a positive role model	1. Guides and co-ordinates the activities of the multiprofessional team 2. Initiates and changes patient/client care through practice development 3. Takes responsibility for policy and guideline development and implementation 4. Introduces and develops patient/client care services 5. Changes clinical practice through formal education of the multiprofessional team 6. Mentors and coaches the multiprofessional team in clinical practice 7. Acts as a positive role model for autonomous clinical decision making and ongoing professional development	1. **Capacity and capability of the MDT** – increased number of MDT members with new knowledge or clinical skills for specialist patient care due to advanced practitioners' education interventions and facilitation which increase MDT motivation to engage in advancing their professional and practice development 2. **Measure of esteem** – positive evaluation of the advanced practitioners' contribution to improved delivery of patient care and healthcare services. Formal recognition of clinical expertise and ability to lead profession by being invited to act as member of national/international committees responsible for policy, procedures and strategic planning 3. **New initiatives for clinical practice and healthcare delivery** – advanced practitioner-led project development within healthcare organisations for introduction of new patient services, new clinical practices, new healthcare processes and new support measures leading to improved patient services 4. **Clinical practice based on evidence** – increased use of research-based evidence to inform guideline development and clinical practice. Advanced practitioner-led evaluation of patient care for quality assurance mechanism and benchmarking against national standards and for service development. Advanced practitioner-led research initiatives leading to knowledge generation by research
Professional leadership activities – externally focused, crossing boundaries of the local service into national and international arenas, shaping and influencing healthcare and healthcare reform, contributing to the development of the profession	1. Develops policy at national and international level 2. Engages in education outside the service at national and international level 3. Engages in professional organisations at national and international level	

Manley and Jackson (2020) present the Venus model for workforce transformation. Developed from four mixed-method studies and embracing workforce transformation, safety culture, integration and continuous professional development, the Venus model describes the most influential strategies, skills and know-how required to support frontline teams to transform practice through

TABLE 20.7 Four elements of cultures for innovation.

Element	Description
1. Inspiring vision and strategy	Teams and organisations that have an inspiring vision and strategy focused on high-quality, continually improving, compassionate care are likely to innovate in pursuit of that vision and strategy through identified priorities and clearly aligned and agreed goals for all teams
2. Enthusiastic team and cross-boundary working	Compassionate leadership encourages connections across boundaries and team members to listen carefully to each other, understand all perspectives and help and support each other
3. Positive inclusion and participation	Compassionate leadership ensures that all voices are heard in the process of delivering and improving care, creates psychological safety and encourages listening to develop mutual understanding and support to create safe team environments and higher levels of learning, creativity in decision making and innovation. Includes stakeholder involvement
4. Support and autonomy for all staff to innovate	Compassionate leaders create a positive emotional climate for staff, including helping them cope with negative experiences. Leaders promote positive emotions among staff and leader positivity leads to higher levels of team creativity and innovation

Source: Adapted from West (2021).

interprofessional learning, development, improvement and innovation, alongside the essential organisational and system factors required to enable this. The model includes five stems and identifies key skill sets identified as pivotal to successful transformation, summarised in Table 20.8. This model may provide advanced practitioners with a helpful framework for developing the range of knowledge and skills for progressing improvement and innovation in their practice as identified in Table 20.1 aligned to team and practice development, quality improvement and innovation at micro-, meso- and macro-system levels.

TABLE 20.8 Summary of Venus model.

Skilled facilitation	Being able to facilitate an integrated approach to learning, development, improvement, knowledge translation, inquiry and innovation drawing on the workplace as an influential resource through: • growing the workforce within and across the system through systems leadership • helping the workforce achieve role clarity and career progression through CPD • working as high-performing teams capable of adapting to changing context to meet health needs, knowledge translation and culture change. The scope and range of facilitation activities include facilitating individuals and groups through to organisation and systems across activities from developing skills and competencies to translating knowledge into practice, improvement and innovation. • Facilitation strategies include: • building good relationships that enable shared values and meanings, challenge, new ideas for improvement • creating safe spaces for conversations and reflection • enabling service user feedback • positivity.

TABLE 20.8   (Continued)

Leadership	Need for leadership expertise and skills at every level of the system to support transformation involving: • leadership that is facilitative and people centred, enabling empowerment of teams and creative solutions to sustainable system change • leadership expertise that is enabling across boundaries, for others to grow and for transformation • leadership that supports sustainable person-centred transformation at micro, meso, and macro levels.
Practice development	Focusing on collaborative, inclusive and participative approaches with stakeholders to develop person-centred, safe and effective cultures and sustainable practice change using the principles of practice development in Table 20.5.
Improvement	Involves need for improvement skills to support person-centredness, holism, safety and effectiveness combined with the processes of practice development. Requires a collective leadership approach: • using improvement approaches that use measurement wisely to focus on measuring what is valued and evaluating positive progress • consistent in the use of improvement approaches, the effective use of data, a focus on relationships and culture • enabling and supportive engagement of frontline staff • working as a system involving patients and service users. At micro level requires: • knowledge of improvement tools and which to use, how to use them, what results mean and how to act on the results, e.g. PDSA cycles. At meso level requires: • commitment to culture of safety with widespread deployment of process improvement tools and small-scale change processes. At macro level requires: • understanding of population health and characteristics and clinical systems leadership skills that integrate improvement to enable the system to understand what needs to improve and how to improve.
Culture change	Culture is about 'the way things are done around here' underpinned by values, beliefs and assumptions which will influence whether any transformation can be achieved. Individual enablers of role clarity, transformational leadership and skilled facilitation are essential for culture change and facilitating culture change at the micro-systems level for person-centred, safe and effective care

Source: Adapted from Manley and Jackson (2020).

Advanced practitioners may also find a range of NHS resources related to improvement, innovation and change helpful in providing for additional information, including the following.

• NHS England (2018) The Change Model Guide. The Change Model provides a framework to enable effective and sustainable change that delivers benefits for staff, patients and communities. The Change Model is for anyone who wants to make a difference –in a clinical or support role at any level of an organisation. www.england.nhs.uk/wp-content/uploads/2018/04/change-model-guide-v5.pdf

- NHS England (2018) Leading Large Scale Change: A Guide to Leading Large Scale Change Through Complex Health and Social Care Environments. A Practical Guide. www.england.nhs.uk/sustainableimprovement/leading-large-scale-change
- NHS England (2017) Thinking Differently. This book provides a range of practical approaches and tools that many NHS leaders and frontline teams have used to fundamentally rethink pathways of care and service delivery. This guide describes how to improve and transform services. www.england.nhs.uk/improvement-hub/publication/thinking-differently
- NHS Improvement (2014) First Steps Toward Quality Improvement: A Simple Guide to Improving Services. This provides the information for first steps towards making quality improvements, including a blend of project management and improvement tools, combined with practical know-how and first-hand experience gained from working with NHS teams. www.england.nhs.uk/improvement-hub/wp-content/uploads/sites/44/2011/06/service_improvement_guide_2014.pdf
- NHS England and NHS Improvement (2014) Plan, Do, Study, Act (PDSA) Cycles and The Model for Improvement. www.england.nhs.uk/wp-content/uploads/2022/01/qsir-pdsa-cycles-model-for-improvement.pdf
- NHS Scotland Model for Improvement (n.d.). https://learn.nes.nhs.scot/2959/quality-improvement-zone/qi-tools/model-for-improvement
- Bauer M, Damschroder L, Hagedorn H et al. (2015) An introduction to implementation science for the non-specialist. BMC Psychology (2015) 3: 32.
- Bryant-Lukosius D, Spichiger E, Martin J et al. (2016) Framework for evaluating the impact of advanced practice. Journal of Nursing Scholarship 48(2): 201–209.

Learning Event 1

In collaboration with clinical team colleagues, facilitate a discussion exploring opportunities for practice development, improvement and innovations in your practice, clinical team or service, including identifying the potential barriers, enablers and support needed from service leaders to initiate.

Learning Event 2

Consider the principles of practice development in Table 20.5 and the Venus Model in Table 20.8 to reflect on your own knowledge and skills, identifying any areas for development and support for inclusion in your personal development action plan.

Learning Event 3

The findings from Fothergill et al. (2022) highlight the challenges and barriers to engaging with the educational, leadership and research pillars of the HEE Multi-professional Framework for Advanced Clinical Practice and identify a number of recommendations including: (i) a need to highlight the value and importance of each of the four pillars of practice to employers, to encourage the allocation of adequate resources and support for APs to work across all four pillars; (ii) the need for increased efforts to support APs with national and international research engagement to support professional development and share best practice. Develop a plan for how you might take these recommendations forward for your role within your organisation.

Learning Event 4

Review the PEPPA-PLUS framework (Bryant-Lukosius et al. 2016) and analyse opportunities to evaluate your APs role, practice or service. Identify the aims of the evaluation and potential methods to achieve this.

CONCLUSION

Innovation has significance for advanced-level practice and advanced practitioners. This has been examined in two ways. The first, with advanced practice as an illustration of innovation in workforce transformation globally and nationally. Second, by focusing on the expectations of the advanced practitioner and their enactment as a clinical and professional leader facilitating and leading practice development, continuous improvement and innovation at individual, team, wider organisational and system levels. Advanced practitioners are expected to lead at different levels, working collaboratively at micro (clinical team), meso (organisational), and macro (systems) levels, and to use their expert knowledge, skilled facilitation and leadership strategies, practice development, improvement skills and tools, and culture change skills to promote and support innovation in healthcare.

Each of these levels of leadership requires a particular leadership strategy, knowledge and skill set to achieve success as clinical systems leaders focus on the cultural outcomes associated with quality care in the workplace. Models and frameworks for examining facilitation and leadership strategies have been published to enable advanced practitioners to systematically implement, evaluate and, importantly, disseminate their progress in supporting practice development, improvement and innovation across the health system.

Take Home Points

- Innovation has significance for advanced practice and advanced practitioners. First, advanced practice is a key systems innovation in global and national workforce transformation. Second, advanced practitioners, as clinical and professional leaders, have a pivotal role in facilitating and leading practice development, improvement and innovation at individual, team, organisation and systems levels.

- There is a need to continue to evaluate advanced practice and the implementation and impact of national frameworks and advanced practice roles.

- Leading practice development, continuous improvement and innovation to enhance patient care, service and system delivery are key parts of the AP role. Each requires a particular leadership strategy, knowledge and skill set to achieve success.

REFERENCES

Beech, J., Bottery, S., Charlesworth, A. et al. (2019). *Closing the Gap. Key Areas for Action on the Health and Care Workforce*. The Health Foundation www.nuffieldtrust.org.uk/files/2019-03/heaj6708-workforce-full-report-web.pdf.

de Bont, A., van Exel, J., Coretti, S. et al. (2016). Reconfiguring health workforce: a case-based comparative study explaining the increasingly diverse professional roles in Europe. *BMC Health Services Research* 16: 637.

Bryant-Lukosius, D., Spichiger, E., Martin, J. et al. (2016). Framework for evaluating the impact of advanced practice nursing roles. *Journal of Nursing Scholarship* 48 (2): 201–209.

Elliott, N., Higgins, A., Begley, C. et al. (2012). The identification of clinical and professional leadership activities of advanced practitioners: findings from the Specialist Clinical and Advanced Practitioner Evaluation study in Ireland. *Journal of Advanced Nursing* 69 (5): 1037–1050.

Elliott, N., Begley, C., Kleinpell, R., and Higgins, A. (2014). The development of leadership outcome-indicators evaluating the contribution of clinical specialists and advanced practitioners to health care: a secondary analysis. *Journal of Advanced Nursing* 70 (5): 1078–1093.

Elliott, N., Begley, C., Sheaf, G., and Higgins, A. (2016). Barriers and enablers to advanced practitioners' ability to enact their leadership role: a scoping review. *International Journal of Nursing Studies* 60: 24–45.

Evans, C., Poku, B., Pearce, R. et al. (2020a). Characterising the evidence base for advanced clinical practice in the UK: a scoping review protocol. *BMJ Open* 10: e036192.

Evans, C., Pearce, R., Greaves, S., and Blake, H. (2020b). Advanced clinical practitioners in primary care in the UK: a qualitative study of workforce transformation. *International Journal of Environmental Research and Public Health* 17: 4500.

Fothergill, L.J., Al-Oraibi, A., Houdmont, J. et al. (2022). Nationwide evaluation of the advanced clinical practitioner role in England: a cross-sectional survey. *BMJ Open* 12: e055475.

Gerrish, K., Guillaume, L., Kirshbaum, M. et al. (2011). Factors influencing the contribution of advanced practice nurses to promoting evidence-based practice among front-line nurses: findings from a cross-sectional survey. *Journal of Advanced Nursing* 67 (5): 1079–1090.

Health Education England (2017). Multi-professional Framework for Advanced Clinical Practice in England. www.hee.nhs.uk/sites/default/files/documents/multi-professionalframeworkforadvancedclinicalpracticeinengland.pdf

Higgins, A., Begley, C., Lalor, J. et al. (2014). Factors influencing advanced practitioners' ability to enact leadership: a case study within Irish healthcare. *Journal of Nursing Management* 22: 894–905.

Lawler, J., Maclaine, K., and Leary, A. (2020). Workforce experience of the implementation of an advanced clinical practice framework in England: a mixed methods evaluation. *Human Resources for Health* 18: 96.

Leary A (2019). The healthcare workforce should be shaped by outcomes, rather than outputs. https://blogs.bmj.com/bmj/2019/05/31/alison-leary-the-healthcare-workforce-should-be-shaped-by-outcomes-rather-than-outputs

Leary, A. and MacLaine, K. (2019). The evolution of advanced nursing practice: past, present and future. *Nursing Times* 115 (10): 18–19.

Leighann, K. and Massoud, R. (2017). What do we mean by innovation in healthcare? *EMJ Innovation* 1 (1): 89–91.

Lockwood, E.B., Lehwaldt, D., Sweeney, M.R., and Matthews, A. (2020). An exploration of the levels of clinical autonomy of advanced nurse practitioners: a narrative literature review. *International Journal of Nursing Practice* 28: e12978.

Manley, K. (1997). A conceptual framework for advanced practice: an action research project operationalising an advanced practitioner/consultant nurse role. *Journal of Clinical Nursing* 6 (3): 179–190.

Manley, K. and Jackson, C. (2020). The Venus model for integrating practitioner-led workforce transformation and complex change across the health care system. *Journal of Evaluation in Clinical Practice* 26: 622–634.

Manley, K., Sanders, K., Cardiff, S., and Webster, J. (2011). Effective workplace culture: the attributes, enabling factors and consequences of a new concept. *International Practice Development Journal* 1 (2): 1–29.

Manley, K., O'Keefe, H., Jackson, C. et al. (2014). A shared purpose framework to deliver person-centred, safe and effective care: organisational transformation using practice development methodology. *International Practice Development Journal* 41 (1): Article 2.

McCormack, B., Manley, K., Kitson, A., and Harvey, G. (1999). Towards practice development – a vision in reality or a reality without vision? *Journal of Nursing Management* 7: 255–264.

NHS Employers (2021). Advanced and Enhanced Clinical Practice. www.nhsemployers.org/articles/advanced-and-enhanced-clinical-practice

NHS England (2015). Five Year Forward View. www.england.nhs.uk/wp-content/uploads/2014/10/5yfv-web.pdf

NHS England (2016). Innovation into Action: Supporting Delivery of the NHS Five Year Forward View. www.england.nhs.uk/wp-content/uploads/2015/10/nhs-inovation-into-action.pdf

NHS England (2019). The NHS Long Term Plan. www.longtermplan.nhs.uk

NHS England (2020). We Are The NHS: People Plan 2020/21 – Action For Us All. www.england.nhs.uk/wp-content/uploads/2020/07/We-Are-The-NHS-Action-For-All-Of-Us-FINAL-March-21.pdf

NHS Institute for Innovation and Improvement (2007). Thinking Differently. www.england.nhs.uk/improvement-hub/publication/thinking-differently

Omachonu, V.K. and Einspruch, N.G. (2010). Innovation in healthcare delivery systems: a conceptual framework. *Innovation Journal* 15 (1): Article 2.

Rogers, E.M. (1983). *Diffusion of Innovations*, 3e. London: Macmillan/Free Press.

The Health Foundation (2021). Quality improvement made simple: what everyone should know about health care quality improvement. http://health.org.uk/publications/quality-improvement-made-simple

The King's Fund (2017). Caring to change: how compassionate leadership can stimulate innovation in healthcare. www.kingsfund.org.uk/publications/caring-change

Varkey, P., Horne, A., and Bennet, K.E. (2008). Innovation in health care: a primer. *American Journal of Medical Quality* 23: 382–388.

West, M.A. (2021). *Compassionate Leadership: Sustaining Wisdom, Humanity and Presence in Health and Social Care*. UK: Swirling Leaf Press.

West, M.A. and Farr, J.L. (1990). *Innovation and Creativity at Work: Psychological and Organizational Strategies*. New York: Wiley.

World Health Organization 2016 Global Strategy on Human Resources for Health: Workforce 2030. https://apps.who.int/iris/bitstream/handle/10665/250368/9789241511131-eng.pdf

SELF-ASSESSMENT QUESTIONS

1. Define practice development and innovation, and identify the similarities and differences between them.
2. Explain what micro, meso, and macro levels refer to.
3. What are audit, service evaluation and research (see `https://nspccro.nihr.ac.uk/working-with-us/research-service-evaluation-or-audit`)?
4. What are the differences between clinical and professional leadership?

GLOSSARY

Clinical leadership Involves promoting change in the organisation or micro-system. Acting as a positive role model (Elliot et al. 2012).

Innovation Involves new, better or more effective ways of solving challenges or problems that confront people, teams, organisations or communities in healthcare (The King's Fund 2017).

Practice development A continuous process of improvement towards increased effectiveness in person-centred care achieved through the enabling of healthcare teams to transform the culture and context of care (McCormack et al. 1999).

Professional leadership Externally focused, crossing boundaries of the local service into national and international arenas to shape and influence healthcare and healthcare reform, and contribute to the development of the profession (Elliot et al. 2012).

CHAPTER 21

Professional Development and Transition

Vikki-Jo Scott and Esther Clift

> **Aim**
>
> The aim of this chapter is to explore and develop understanding of key concepts in relation to professional development for people currently working in or training for advanced clinical practice roles. This includes aspects relating to transition to, within, and beyond AP roles.

LEARNING OUTCOMES

After reading this chapter the reader will:

1. recognise the importance of ongoing personal professional development for advanced practice and its impact on addressing evolving and novel aspects of population need and its contribution to patient safety
2. understand the contribution that can be made by advanced practitioners (APs) to developing a team to work effectively, including role negotiation, embracing diversity, and driving quality improvement
3. be aware of the contribution that can be made to development of advanced practice beyond the local context
4. be able to plan the next steps in their professional development, including towards consultant level.

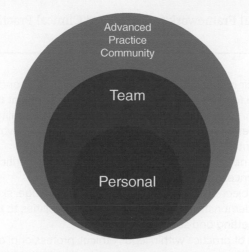

FIGURE 21.1 Layers of professional development and transition in advanced practice.

INTRODUCTION

The goal of advanced practice roles is to manage clinical care in partnership with individuals, families and carers. It includes the analysis and synthesis of complex problems across a range of settings, enabling innovative solutions to enhance people's experience and improve outcomes. Transition into an autonomous role as an advanced practitioner is both daunting and a cause for celebration (Skills for Health 2020).

When considering professional development and transition in advanced practice, it is important to recognise that this goes beyond just the development of the individual. Advanced practitioners are rarely 'sole operators' and commonly work within a multi-professional team that has an overarching employing organisation. The individual's development will impact the broader team and organisation in which they work. At an advanced level of practice, it is also expected that individuals will contribute to the broader development of the advanced practice profession, which is diverse, multiprofessional, and evolving fast. It is therefore helpful when looking at this topic to consider the 'personal', the 'team' and the 'AP community' and how the development of one will radiate out to the other layers (Figure 21.1).

As described in Table 21.1, the Multi-professional Framework for Advanced Clinical Practice (HEE 2017) provides helpful guidance on the expectations for APs at each layer of professional development.

PERSONAL PROFESSIONAL DEVELOPMENT

Personal professional development is lifelong. We never stop learning and the nature of AP is that it is evolving, adapting to population needs. It is an innovative role often moving into uncharted territories which require that we use new or unfamiliar approaches or apply knowledge, skills, and behaviours in novel contexts.

In order to develop, you need to remember where you have developed from and recognise how much was learnt along the way to provide confidence and a direction for future development.

While it might be useful to think about this as a journey as depicted in Figure 21.2, where you set a goal, work towards it and then step on the podium at the end and take your medal, actually the race is

TABLE 21.1   Multi-professional Framework for Advanced Clinical Practice: guidance for professional development.

Personal:
1.1 Practise in compliance with their respective code of professional conduct and within their scope of practice, being responsible and accountable for their decisions, actions and omissions at this level of practice.
1.2 Demonstrate a critical understanding of their broadened level of responsibility and autonomy and the limits of own competence and professional scope of practice, including when working with complexity, risk, uncertainty and incomplete information.
1.3 Act on professional judgement about when to seek help, demonstrating critical reflection on own practice, self-awareness, emotional intelligence, and openness to change.
1.11 Evidence the underpinning subject-specific competencies i.e. knowledge, skills and behaviours relevant to the role setting and scope, and demonstrate application of the capabilities to these, in an approach that is appropriate to the individual role, setting and scope.
2.11 Negotiate an individual scope of practice within legal, ethical, professional and organisational policies, governance and procedures, with a focus on managing risk and upholding safety.
3.1 Critically assess and address own learning needs, negotiating a personal development plan that reflects the breadth of ongoing professional development across the four pillars of advanced clinical practice.
3.2 Engage in self-directed learning, critically reflecting to maximise clinical skills and knowledge, as well as own potential to lead and develop both care and services.

Team:
2.4 Actively engage in peer review to inform own and other's practice, formulating and implementing strategies to act on learning and make improvements.
3.4 Advocate for and contribute to a culture of organisational learning to inspire future and existing staff.
3.6 Identify further developmental needs for the individual and the wider team and supporting them to address these.
3.7 Supporting the wider team to build capacity and capability through work-based and inter- professional learning, and the application of learning to practice

Advanced Practice Community:
4.8 Facilitate collaborative links between clinical practice and research through proactive engagement, networking with academic, clinical and other active researchers

Source: Adapted from HEE (2017).

FIGURE 21.2   The professional development journey.

never over! For the duration of our working lives, there are always new goals that we can choose to reach for. Sometimes this is because we want to push ourselves in a different direction, and sometimes it is because the world around us has changed and to keep up with this change, we need to 'adjust our sails' and set new goals.

It is important to remember, however, that we are never starting from scratch each time a new goal is set. All your learning and experiences to date will have shaped what you are, and often lessons learnt from these can be applied or adapted to help you in achieving your next goal. Often, however, the hard part is remembering what we have learnt along the way.

Think about how difficult it is to explain to someone a task that you do now unconsciously. To be successful at this, you need to break it down into its constituent parts or stages of the process. Some will seem familiar and easily transferable to a new skill, and others appear quite specialised which took practice or different approaches, resources or knowledge to master . . . but you did get there in the end!

As an advanced practitioner, you will have started in a particular profession. You will have learnt the skills relevant to this profession, applying the knowledge and evidence base to underpin your actions, and have continued to build upon these through experience. All professions that work within the definition of 'advanced practice' are regulated. This means that educational standards have been set for approval of an individual to enter that profession and a monitoring and revalidation process is required for them to continue to practise. All regulatory requirements for healthcare professions provide scope for and requirement to continually develop and enhance practice. AP development is therefore not outside or in addition to the requirements of professional revalidation; it is the way in which you can demonstrate how you are encompassing the requirements of your profession-specific regulatory body to continually develop.

For example, the Nursing and Midwifery Council (2020) requires that registrants:

- 6.2 maintain the knowledge and skills you need for safe and effective practice
- 9.2 gather and reflect on feedback from a variety of sources, using it to improve your practice and performance
- 13.5 complete the necessary training before carrying out a new role
- 19.2 take account of current evidence, knowledge and developments in reducing mistakes and the effect of them and the impact of human factors and system failures
- 22.3 keep your knowledge and skills up to date, taking part in appropriate and regular learning and professional development activities that aim to maintain and develop your competence and improve your performance.

The Health and Care Professions Council (2022) requires that registrants:

1. maintain a continuous, up-to-date and accurate record of their CPD activities
2. demonstrate that their CPD activities are a mixture of learning activities relevant to current or future practice
3. seek to ensure that their CPD has contributed to the quality of their practice and service delivery
4. seek to ensure that their CPD benefits the service user.

Learning Event

- Consider what evidence you need to collect, review, evaluate, and act upon to demonstrate ongoing development to meet your relevant regulatory body standards.

This evidence should relate to your current job, specialist field, and level of practice. As a starting point, you might find it helpful to look at your job description or the job description of a role you are aiming for. This is likely to give you particular expectations around your role, including relevant competencies and capabilities, tasks and responsibilities. These can then be mapped to the expectations around advanced practice by looking at the capabilities in the Multi-professional Framework (HEE 2017).

You might also have particular standards and expectations to provide assurance of your ability to continue to work at a specific level of practice. For example, each of the regulatory bodies has specific requirements regarding periodic submission of evidence of continuing professional development (CPD).

Professional bodies (e.g. Royal College of Occupational Therapy, Chartered Society of Physiotherapy) will supplement the more generic standards expected by the regulatory body (the HCPC), giving more specific direction on the expectations for your profession.

In addition, standards may have been set for a particular specialism or context of practice. These are commonly referred to as 'credentials'. The two longest established of these are intensive and emergency care which are governed by the Faculty of Intensive Care Medicine (FICM 2015, 2022)and Royal College of Emergency Medicine (RCEM 2017) (commonly referred to as 'credentialling bodies' in advanced practice). Work is also under way through the Centre for Advancing Practice to develop, validate and publish credentials for particular specialisms. You should continue to look out for credentials that are relevant to your field of practice and think about what evidence you can provide or need to gain to demonstrate that you meet the expectations for the specialism in which you work.

Accreditation Considerations

You can find out more about the work that the Centre for Advancing Practice is undertaking with regard to 'credentials' for particular fields of practice here: https://advanced-practice.hee.nhs.uk/credentials

Credentials are described as 'standardised, structured units of assessed learning that are designed to develop advanced-level practice capability in a particular area'. (HEE 2022) The Centre for Advancing Practice refers to a 'credential specification' to describe the document that sets out the learning experience and outcomes (including the AP area-specific capabilities) that a credential should develop and assess. As Centre endorsement for a credential is confirmed and documents finalised, each resource will be launched as a Centre-endorsed credential specification. Regular updates on Centre-endorsed credential specifications will be provided on the credentials webpage.

For example, currently there are credentials available for those APs working in acute medicine (co-produced with the Royal College of Physicians), mental health, or for APs who work with older people, and other areas are listed as endorsed or currently undergoing development. All Centre-endorsed credentials are expected to reflect the four pillars and capabilities in the Multi-professional Framework for Advanced Clinical Practice (HEE 2017) and therefore will include an expectation regarding ongoing professional development within the relevant field of practice.

In the acute medicine curriculum framework, expected capabilities for this field of practice are split into core, generic, and specialty. All are linked back to the Multi-professional Framework, and examples of evidence that can be used to inform the decision as to whether someone can demonstrate the capability is listed.

A learning outcome for acute medicine is 'Developing within the context of advanced level practice as a learner, teacher, and supervisor'. This is expressed in a *core* capability in practice as 'critically reflects on their own learning needs and develops an individualised learning plan, seeking out or creating opportunities for their own development'. In the *generic* clinical capabilities in practice relating to advanced clinical assessment and decision making, this is noted as 'critically reflects on their assessment, diagnostic and decision-making skills, identifies areas for future development and seeks out opportunities to address these development needs'. In the *specialty* clinical capabilities in practice relating to prioritisation and selection of patients according to severity of illness and escalation of care, APs in acute medicine 'critically reflect on their management of the unwell patient and use this process to identify development needs and seek out opportunities to address these'. Suggested examples of evidence for demonstration of these core, generic, and speciality capabilities are a work-place supervisor report, a Professional Development Plan, and reflective log.

The Faculty of Intensive Care Medicine provide a curriculum that sets out the expectations regarding recognition by them to practice as an Advanced Critical Care Practitioner (ACCP). Within their handbook they note that the outcome from their training programme 'is such that mastery of the specialty to the level required to commence autonomous practice in a specific post is achieved by the end of training as knowledge, skills, attitudes, and behaviours metaphorically spiral upwards. Following qualification, the continuing professional development of the ACCP will follow the same model'. Their ACCP advisory group has also produced a CPD and appraisal pathway by which ACCPs can plan, institute, maintain, and evidence their ongoing clinical academic, and professional learning. www.ficm.ac.uk/careersworkforceaccps/accp-cpd-and-appraisal

They note this is in addition to regulatory body requirements regarding re-validation (with the NMC or HCPC) and includes a 'medical style' appraisal, as clinical supervision of ACCPs rests with the Consultant Medical Staff in Critical Care and clinical leads for ACCPs.

In the Royal College of Emergency Medicine 'Emergency Care Advanced Clinical Practitioner Curriculum (Adult and Paediatric)' (p. 29) they also note the need to address the requirements for CPD as set out by the relevant regulatory body that apply to the particular profession you originally registered in (NMC or HCPC). In the 'common competencies' they also make reference to particular behaviours that are expected. This includes the need to 'Keep up to date with national reviews and guidelines of practice (e.g. NICE and SIGN)' under the 'common competency for Evidence and Guidelines, (page 90). https://rcem.ac.uk/emergency-care-advanced-clinical-practitioners

So when starting out on your own personal professional development, it is helpful to identify:

- the expectations you should be working to
- who governs these expectations
- how you can/must demonstrate that you meet these expectations.

Requirements for CPD within regulatory, professional, or credentialling bodies are often linked to expectations around supervision. Successful professional development is much more likely to be achieved where an individual is supported and guided in their practice, with opportunities for assessment, feedback and discussion. Certain criteria may be set down by your employer or your regulatory, professional, or credentialling body regarding:

- what type, model and volume of supervision should be expected
- who can act as an appropriate supervisor
- whether they have a role to play in assessing and confirming your progress and achievement.

Establishing an effective supervisory relationship is key to success. It can have a significant influence on your development and your experience of the process, which may in turn affect how well you feel able to support others. You may or may not have some choice about who your supervisor will be. Getting the right balance between someone you feel you can talk to easily and someone that you feel will be honest without repercussions on friendship or working relations can be difficult! Be aware of the professional relationship status that supervision holds, know what to expect, and know who else you can turn to if the supervision is not working as it should.

Coaching may or may not be an approach taken within your supervision, but is strongly encouraged as a reflective challenge for your practice and to develop your leadership capability. Many employers will have a people development team with some leadership coaches who would be happy to support you.

However, remember that you are the person who is most invested in your development. Others (including employers, supervisors and coaches) will have their own agenda and will not necessarily appreciate the complexity of your journey to where you are today and the rich texture of how you perform at your best. A key expectation of advanced practice is developing autonomy – taking personal responsibility for driving your progress forward in the way that works best for you is a necessary adjunct to effective supervision.

CONTINUING PROFESSIONAL DEVELOPMENT AND ROLE TRANSITION

Healthcare and population needs are always changing, so, as with CPD, transition into the role of advanced practice may never feel like it ends as there are always going to be new knowledge and skills to learn. However, by setting clear objectives for your development and career aspirations, targets and goals, you will be presented with more opportunities to make a conscious decision about what changes you want, rather than just being dragged along with the flow of change. To do this, establish what the barriers or facilitators to change are and identify allies who will help you to facilitate your development. You should also take time to understand how your objectives align with intrinsic motivators (e.g. what gives you meaning, a sense of belonging or self-esteem) and extrinsic motivators (e.g. rewards, competition, how you are seen by others) as well as organisational strategic objectives.

Every organisation should undertake an annual review or appraisal for all staff. This provides a golden opportunity to articulate and negotiate your achievements and aspirations, and to seek endorsement from your line manager for your plans. As you develop as an advanced practitioner, you should use this to synthesise your personal aspirations, your organisational objectives, and the required actions to grow in your advanced practice capabilities.

To help you with this, there a number of skills and tools you can use to identify, plan, and sustain your learning.

- Undertaking a learning needs assessment will provide dedicated time and space to decide what you need to focus on for your development. From this, you can be more targeted on the actions you choose to undertake to address your learning needs. Within learning needs analysis, it helpful to get a variety of perspectives on the areas you may need to consider as a development goal. Using a self-assessment tool alongside gathering feedback (perhaps through a 360 appraisal) can help to discern what is needed. We are not always the best judge of how we are perceived by others and tend to over- or underemphasise our strengths and weaknesses. Learning needs analysis does not need to be complicated; asking simple questions such as what are your goals, what are your desired outcomes, what knowledge/ skills do you already have and what do you need, can help to identify the gaps and prioritise actions.
- Using a goal-setting tool such as 'SMART' can also help to clearly and concisely identify objectives and the actions, resources and time scale needed to achieve them. Think about, write out, and where possible discuss and agree these with your supervisor.

S Specific – write a clear aim and why it is significant. Try to keep it simple (you can break down complex aims into smaller chunks to help to keep them specific enough for actions to be set).

M Measurable – how are you going to meaningfully measure achievement of your aim? What will tell you that you have been successful?

A Action – what are the achievable and agreed actions you are going to undertake to address your aim?

R Resources – what resources are you going to need to achieve your goal (these could be money, people, or access to a resource such as a course or online learning)? Consider whether these are realistic (if not, you may need to adjust your goal or actions), and be clear about how these will help you to achieve your goal.

T Time – set a date by which you expect to achieve your goal. This may include setting dates for interim points for when actions need to be carried out and when review is needed to check you are on track (or if you need to adjust your plan). This could be linked with a job plan, which is a helpful way of laying out time to facilitate your own development and ensure that you are meeting all four pillars of advanced practice.

- Other planning tools such as a Gantt chart can also be helpful to clearly set out timelines and actively plan for regular review points. Passively relying on annual review may mean momentum is lost or changes in circumstances may derail your goals rather than adjusting to the circumstances while still keeping the ultimate goal in mind. These tools are also helpful as they encourage you to break a 'master plan' or overarching goal into smaller, more manageable steps. At different times, you may need to break your actions down to smaller ones to keep moving forward. For example, what can you do to move towards your goal in the next 15 minutes rather than in the next month?

- Reflective tools or models are well known and used in healthcare, particularly within initial training or more formal education. You could try a few different ones to find one that feels the best fit for you and until it feels familiar and easy to use. A key principle of reflection is that it is an active rather than passive process, where you set aside time and head space to engage with your experience and consider how that may help you for the future. All reflective models will encourage you to not just keep your reflective thoughts in your head. Writing them down and discussing them with someone else helps to expose your thoughts; this can provide a definite frame of reference for your goals and plans, and from this give you the driving force to turn this into a tangible physical action.

- You may find using the NHS leadership model alongside the above or as a structure for reflection helpful. It provides prompts to explore different aspects of leadership (which is a key pillar of AP) and provides tools for self and peer assessment and a way in which to record your experiences, plan your development and track your progress. `www.leadershipacademy.nhs.uk/resources/healthcare-leadership-model`

- Quality improvement methodology can help develop an iterative approach to recognising where improvements can be made to any area. This may be training and development, specific patient safety issues or service efficiencies. Quality improvement tools are data-driven accessible tools which quantify process and plans, such as driver diagrams and Plan Do Study Act (PDSA) cycles. These can be really powerful to manage change. NHS England (2022) provides access to a range of quality, service improvement and redesign tools for useful reference.

Your attitude to learning can also have an impact on success. Studies that talk about a 'growth mindset' noted that people who believed that if they worked hard they could learn and achieve more were actually more successful. Although the research has largely been based on children, this can also apply to adults. (Take a look at Carol Dweck's TED talk 'The power of believing that you can improve': www.ted. com/talks/carol_dweck_the_power_of_believing_that_you_can_improve?language=en.)

By remaining open to learning and believing that putting some effort into learning can help you achieve your goals, you are more likely to achieve what you are aiming for. Being passive and expecting the 'learning to come to you' are much less likely to be successful.

This is one of the reasons why there has been a shift away from using lectures as the primary way of delivering education. Just being present in a lecture theatre or gathering together a folder of attendance certificates will not automatically guarantee that learning has been achieved – it requires some active engagement by the learner for the transfer of knowledge from one person or source to another to happen. Verification of learning and capability in advanced practice takes note of this.

For example, in the AP Apprenticeship Standards for End Point Assessment, and in the Centre for Advancing Practice e-portfolio route for evidencing that a person adequately meets the capabilities expected for working at this level of practice, a range of evidence is required. The portfolios and assessments used will expect not just a collection of certificates but articulation of how a particular learning event or experience has contributed to your development and can be evidenced in your practice as an AP. This requires engagement with reflection on learning and within this, clear articulation of how this applies to your practice as an AP. For this reason, you will need to engage with a range of work-based assessment which includes external observation and endorsement of your capability as well as use of case studies to provide examples of how learning has been applied, and the expected outcomes of learning achieved. Within this process and noting the 'growth mindset' approach, this requires that you acknowledge weaknesses as well as strengths, drawing upon both positive and negative feedback and experiences to plan and then demonstrate your development.

There is also a temptation to feel you have to do everything to a perfected level before pushing yourself forward into new roles/ tasks/ contexts, but in reality we are continually developing; you can never be fully and perfectly prepared, but you can be open to learning along the way, adapting as needed. Sometimes you do need to 'just go for it'. Opportunities come by every now and again and if you do not allow time away from the day-to-day tasks, you may miss these opportunities.

Finally, when considering your personal development, remember to look after yourself! Research has shown that healthcare worker well-being, organisational change, and patient safety are linked (Montgomery et al. 2020). There has been significant discussion of 'building resilience' and efforts to reduce burnout in healthcare workers, with the COVID-19 pandemic particularly highlighting the negative long-term impact this can have. APs are not immune to this! In fact, they may be more at risk due to the emerging nature of AP roles where established support networks and a clear role identity, scope of practice and legitimised autonomy can be a challenge. A (usually unjustified) sense of needing to prove yourself due to imposter syndrome has been noted to be a common feature of people's experience, particularly where they are working in innovative ways or in new teams or services. Investing time in your own development and well-being is consequently worthy of attention, not least because it contributes to patient safety. This is, of course, a priority all can agree on as important.

SUPPORTING PROFESSIONAL DEVELOPMENT WITHIN A TEAM

It is unlikely that as an AP you will be working in isolation. Commonly, APs work within a multidisciplinary team. Within this environment, it is important that as part of your CPD, you develop your professional identity. Team members are not expected to work the same or bring the same knowledge, skills, and experience to the role they play within a team. Each team member should be encouraged to draw on others' strengths to complement what they contribute, thus allowing the service to adapt to address the needs of the patients, carers, and organisations they work with.

From the team perspective of professional development, it is important therefore to recognise the strengths of others. You should take a facilitatory approach to identify where individuals may need support to develop their contribution/expertise, as well as identifying where as a team there may be areas that need developing. As an advanced practitioner, you are also likely to be leading a team and supporting trainees.

Having identified potential areas for development within your team, the focus should move on to identifying potential actions or solutions to the deficits identified. Taking a team-based, co-design approach to this part of the process will reflect the expected values and capabilities of advanced practice, as well as being more likely to be successful.

Ask team members both what they see as potential weaknesses or challenges (e.g. through a learning needs assessment and evaluation of feedback) and what the potential actions to address these are. This will help to reveal issues you may not be aware of and draw on the collective creativity of the team to establish workable development plans that are not the sole responsibility of one person to address. This will allow you to demonstrate that you are taking an active role in the development of others, and that you recognise that 'one size does not fit all'; different approaches and focus will be needed for different team members at different times.

Some examples of case studies from different fields of practice are given below. We suggest you use these as learning events to think about how professional development and transition could relate to advancing practice within your own team.

Learning Event

Consider the case studies in the boxes below. Then try to write a case study for yourself using the trigger questions.

- If you were to describe your role within your field of practice, how would you explain the particular knowledge, skills, and experience you contribute to the team and service in which you work?
- How could this be/ is this complemented by others in the team?
- Where does this create a gap or conflict within your team?
- What models, tools or techniques and forums or routes of communication could you use to identify and address any gaps in the team? (You might find referring to the QSIR tools presented by NHS England useful here: www.england.nhs.uk/sustainableimprovement/qsir-programme/qsir-tools).

Field of Practice – Paediatrics/Learning Disabilities

James is based in a community paediatric service, working with young people with a learning disability, often in the early stages of their journey through diagnosis and support. This draws on his background as a learning disability nurse but allows him to utilise more advanced skills and knowledge.

James is able to provide support within a clinic setting; this can encompass concerns such as difficulties with sleep, building awareness of diagnosis or unpicking behaviours which challenge. He also advocates for annual health checks when young people reach 14 years of age and supports transition when moving to adult services. As part of his role, he provides a clinic within a special school for young people with learning disabilities.

James also supports the wider team in their understanding of learning disabilities through training and supervision. He represents his service at an operation level with colleagues across the integrated care system, ensuring strong interagency working.

He is considering where developing his role as an AP could take him next, but also how he might be able to contribute to develop the service he is in. James has decided that undertaking a 360 self-assessment, alongside undertaking a learning needs assessment of his team, would help with this. He plans to use a stakeholder SWOT analysis (strengths, weakness, opportunities, and threats) to determine a project the team can work on to improve the experience of children with learning disabilities and their families who come under his service.

Field of Practice – Mental Health

Andrea works as an advanced practitioner in an older people's mental health service. She is responsible for supporting people who are acutely unwell and admitted to a bedded unit for their care.

She supports the ward with training in therapeutic interventions, as well as formulations and assessments while on the ward. She also supports people at home, to enable continuity of care, and facilitate clinical monitoring as required.

Her background as an occupational therapist means that she sometimes takes a different approach to other colleagues in her team, with a particular focus on what occupation means to and how it is valued by the individual, rather than being driven by the particular patient pathway or environment that the person finds themselves in at the time that she encounters them.

Andrea is thinking about how she can use her background as an OT and her role as an AP to better facilitate the transition of patients from the inpatient bedded unit to their return home within her older people's mental health service. She decides to ask colleagues to help her draw up a process map and fishbone diagram for a typical journey a client would normally take through their service. She then uses the 'Six Thinking Hats' approach with the rest of her team to generate ideas for improvement, and responsibility charting to agree who is doing what (drawing on their particular strengths and sphere of influence).

De Bont et al. (2016) and Thompson et al. (2019) discuss how the perception and understanding of the AP role, particularly by physicians and employers, had a major influence on how, what and where AP roles were developed. They noted that this occurred even in situations where specific policy or protocols were in place to ensure consistency. Personal relationships can therefore be key to the extent to which your development as an autonomous advanced practitioner is fostered. Trust is required between professions to allow the sharing, reallocation, or shaping of healthcare services, roles and tasks. Effective relationships within teams may require a long time to build up. Investing time in building relationships within your team can therefore be useful for your own, as well as others' development and ability to transition roles towards greater autonomy. Taking a stakeholder analysis approach can assist with this, as it opens the opportunity to hear and try to understand from different perspectives, and then to take account of these in any plans you make.

Whilst advanced practice roles have been in existence for a considerable time, APs, or aspiring APs, are often in a position where they need to make the case for an AP role to be included in a team or service. For this to occur, you will need to establish the need for a role that goes beyond the boundaries of individual expertise. You will need to make a sustainable case for the role to continue even if the individual who makes the business case is no longer there. Gathering data, feedback, evidence of impact and the perspective of key stakeholders can be influential in making a sound financial business case. Taking time to gather information about population needs, the current service, team members' strengths and challenges, and examples of beneficial impact can be the key to opening the door for professional development and role transition and AP role formation at a team level.

CONTRIBUTION TO BROADER DEVELOPMENT OF ADVANCED PRACTICE

Within the Multi-professional Framework for Advanced Clinical Practice in England (HEE 2017), a core capability of the 'research' pillar is that APs are engaging and using networks to support their practice. This should be seen as your wider community of practice (beyond those you directly work with).

There are a number of organisations developing in specific areas, such as the British Geriatrics Society for all professions working with older people, the Advanced Practice Physiotherapy Network and many others. A community of practice (COP) is defined as a group of people who share a concern or a passion for something they do, and learn how to do it better as they interact regularly (Wenger 2000). They usually have an agreed domain or identity shared by an area of interest, an agreed community in order to build relationships to learn from each other, and share resources on their practice.

Identifying and engaging with a community of practice is likened to 'finding your tribe' – somewhere you feel you belong. It can be an incredibly helpful resource for shaping and supporting professional development and role transition at personal and team levels. It can help to 'calibrate' your ideas about what advanced practice is, what it can achieve and what further opportunities there are to explore in this exciting field of practice.

A particular feature of advanced practice is that it is diverse and often shaped by the local context. This can lead to a belief that the local way to operate is the only way, but by tapping into the diverse population of advanced practice, you can draw upon their experiences to open up the potential options available. Due to the types of work that APs engage with and the position that this role affords, APs are often in the position of being trailblazers and innovators, having to create new solutions or deal with new problems to solve. This provides an opportunity to view the situation beyond the boundaries of your particular experience to date, your profession, team, or service.

In many large organisations (including at integrated care system level), there are opportunities being created for leadership in advanced practice. It may seem tempting to see working as an AP as an ultimate destination for role transition. However, taking a lead AP role can allow you to continue to develop and influence others at a broader organisational or COP level.

A fundamental feature of leadership is that you are supporting others to take their journey of development and hopefully make it a positive experience for them. This requires that you share your knowledge, skills, and experiences. Actively looking for ways in which to disseminate the work you are doing as an AP should therefore always be a part of your development plan.

Sharing your experience (e.g. through publication, presentation at conference or network meetings, and reporting at a higher organisational level) can significantly increase the impact of the work you do across many different fields of practice. Through engaging with dissemination activities at a COP level, you will find this is paid back in kind through the connections and networks you make, which will help to sustain your development as an AP. As an example, the Centre for Advancing Practice runs an annual conference for sharing good practice, submitting posters and learning how others are continuing with CPD.

WHAT NEXT?

Working as an experienced AP may be the height of your career aspirations, but there are growing opportunities to move into consultant roles. Consultants work within the four pillars of advanced practice but develop a fifth pillar in consultancy, which relates to a wider level of influence, at national or international level (Gerrish et al. 2013).

Consultant practitioners continue to provide a component of face-to-face clinical care in their area of expertise, but they also hold a portfolio of other areas of senior leadership, in research, systems leadership or education, but usually contributing to all four pillars. Consultants may vary their focus of expertise through their career, for example with lecturing posts, systems leadership posts, and national clinical leadership roles.

Governance for clinical roles lies within the profession-specific capabilities, individual roles and local governance guidelines.

Some regions have their own consultant development pathways, which are multiprofessional communities of practice and offer some funding to support level 8 learning for professional doctorates or PhDs.

CONCLUSION

This chapter has promoted personal professional development for advanced practitioners, highlighting its direct and indirect impact as it addresses developing and innovative aspects of population need. Active involvement is key to successful development; it is essential to plan professional development as the practitioner transitions into an autonomous and meaningful role.

Continued professional and personal development provides the opportunity for advanced practitioners to access educational activity to support improvements in patient outcomes; it can also help staff to develop confidence and competence in new interventions and techniques. Professional development is a continuous process, and should be directed at a personal, team, and community level. Bespoke, individualised plans for transition and development are needed, reflecting the significant diversity that is associated with advanced practice.

Personal and professional development has an impact on quality improvement, the safety of patients, effective team working and service delivery; its value should not be underestimated or neglected. The advanced practitioner is required to be personally active in the process of development and role transition.

Take Home Points

- Professional development is a continuous process and should be addressed at a personal, team, and community level.
- There is significant diversity in advanced practice; bespoke, individualised plans for transition and development are needed.
- As an advanced practitioner, you need to be personally active in the process of development and role transition.
- The impact of personal well-being and professional development on quality improvement, patient safety, team working and service delivery should not be underestimated or neglected.

REFERENCES

De Bont, A., Van Exel, J., Coretti, S. et al. (2016). Reconfiguring health workforce: a case-based comparative study explaining the increasingly diverse professional roles in Europe. *BMC Health Services Research* 16: 637.

Faculty of Intensive Care Medicine (2015). Curriculum for Training for Advanced Critical Care Practitioners Handbook, Edition 1, v1.1, Page I-9. www.ficm.ac.uk/careersworkforceaccps/accp-curriculum

Faculty of Intensive Care Medicine (2022). ACCP CPD and Appraisal. www.ficm.ac.uk/careersworkforceaccps/accp-cpd-and-appraisal

Gerrish, K., McDonnell, A., and Kennedy, F. (2013). The development of a framework for evaluating the impact of nurse consultant roles in the UK. *Journal of Advanced Nursing* 69 (10): 2295–2308.

Health and Care Professions Council (2022). Standards of Continuing Professional Development. www.hcpc-uk.org/standards/standards-of-continuing-professional-development

Health Education England (2017). Multi-professional Framework for Advanced Clinical Practice in England. www.hee.nhs.uk/sites/default/files/docuemtns/HEE%20ACP%Framework.pdf

Health Education England (2022). Credentials. https://advanced-practice.hee.nhs.uk/credentials

Montgomery, A., van der Doef, M., Panagopoulou, E., and Leiter, M.P. (2020). *Connecting Healthcare Worker Well-Being, Patient Safety and Organisational Change – The Triple Challenge.* Cham: Springer.

NHS England (2022). Quality, service improvement and redesign (QSIR) tools. www.england.nhs.uk/sustainableimprovement/qsir-programme/qsir-tools

Nursing and Midwifery Council (2020). The Code: Professional standards of practice and behaviour for nurses, midwives and nursing associates. www.nmc.org.uk/standards/code

Royal College of Emergency Medicine (2017). Emergency Care Advanced Clinical Practitioner Curriculum (Adult and Paediatric) Version 2.0. https://rcem.ac.uk/emergency-care-advanced-clinical-practitioners

Skills for Health (2020). Advanced Clinical Practice: Capabilities framework when working with people who have a learning disability and/or autism. www.skillsforhealth.org.uk/images/services/cstf/ACP%20in%20LDA%20Framework.pdf

Thompson, J., McNall, A., Tiplady, S. et al. (2019). Whole systems approach: advanced clinical practitioner development and identity in primary care. *Journal of Health Organization and Management* 33: 443–459.

Wenger, E. (2000). *Communities of Practice. Learning, Meaning and Identity.* Cambridge: Cambridge University Press.

FURTHER READING

Health Education England. Advanced Practice Toolkit. www.e-lfh.org.uk/programmes/advanced-practice-toolkit

Health Education England Advanced Practice Workplace Supervision Minimum Standards for Supervision. https://healtheducationengland.sharepoint.com/sites/APWC/Shared%20Documents/Forms/AllItems.aspx?ga=1&id=%2Fsites%2FAPWC%2FShared%20Documents%2FResources%20and%20News%2FAdvanced%20practice%20workplace%20supervision%2FAdvanced%20practice%20workplace%20supervision%2D%20Minimum%20standards%20for%20supe

rvision%2Epdf&parent=%2Fsites%2FAPWC%2FShared%20Documents%2FResources%20and%20
News%2FAdvanced%20practice%20workplace%20supervision

NHS England. The Centre for Advancing Practice. https://advanced-practice.hee.nhs.uk/

SELF-ASSESSMENT QUESTIONS

1. What policy documents should you refer to when planning your development as an AP?
2. What tools can you use to plan and structure professional development?
3. Who will play a role in influencing the effectiveness of a team containing APs (i.e. who are your key stakeholders)?
4. What networks/forums should you access to contribute and learn from the development of AP at a regional, national or international level?

GLOSSARY

Coaching   A process aiming to improve performance, focusing on the here and now as opposed to the distant past or future. There are a number of different models of coaching; the coach acts as a facilitator of learning.

Community of practice   Organised groups of people who have a common interest in a specific clinical domain. Communities of practice collaborate regularly, sharing information, improving their skills and actively working on advancing their sphere of practice.

Credentials   Standardised, structured units of assessed learning that have been designed to develop advanced-level practice capability in a specific field.

Extrinsic motivators   Motivators that involve engaging the individual in behaviours so as to earn external rewards or avoid penalties.

Intrinsic motivators   Behaviours that are driven by internal rewards. The person is performing an activity for its own sake rather than from the need for some external reward. The behaviour itself is its own reward.

Lifelong learning   Also know as continuous learning. Continually learning throughout the clinician's career and their personal life.

Professional development plan   Professional development plans identify clear, achievable goals to meet the individual's professional development needs, usually aligned to the department's or organisation's objectives. The plan is a structured method of recording identified professional development goals that are discussed and agreed with the line manager, providing an opportunity for acknowledgement of the clinician's strengths and accomplishments while identifying their future development needs.

Professional portfolio   A structured collection of carefully selected materials, providing credible evidence of a clinician's employment, education and professional development over time. Portfolios evidence achievements, demonstrate professional development and can help in career planning.

Revalidation   An evaluation of a clinician's fitness to practise, sometimes through appraisal. Revalidation confirms the continuation of a clinician's licence to practise.

Supervision   A process of professional support and learning, it is undertaken through a variety of activities. Supervision enables individual clinicians to develop their knowledge and competence, take on responsibility for their own practice and enhance quality of care provision and ensure patient safety.

Index

The Advanced Practitioner: A Framework for Practice, First Edition. Edited by Ian Peate,
Sadie Diamond-Fox, and Barry Hill.
© 2024 John Wiley & Sons Ltd. Published 2024 by John Wiley & Sons Ltd.